Acute Trauma-Induced Coagulopathy

Trauma-induced coagulopathy (TIC) is a life-threatening complication affecting severely injured patients. This text covers TIC's pathophysiology, risk factors, TBI-associated coagulopathy, diagnostic tools, transfusion prediction scores, and management strategies along with insights into cutting-edge diagnostic approaches. Looking toward the future, it discusses emerging innovations in trauma care and concludes with valuable lessons from a retrospective analysis offering both a regional perspective and global implications for improving trauma care protocols and patient survival for clinicians, trauma surgeons, emergency physicians, and healthcare researchers.

Key Features

- Offers an in-depth analysis of TIC, including its mechanisms, diagnostic tools, and management strategies, and serves as a comprehensive reference for improving trauma outcomes.
- TIC is a major contributor to preventable trauma deaths, and this resource addresses the growing need for targeted, evidence-based approaches among trauma care professionals.
- Includes a rare retrospective review drawing on data from national and international experience and perspectives to inform trauma care practice.

Acute Trauma-Induced Coagulopathy

Mechanisms, Diagnostics, and Management Strategies

Edited by
Venencia Albert, Arulselvi Subramanian,
Deepak Agrawal

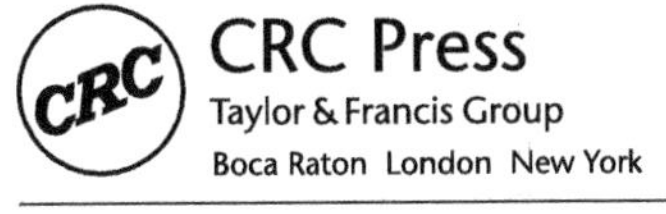

CRC Press
Taylor & Francis Group
Boca Raton London New York

CRC Press is an imprint of the
Taylor & Francis Group, an **informa** business

Designed cover image: Shutterstock: Ms. Deanne Fernandes

First edition published 2027
by CRC Press
2385 NW Executive Center Drive, Suite 320, Boca Raton FL 33431

and by CRC Press
4 Park Square, Milton Park, Abingdon, Oxon, OX14 4RN

CRC Press is an imprint of Taylor & Francis Group, LLC

ISBN: 978-1-041-19299-2 (hbk)
ISBN: 978-1-041-17406-6 (pbk)
ISBN: 978-1-003-71107-0 (ebk)

DOI: 10.1201/9781003711070

Typeset in Minion Pro
by KnowledgeWorks Global Ltd.

DEDICATION

To the patients whose clinical manifestations initially highlighted the fundamental questions in trauma-induced coagulopathy.

To the multidisciplinary teams in trauma care and laboratory medicine whose continuous efforts are advancing the field of trauma care and innovation.

To our collaborators and trainees, whose contributions transformed concepts into data, methods, and meaningful outputs.

To the mentors and colleagues whose guidance shaped the research path that led to this collaborative volume.

Venencia Albert, Arulselvi Subramanian, Deepak Agrawal

CONTENTS

FOREWORD

It is my distinct pleasure to write the Foreword for the book, *Acute Trauma-Induced Coagulopathy: Mechanisms, Diagnostics, and Management Strategies.* Trauma-induced coagulopathy is a crucial topic, profoundly impacting the mortality and morbidity of severely injured patients. It stands as an independent risk factor not only for clinical outcomes but also for resource utilization and the cost of care.

In my 25 years as a trauma surgeon, I have devoted much of my career to discovery-based research, serving as a principal investigator on National Institutes of Health (NIH) and National Science Foundation (NSF)-funded projects. Yet the realities of trauma medicine are never theoretical. Just two months ago, I cared for a young, 24-year-old patient who had sustained catastrophic injuries in a head-on collision. Intubated at the scene for a low Glasgow Coma Scale score, he arrived in the trauma bay with severe traumatic brain injury. Bleeding from his airways and intravenous sites, accompanied by marked lactic acidosis and altered coagulation parameters, illustrated the devastating consequences of trauma-induced coagulopathy. Despite maximal resuscitative efforts, we were unable to save him; his condition epitomized how coagulopathy can amplify the severity of primary injuries and complicate management.

This book arrives at a timely moment, providing essential insight and guidance on this complex subject. I have had the privilege of knowing Drs. Subramanian, Agrawal, and Albert for over a decade. Their choice of topics, each clinically relevant and thoughtfully curated, demonstrates their commitment to advancing trauma care. The book delves into critical basic science underlying coagulopathy, thoroughly exploring prevention and intervention strategies. Particularly noteworthy is the discussion on the interplay between traumatic brain injury and coagulopathy, as well as the inclusion of massive transfusion protocols and real-world clinical scenarios.

The illustrations and diagrams that accompany each chapter are clear and accessible, benefiting not only seasoned clinicians but also medical students, residents, and researchers. I commend the authors for their dedication and hard work in producing this comprehensive resource. I am confident that this book will be a significant and lasting contribution to the field.

Dr. Krishnan Raghavendran, MBBS, FACS
Professor of Acute Care Surgery
Emeritus Director and Founder Michigan Center for Global Surgery
Department of Surgery
University of Michigan, Ann Arbor, Michigan, USA

PREFACE

The genesis of this book lies in our work on early markers of trauma-induced coagulopathy (TIC) in isolated severe traumatic brain injury. The research was carried out at the All India Institute of Medical Sciences, New Delhi, and supported by the Indian Council of Medical Research and the Department of Biotechnology. We observed complex interplay between coagulation abnormalities, endothelial dysfunction, and secondary brain injury. These observations pointed to the need for integrated, mechanism-based approaches to the diagnosis and management of trauma-induced coagulopathy and form the foundation of this book.

The scope and direction of the book reflect our combined experience in neurosurgery, laboratory medicine, and translational trauma research. The aim was to link mechanisms with bedside practice. Trauma-induced coagulopathy is not confined to one specialty. It cuts across disciplines, and patient care improves when those boundaries are bridged.

The chapters bring together national and international contributors from laboratory medicine, hematology, anesthesiology, neurosciences, emergency medicine, trauma surgery, and transfusion medicine. They present current evidence, emerging ideas, and practical considerations, highlighting the multidisciplinary nature of modern trauma care.

This book is intended for clinicians, researchers, and trainees involved in trauma care. We hope it supports clearer thinking, stronger collaboration, and more informed management of trauma-related coagulopathy.

Venencia Albert
Arulselvi Subramanian
Deepak Agrawal

ACKNOWLEDGMENTS

We thank the All India Institute of Medical Sciences, New Delhi, for the strong clinical and research environment and support that shaped this work.

We are also grateful to all the organizations and experts worldwide whose contributions strengthened the scientific depth of this book.

ABOUT THE EDITORS

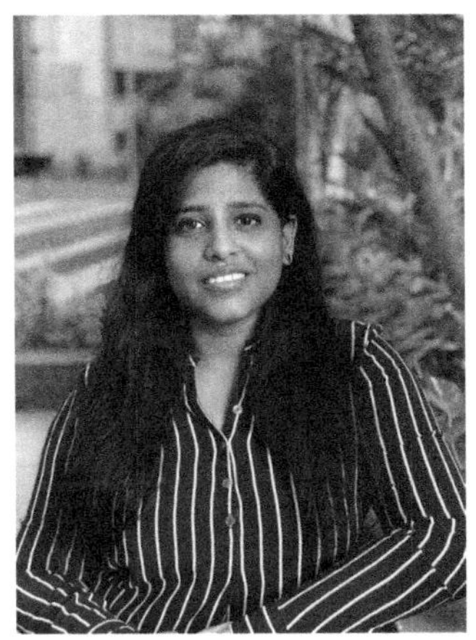

Venencia Albert is a research scientist at the Division of Laboratory Medicine, Jai Prakash Narayan Apex Trauma Center, All India Institute of Medical Sciences. Her work focuses on trauma care, coagulation disorders, neurosurgery, and infectious disease epidemiology. She earned her PhD in laboratory medicine, studying early markers of trauma-induced coagulopathy in severe traumatic brain injury and contributing to the understanding of early coagulation changes after brain injury. She has published widely in peer-reviewed journals and presented her work at international forums, including the World Congress of Neurology. She has received several recognitions, including a young researcher award and multiple travel fellowships. Dr. Albert has been involved in national research initiatives under the Indian Council of Medical Research, including fungal disease registries and foodborne pathogen surveillance. She has contributed to scientific publishing through the *Indian Journal of Medical Research*, served as guest editor for a special issue in *Clinical and Applied Thrombosis/Hemostasis (CATH)*, *SAGE Journals*, and is currently the associate editor for the *Journal of Pediatric Neurosciences*. Her interests include diagnostics, translational medicine, and predictive analytics to improve trauma care and public health.

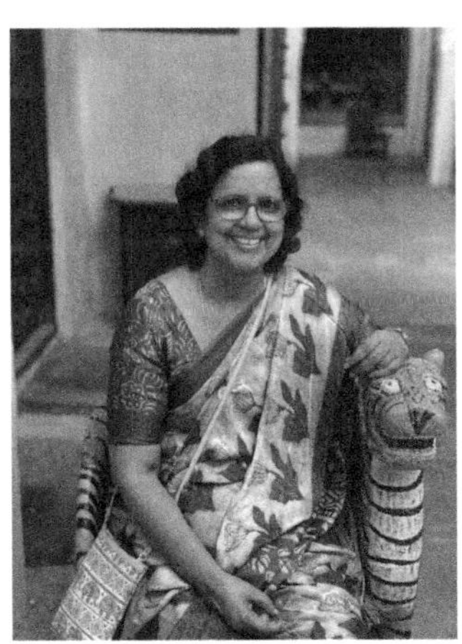

Arulselvi Subramanian is a distinguished professor and researcher in the field of laboratory medicine, with a specialization in pathology. Her research interests also include post-trauma cognitive changes, trauma immunology, and pathology. She currently serves as Head of the Division of Trauma Laboratory Medicine and In-charge of the Blood Center, Unit of Pathology/Laboratory Medicine, at the Jai Prakash Narayan Apex Trauma Centre, AIIMS, New Delhi.

With over 20 years of academic and research experience, she has contributed extensively to understanding coagulation abnormalities and transfusion practices in trauma and critical care. She has authored more than 200 peer-reviewed publications covering hemostatic disorders, blood component therapy, and diagnostic advances in coagulation testing. She has played an active role in developing clinical guidelines for coagulopathy management and transfusion optimization. She is a committed mentor to postgraduate students and research fellows and is a key investigator in several national and international trauma research collaborations.

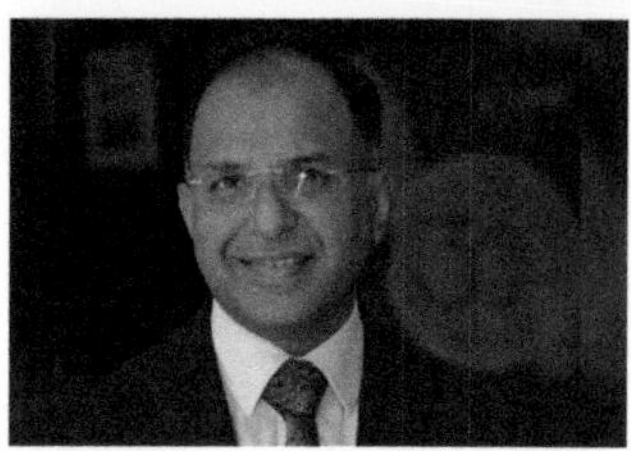

Deepak Agrawal is currently a professor of Neurosurgery and Gamma-Knife at the All India Institute of Medical Sciences (AIIMS), New Delhi. Dr. Agrawal has a keen interest in research and innovation and is co-inventor of the world's cheapest and smallest ventilator, named AgVa. He has ten patents to his credit. He has executed more than 1000 GK procedures and introduced several innovations in the GK unit at AIIMS.

He has won several national and international awards for his research, including the American Congress of Neurosurgeons (CNS) Young Neurosurgeon of the Year award and the DST BIG grant. He has more than 300 indexed publications and has been the principal investigator in several multicentric projects, including receiving an RO3 grant from the National Institutes of Health (NIH).

He has been the editor of the *Journal of Peripheral Nerve Surgery (JPNS)* and the *Indian Journal of Neurotrauma (IJNT)* and has been credited with improving the impact factor of these journals. Recently, he has become the editor of the *Journal of Pediatric Neurosciences (JPN)*.

CONTRIBUTORS

Deepak Agrawal
Department of Neurosurgery & Gamma-Knife
Jai Prakash Narayan Apex Trauma Centre
All India Institute of Medical Science
New Delhi, India

Venencia Albert
Division of Trauma Laboratory Medicine
Jai Prakash Narayan Apex Trauma Centre
All India Institute of Medical Science
New Delhi, India

Ajay Ambalakkatte
Department of Emergency Medicine
All India Institute of Medical Science
Nagpur, India

V. T. Amrithanand
Department of Emergency Medicine &
    Trauma
Jawaharlal Institute of Postgraduate
    Medical Education & Research
Pondicherry, India

S. Anukarthika
Department of Emergency Medicine
    & Trauma
Jawaharlal Institute of Postgraduate
    Medical Education & Research
Puducherry, India

Andrea Capponi
Department of Medical and Surgical
    Critical Care
University of Florence
Florence, Italy

Vineeth Chandran K P
Department of Emergency Medicine
All India Institute of Medical Science
New Delhi, India

Richa Chauhan
Department of Hematology
All India Institute of Medical Science
New Delhi, India

Nishtha Chawla
Department of Psychiatry & Jai Prakash
    Narayan Apex Trauma Centre
All India Institute of Medical Science
New Delhi, India

Hemant Choudhary
Department of Psychiatry
All India Institute of Medical Science
New Delhi, India

Thomas E. Croley II
Great Lakes Environmental Research
    Laboratory
National Oceanic and Atmospheric
    Administration
Ann Arbor, Michigan

Jasmita Dass
Department of Hematology
All India Institute of Medical Science
New Delhi, India

Amit Gupta
Department of Trauma Surgery & Critical
    Care
Jai Prakash Narayan Apex Trauma Centre
All India Institute of Medical Science
New Delhi, India

Babita Gupta
Department of Trauma Anaesthesia
    & Critical Care
Jai Prakash Narayan Apex Trauma Centre
All India Institute of Medical Science
New Delhi, India

Joses Dany James
Department of Trauma Surgery
Christian Medical College
Vellore, India

Sruthi Kandaswamy
Department of Pathology
Pondicherry Institute of Medical Sciences
Puducherry, India

Aparna Krishna
Department of Transfusion Medicine
Jawaharlal Institute of Postgraduate
    Medical Education & Research
Puducherry, India

Vignesh Kumar
Department of General Surgery
Pondicherry Institute of Medical Sciences
Puducherry, India

Nistha Malik
Department of Anesthesiology
Pain Medicine & Critical Care
Jai Prakash Narayan Apex Trauma Centre
All India Institute of Medical Science
New Delhi, India

Radheshyam Meher
Department of Transfusion Medicine
Jai Prakash Narayan Apex Trauma Centre
All India Institute of Medical Science
New Delhi, India

Sharmishtha Pathak
Department of Trauma Anaesthesia &
    Critical Care
Jai Prakash Narayan Apex Trauma
    Centre
All India Institute of Medical Science
New Delhi, India

Abhishek Satapathy
Division of Trauma Laboratory Medicine
Jai Prakash Narayan Apex Trauma Centre
All India Institute of Medical Science
New Delhi, India

Tushar Sehgal
Department of Laboratory Medicine
All India Institute of Medical Science
New Delhi, India

Abhishek Singh
Department of Anaethesia and Critical
    Care
Jai Prakash Narayan Apex Trauma
    Centre
All India Institute of Medical Science
New Delhi, India

Arulselvi Subramanian
Division of Trauma Laboratory Medicine
Unit of Pathology/Laboratory Medicine
Jai Prakash Narayan Apex Trauma Centre
All India Institute of Medical Science
New Delhi, India

Nitin Tiwari
Division of Trauma Laboratory Medicine
Jai Prakash Narayan Apex Trauma Centre
All India Institute of Medical Science
New Delhi, India

ABBREVIATIONS

AA	Arachidonic acid
ACT	Activated clotting time
ADP	Adenosine diphosphate
AIS	Abbreviated Injury Scale
aPC	Activated Protein C
aPTT	Activated partial thromboplastin time
AT	Antithrombin
ATC	Acute traumatic coagulopathy
ATIC	Acute trauma-induced coagulopathy
BBB	Blood–brain barrier
BD	Base deficit
BDMP	Brain-derived microparticles
CCT	Conventional coagulation test
CI	Confidence interval
CK	Citrated kaolin
CRT	Citrated RapidTEG
CSF	Cerebrospinal fluid
CT	Computed tomography
DAI	Diffuse axonal injury
DIC	Disseminated intravascular coagulation
DTICH	Delayed traumatic intracranial hemorrhage
ED	Emergency Department
EDH	Epidural hematoma
eFAST	extended Focused Assessment with Sonography in Trauma
EGL	Endothelial glycocalyx layer
ELISA	Enzyme-linked immunosorbent assay
EMP	Endothelial-derived microparticle
EoT	Endotheliopathy of trauma
EPCR	Endothelial protein C receptor
FDP	Fibrin degradation product
FFP	Fresh frozen plasma
FLEV	Level of fibrinogen in plasma
FSC	Forward scatter
GCS	Glasgow Coma Scale
GP	Glycoprotein
Hb	Hemoglobin
Hct	Hematocrit
HF	Hyperfibrinolysis
ICH	Intracranial hemorrhage
ICP	Intracranial pressure
IL	Interleukin
INR	International normalized ratio
ISS	Injury severity score
iSTBI	Isolated severe traumatic brain injury
ISTH	International Society of Thrombosis and Hemostasis
K-time	Kinetics time

LY30	Percent lysis 30 minutes after maximum amplitude
MA	Maximum amplitude
MODS	Multiorgan dysfunction syndrome
MP	Microparticle
mtMP	Mitochondrial microparticles
PAI-1	Plasminogen activator inhibitor-1
PC	Protein C
PCI	Percutaneous coronary intervention
PF1+2	Prothrombin fragment 1+2
PHI	Progressive hemorrhage injury
PMP	Platelet-derived microparticle
POCT	Point-of-care test
PPH	Postpartum hemorrhage
PRBC	Packed red blood cells
PRP	Platelet-rich plasma
PS	Protein S
PT	Prothrombin time
ROC	Receiver operating curve
ROTEM	Rotational thromboelastometry
RTA	Road traffic accident
rTEG	Rapid thromboelastography
SAC	Systemic acquired coagulopathy
SAH	Subarachnoid hemorrhage
SBP	Systolic blood pressure
SDH	Subdural hematoma
SGOT	Serum glutamic oxaloacetic transaminase
SMP	Soluble fibrin monomer (sFM)
SNS	Sympathetic nervous system
SOFA	Sequential Organ Failure Assessment Score
SSC	Side scatter
Syd-1	Syndecan-1
TAFI	Thrombin activatable fibrinolysis inhibitor
TASH	Trauma-associated severe hemorrhage
TAT	Thrombin/Antithrombin complex
TAVR	Transcatheter aortic valve repair/replacement
TBI	Traumatic brain injury
TEG	Thromboelastography
TF	Tissue factor
TFPI	Tissue factor pathway inhibitor
TM	Thrombomodulin
TNFα	Tumor necrosis factor α
tPA	Tissue plasminogen activator
TXA	Tranexamic acid
VHA	Viscoelastic hemostatic assays
vWF	von Willebrand factor
WHO	World Health Organization

Chapter 1

INTRODUCTION TO TRAUMA-INDUCED COAGULOPATHY

Tushar Sehgal, Venencia Albert, Babita Gupta,
and Arulselvi Subramanian

DOI: 10.1201/9781003711070-1

INTRODUCTION

Trauma is one of the leading causes of mortality globally. As per World Health Organization (WHO) data from 2019, road traffic accidents (RTAs) are ranked as the seventh leading global cause of mortality, in order of number of lives lost. Amongst the various reasons leading to mortality of a victim of RTA, exsanguination is a predominant factor, second only to central nervous system (CNS) injury.[1,2]

Post-traumatic haemorrhage is caused by two main mechanisms. The first is exsanguination caused due to direct injury of blood vessels. In cases of injury of large-calibre arterial vessels, there is profuse haemorrhage with shock. The second mechanism is bleeding secondary to development of trauma-induced coagulopathy (TIC), which involves secondary bleeding from a widespread microvascular haemorrhage that is not localized to the site of the trauma. The term *"trauma-induced coagulopathy" was introduced to describe a process that impairs blood coagulation and increases blood loss by a possible deregulation of the intrinsic coagulation system in trauma patients.*[3]

Approximately 30% of patients with massive trauma develop TIC upon arrival in the emergency department (ED). Although it was once believed that TIC begins hours or even days after the traumatic event, it is currently clear that it begins at the moment of trauma, and the associated mortality is about 35–50%. The occurrence and frequency of TIC in children is less as compared to adults. Older adults are more likely to develop TIC than younger adults. Thus, a systematic diagnostic and therapeutic approach is required to reduce the number of preventable deaths attributable to traumatic injury.[4–6]

The normal coagulation response is initiated with injury to vascular endothelium. This activates platelets, which adhere to the injury site, forming the initial clot, and the coagulation cascade, amplified by activated platelets, leading to a thrombin burst that cleaves fibrinogen into fibrin[7] (Figure 1.1). Fibrin monomers then crosslink onto the aggregated platelets, further stabilizing the clot. In normal conditions, anticoagulation and fibrinolytic processes limit excessive clot formation to maintain vascular patency.[8]

The term "haemostasis," which means "physiological process that stops bleeding," is derived from the Greek words "heme" (blood) and "stasis" (to stop).[9] The series of events that result in haemostasis is known as the coagulation pathway. Injury to the vasculature, whether mechanical, chemical, or electrical, is traditionally considered the primary trigger for coagulation.[10] The endothelium, platelets, and white cells are among the major components needed for the start of coagulation. The coagulation cascade is the successive activation of each coagulation zymogen caused by these components adhering to the surface in close geographic proximity.[10] This complex mechanism prevents spontaneous bleeding. The common pathway is the point at which the intrinsic and extrinsic paths converge after starting independently. This further results in the activation of fibrin and the synthesis of thrombin, prompting platelet aggregation, forming and stabilizing a fibrin mesh, and inhibiting fibrinolysis.[11–13]

The fundamental concept of blood coagulation was initially introduced in *Nature* and *Science* publications during the 1960s by Davie, Ratnoff, and Macfarlane. The sequence of proenzymes activated by proteolytic cleavage, which in turn activates "downstream" enzymes, was clarified in these articles. Schematically, the coagulation system is divided into intrinsic and extrinsic pathways. The extrinsic pathway is activated in response to tissue trauma, resulting in the activation of tissue factor (TF). The importance of the intrinsic pathway is less evident *in vivo*. However, it is essential when blood is stimulated by contact with artificial surfaces, such as a cardiopulmonary bypass circuit or a mechanical circulatory support device.[14] Numerous inhibitors control the coagulation process, preventing thrombus formation and limiting clot formation. This critical balance is compromized if the activity of naturally occurring inhibitors is reduced or the procoagulant activity of the coagulation factors increases.[15]

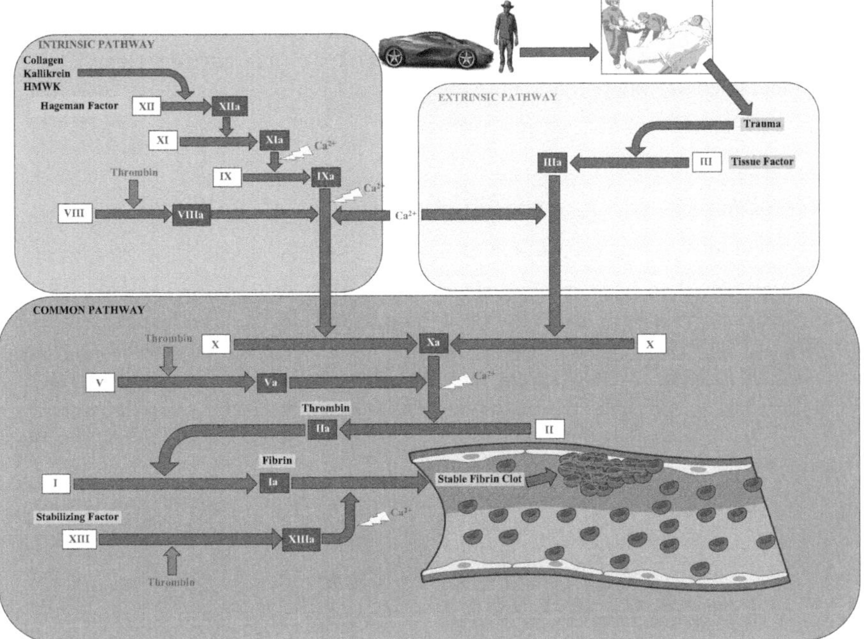

Figure 1.1 Overview of the coagulation cascade. Selected elements were sourced from the National Institute of Allergy and Infectious Diseases (NIAID) of the National Institutes of Health (NIH) BioArt Source (bioart.niaid.nih.gov).

Overview of Coagulation Cascade and Its Regulation

THE COAGULATION CASCADE

Traditionally, it is divided into extrinsic and intrinsic pathways (Figure 1.1). Exposed endothelial collagen following endothelial damage activates the intrinsic pathway, while TF produced by endothelial cells following external damage activates the extrinsic pathway. Both pathways result in factor X activation. Though it ignores the crucial function that cell-based surfaces play in *in vivo*, the traditional cascade of blood coagulation is very helpful for comprehending *in vitro* coagulation testing.[16]

INTRINSIC PATHWAY

Of the two haemostatic pathways, this one is the more extensive one. The partial thromboplastin time (PTT) is a clinical measure of the intrinsic pathway. It starts with prekallikrein, HMW kininogen, and factor XII. After endothelial damage, factor XII, an inactivated serine protease zymogen, is exposed to endothelial collagen and transforms into factor XIIa, or activated serine protease. To convert factor XI into factor XIa, factor XIIa serves as a catalyst. Factor IX is subsequently activated to factor IXa by factor XIa. To activate factor X into factor Xa, activated factor IXa then forms a tenase complex with its cofactor, factor VIII, on a phospholipid surface.[17,18]

EXTRINSIC PATHWAY

The shorter secondary haemostasis pathway is known as the extrinsic pathway. The prothrombin time (PT) is a clinical indicator of the extrinsic route. The pathway is activated by TF, present in the subendothelial tissue. There is minimal contact between TF and plasma procoagulants under physiological settings in a normal vascular endothelium. However, when the vessel is damaged, the endothelial cells produce TF, which binds with calcium and factor VIIa to facilitate the conversion of factor X to Xa. At this stage, intrinsic and extrinsic pathways merge into one.[19,20]

COMMON PATHWAY

This pathway initiates with factor X, which is subsequently activated to factor Xa. The activation of factor Xa triggers a complex response. The complex responsible for converting factor X into factor Xa is known as tenase. There are two forms of tenase: intrinsic, consisting of cofactor factor VIII, factor IXa, a phospholipid, and Ca2+, and extrinsic, which includes factor VII, factor III (TF), and Ca2+. Factor Xa then activates factor II (prothrombin), transforming it into factor IIa (thrombin). Additionally, factor Xa requires factor V as a cofactor to facilitate the cleavage of prothrombin into thrombin. Factor IIa (thrombin) further activates fibrinogen, converting it into fibrin. Thrombin also activates other factors in the intrinsic pathway, such as factor XI, as well as cofactors V and VIII, and factor XIII. Fibrin subunits aggregate to form fibrin strands, while factor XIII acts on these strands to create a fibrin mesh, which serves to stabilize the platelet plug.[17,18,21]

FIBRINOLYTIC SYSTEM

It functions to restrict the size of the clot and is triggered concurrently with the coagulation cascade. Fibrinolysis is an enzymatic process in which plasmin, which is derived from fibrin-bound plasminogen in the liver, breaks down the fibrin clot into fibrin degradation products (FDPs). Urokinase plasminogen activator (uPA) or tissue-type plasminogen activator (tPA), which is secreted from the vascular endothelium, catalyses this process. Tissue occlusion, thrombin, adrenaline, vasopressin, and intense exercise all promote the release of tPA.[22]

Plasmin activity is stringently controlled by its inhibitor, α2 antiplasmin, thereby inhibiting extensive fibrinolysis. The fibrinolytic system's *in vivo* activity is evaluated by measuring the FDPs. The breakdown of cross-linked fibrin produces D-dimers, which are particular markers of fibrinolysis used to diagnose and assess deep vein thrombosis, disseminated intravascular coagulation (DIC), and pulmonary embolism.[22] Plasmin has the potential to break fibrinogen, leading to deleterious consequences; therefore, the fibrinolytic activity is limited by the following factors:

i. Plasminogen activator inhibitor is the primary physiological inhibitor of fibrinolysis and acts by irreversible inhibition of tPA and uPA.

ii. Thrombin-activatable fibrinolysis inhibitor (TAFI) is a plasma proenzyme synthesized by the liver and activated by thrombin. It decreases the affinity of plasminogen to fibrin and augments the action of anti-trypsin in inhibiting plasmin.

iii. Plasmin inhibitors: The glycoproteins α2 antiplasmin and α2Macroglobulin act by inhibiting plasmin.

CURRENT CONCEPT OF COAGULATION

The modern time-based structuring of blood coagulation provides more authentic description of the coagulation process. The classical theories of coagulation provide only a reasonable model of *in vitro* coagulation tests (i.e., aPTT and PT).[22] The contact activation pathway critical for *in vivo* haemostasis does not get support from following observations. Individuals lacking factor XII, prekallikrein, or high-molecular-weight kininogen do not bleed abnormally. Secondly, patients with only trace quantities of factor XI can withstand major trauma without unusual bleeding, and those who completely lack factor XI exhibit mild haemorrhagic disorder. Furthermore, deficiencies of both intrinsic pathway factors such as factor VIII and factor IX (lead to haemophilia A and B, respectively), however the classic description of two pathways of coagulation leave it unclear as to why either type of haemophiliacs cannot not simply clot blood via the unaffected pathway.[22] The current cell-based concept of coagulation is characterized by the initiation, amplification, and propagation phases.

INITIATION

The initiation phase is shown in Figure 1.2. Trauma to the vessel wall is the primary stimulus for coagulation. It activates endothelial cells and translocates P-selectin from Weibel–Palade (WP) bodies to the cell surface. In addition, injury activates platelets, mobilizing P-selectin from the platel*et alp*ha-granules to the platelet's surface. The binding of P-selectin

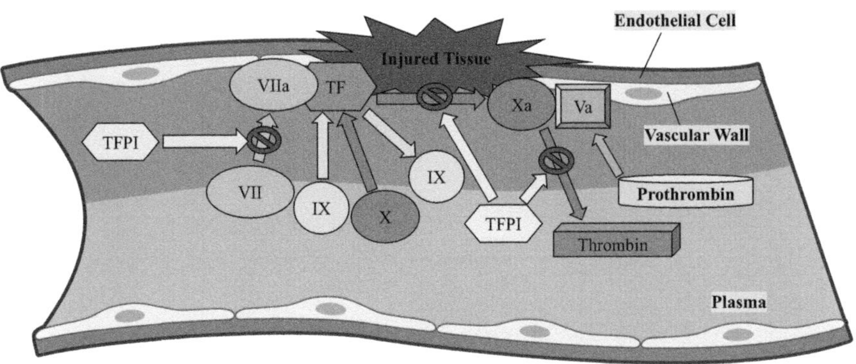

Figure 1.2 Initiation phase of the cell-based model.

to P-selectin glycoprotein ligand-1 results in the rolling of the leukocytes and platelets on the surface of activated endothelial cells to localize thrombus formation.[10] Another protein released from the WP bodies of endothelial cells and the alpha-granules of platelets is the von Willebrand factor (vWF). Under high shear conditions, as in arterial circulation, this protein binds to platelet membrane glycoprotein Ib and to exposed sub-endothelial connective tissue to support the adhesion of platelets at the injury site. In veins with low shear, the vWF released from stimulated endothelium increases the concentration of platelets on the vein wall.[10] Additionally, the vWF binds to platelet glycoprotein IIb/IIIa, enhancing platelet-to-platelet aggregation. Aggregates of platelet-leukocytes on injured endothelium and TF initiate steps leading to fibrin formation. The expression of TF in injured vessels binds factor VIIa to activate factor IX and factor X. This activation of factor IX by the TF-VIIa complex serves as the bridge between classical extrinsic and intrinsic pathways. Factor Xa then binds to factor II to form thrombin (factor IIa). However, only trace amounts of thrombin are formed by this pathway in the initiation phase of coagulation, which can be effectively terminated by the TF pathway inhibitor (TFPI); more significant amounts will be generated during the amplification phase.[10]

AMPLIFICATION PHASE

The amplification phase is shown in Figure 1.3. The insignificant amounts of thrombin generated during the initiation phase further activate platelets, factor V, and factor XI. Activated factor XI is bound to glycoprotein Ib/IX of activated platelets to activate factor IX. Additionally, activated factor IX, previously generated by the TF VIIa complex, diffuses to the surface of activated platelets and binds to the platelet membrane. As previously mentioned, vWF is also bound to glycoprotein Ib/IX. In circulating plasma, thrombin releases factor VIII from vWF and activates it to factor VIIIa. On the platelet surface, factor VIIIa binds factor IXa, and the complex, in the presence of calcium ions, activates additional factor X. This initiates the propagation phase of coagulation.[23]

PROPAGATION PHASE

The propagation phase is shown in Figure 1.4. The "tenase" complex comprises factors VIIIa, IXa, and calcium ions. This complex leads to the large-scale generation of factor Xa. Factor Xa, with factor Va and calcium ions, forms the "prothrombinase" complex that produces the burst of thrombin needed to convert fibrinogen to fibrin. In addition, thrombin activates platelets, factors V, VIII, and XI, thereby catalysing its formation. Furthermore, thrombin activates factor XIII, resulting in clot stabilization, and the TAFI modulates fibrinolysis.[10]

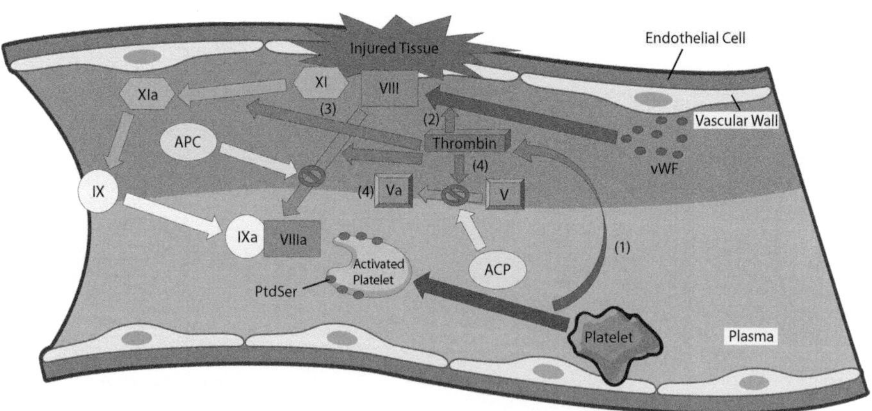

Figure 1.3   Amplification phase of the cell-based model.

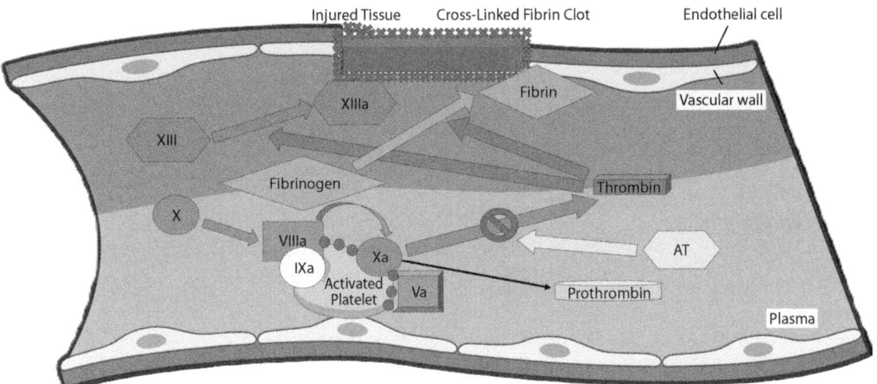

Figure 1.4   Propagation phase of the cell-based model.

REGULATION

The anticoagulant system in our body controls the procoagulant activity in blood and helps to localize the formation of thrombi.[24] The primary natural anticoagulant processes consist of the following.

ANTITHROMBIN

The primary inhibitor of thrombin is antithrombin (AT), formerly known as AT III. It is a serine protease inhibitor and deactivates thrombin, factors IXa, Xa, XIa, and XIIa. In the presence of heparin, the enzymatic activity of AT increases. Heparin sulphate, found on the surface of endothelial cells, binds to AT. AT binds coagulation factors in a ratio of 1:1 forming a complex which is removed by reticuloendothelial cells. Other thrombin inhibitors are heparin cofactor II, $\alpha 2$ macroglobulin and $\alpha 1$ antitrypsin.[22]

TFPI

TFPI is a polypeptide produced by endothelial cells. It acts as a natural inhibitor of the extrinsic pathway by inhibiting TF-VIIa complex.[22]

PROTEIN C ANTICOAGULATION PATHWAY

The propagation phase of the coagulation is inhibited by the protein C pathway (Figure 1.5)[22] that primarily consists of four key elements:

i.   Protein C is a serine protease that has strong anti-inflammatory, profibrinolytic, and anticoagulant effects. With protein S and phospholipids serving as cofactors, it inhibits activated factors V and VIII after being activated by thrombin to create activated protein C (APC).

ii.   Thrombomodulin is a transmembrane receptor on the endothelial cells that prevents the formation of the clot in the undamaged endothelium by binding to thrombin. Endothelial protein C receptor is another transmembrane receptor that plays a vital role in the activation of protein C.

iii.   Protein S synthesized by hepatocytes and endothelial cells, is a glycoprotein that is dependent on vitamin K. Both of its free (40%) and bound (60%) are present in plasma

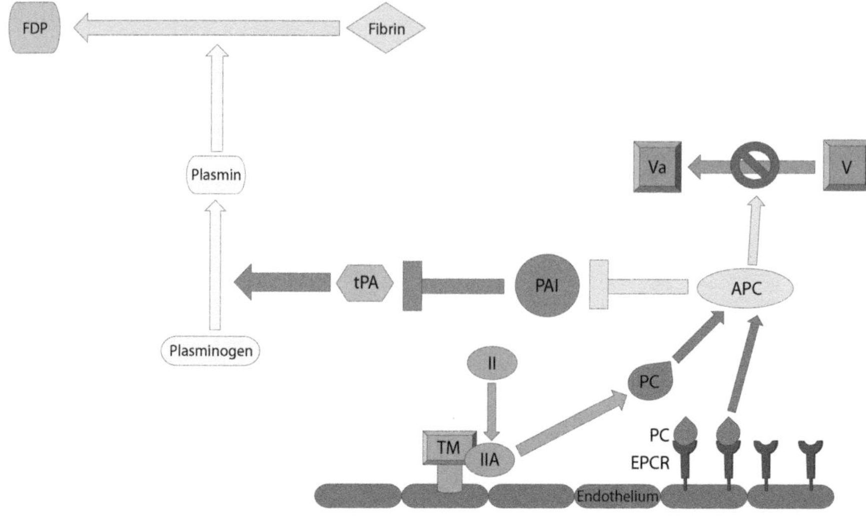

Figure 1.5 Protein C anticoagulation pathway.

(bound to C4b-binding protein). The free form has anticoagulant properties, whereas the bound form inhibits the complement system and is upregulated during inflammatory conditions, which lowers protein S levels and causes a procoagulant state. It helps APC inactivate factor Va and factor VIIIa by acting as a cofactor. It also inhibits the prothrombinase (factor Va–factor Xa) complex directly and reversibly.

iv. Protein Z-dependent protease inhibitor (ZPI) is a protein that, along with its cofactor protein Z (PZ), rapidly inhibits factor Xa on cell surfaces.[22]

TRAUMA-INDUCED COAGULOPATHY (TIC)

TIC has been known by various names, including "severe bleeding tendency," "defibrination syndrome," "consumptive disorder," "bloody vicious cycle," "acute traumatic coagulopathy," and others.[25] The term "trauma-induced coagulopathy" was coined in April 2010 during the National Institutes of Health's Trans-Agency Consortium for Trauma-Induced Coagulopathy Workshop.[26] Because it comprises a wide range of coagulation dysfunctions, TIC lacks rigorous quantitative diagnostic criteria. However, it should be explored when coagulopathy is detected in the context of acute trauma.[27]

HISTORICAL PERSPECTIVE

The first reports of TIC were published in 1954, from studies performed on 11 battle casualties immediately after they had been wounded and resuscitated and during the first days of their convalescence.[28] They documented elevated PT and aPTT in casualties, and their degree of coagulopathy correlated with the number of units of blood received. These findings were interpreted as a state of consumed factors and platelets, exacerbated by dilution derived from fluid administration and blood transfusion. Simmons *et al.*,[29] in 1969, reported cyclic prolongations in PT or PTT accompanied by significant depressions of platelet counts, fibrinogen levels and elevations of fibrinolysis in trauma patients. In 1982, the American Trauma Society suggested that hypothermia and acidosis are complicating factors associated with early mortality in coagulopathic trauma patients.[30] This "bloody vicious cycle" was subsequently replaced by other terms such as "lethal triad," "iatrogenic trauma coagulopathy," and "systemic acquired coagulopathy (SAC)," which suggested that hypothermia, acidosis, and dilution from standard resuscitation can worsen the presenting coagulopathy and perpetuate bleeding.[31] This concept formed the basis of many transfusion protocols and therapies to combat SAC and bleeding in trauma.[32,33] Many authors over the years have rebutted this theory and confirmed that TIC is not merely a systemic response to injury, as patients with early evidence of coagulopathy that is physiologically and mechanistically distinct from SAC.[34-38] In 2003, Brohi *et al.*,[38] in a retrospective study, and MacLeod *et al.*,[39] in a prospective study, reported that TIC presents in 25% of severely injured patients on arrival in the ED.[40] This resulted in the current opinion that coagulopathy in the early stages of trauma, being an acute endogenous response to the injury itself, exists independently and essentially differs from iatrogenic coagulation impairment.[41]

EPIDEMIOLOGY AND BURDEN

TIC is a significant contributor to early morbidity and mortality in trauma patients worldwide. It is believed to affect 25–35% of critically injured patients at the time of hospital admission, with a higher incidence among those arriving with substantial haemorrhage and shock.[39] The incidence of TIC is strongly linked to damage severity, physiological derangement, and the extent of tissue trauma. The reported incidence in India (41–46%) is comparable or greater than in high-income nations, most likely due to delays in pre-hospital care, a lack of structured trauma systems, and a high burden of high-energy injuries such as RTAs.[42] Several studies have documented the epidemiology of TIC across diverse trauma populations,[38,39,43-64] as tabulated in Table 1.1.

In cases of isolated traumatic brain injury (TBI), rates of TIC have ranged widely. Albert *et al.*, in India, reported a 41.6% incidence of TIC in isolated severe TBI.[43] Other studies have reported even higher rates, such as 57% in China[65] and 60% in penetrating TBI cases in the United States.[66] Paediatric populations have also shown a significant burden. Chong *et al.* in Singapore reported a 55.7% frequency of TIC in paediatric TBI patients,[44] whereas Strumwasser *et al.*, in the United States, discovered a 26% incidence of TIC in paediatric trauma.[45] The prevalence of TIC has been shown to vary with demographic parameters. It has been linked to greater mortality in female patients compared to males,[67] and it is more common in elderly adults than in younger adults and children.[26] Children have a lower incidence of TIC than adults. Its incidence rises with injury severity and is linked to poor clinical signs such as low Glasgow Coma Scale scores, high base deficiency, and thrombocytopenia.[38-68] Trauma causes more than five million fatalities worldwide each year and accounts for over 10% of the global disease burden.[69] Haemorrhage accounts for 30–40% of trauma-related mortality, with TIC identified as a major modulator of this outcome.[70] Advances in trauma care in high-income countries, such as structured trauma systems, rapid diagnostic tools, and availability to large transfusion protocols, have contributed to increased survival.[45] Low- and middle-income countries (LMICs), including India, confront continuous issues such as delayed TIC diagnosis, limited access to viscoelastic testing, insufficient blood bank resources, and poor pre-hospital care.[71,72] TIC not only causes premature death, but it also extends intensive care unit hospitalizations, raises healthcare expenses, and causes long-term disability. These findings are especially significant in LMICs because trauma disproportionately impacts young, economically productive people.[26]

Table 1.1   Previously published study size, definition, reported incidence of TIC, and outcomes in trauma patients

Study number	Author	Country	Injury type	TIC%
1	Brohi et al.[38]	UK	Blunt/penetrating trauma	25%
2	MacLeod et al.[39]	USA	Polytrauma	28%
3	Rugeri et al.[46]	France	Blunt trauma	28%
4	Cohen[47]	USA	TBI	28%
5	Zehtabchi et al.[48]	USA	Isolated TBI	17%
6	Talving et al.[49]	USA	Severe TBI	36%
7	Allard et al.[50]	Canada	Severe isolated blunt TBI	35%
8	Lustenberger et al.[51]	USA	TBI	45.7%
9	Lustenberger et al.[52]	USA	Isolated severe TBI	36.4%
10	Wafaisade et al.[53]	Germany	Isolated blunt TBI	22.7%
11	Shaz et al.[60]	USA	Trauma	41.7%
12	Chhabra et al.[55]	India	TBI	46%
13	Greuters et al.[56]	Netherlands	Isolated TBI	24%
14	Sun et al.[65]	China	TBI	57%
15	Franschman[57]	Netherlands	Isolated TBI	Early 34%, delayed 20%
16	Genét[58]	Denmark	TBI	28%
17	Epstein et al.[59]	Australia	Isolated TBI	35.2%
18	Xing Wu[54]	China	Isolated blunt TBI	34.88%
19	de Oliveira Manoel[61]	Canada	TBI	24.3%
20	Dekker[62]	Netherlands	TBI	42%
21	Strumwasser et al.[45]	USA	Trauma (paediatric)	26%
22	Folkerson et al.[66]	USA	Penetrating traumatic brain injury	60%
23	Albert et al.[43]	India	Isolated severe traumatic brain injury	41.6%
24	Böhm et al.[63]	Germany	Isolated traumatic brain injury	20%
24	Chong et al.[44]	Singapore	Traumatic brain injury (paediatric)	55.7%
26	Du et al.[64]	China	Trauma	25.4%

DEFINING TRAUMA-INDUCED COAGULOPATHY

Multiple definitions of TIC have been proposed, and the defining criterion varies considerably, owing to over 20 different proposed parameters of coagulopathy. These parameters include elevated INR, PT, PTT or D-dimer, decreased fibrinogen or factor XIII, higher DIC score, modified DIC score or modified coagulopathy score, and lower α2AP. However, there remains no consensus regarding a standard laboratory definition for TIC. In 1954 Scott et al. identified trauma associated with coagulopathy as a 50% decline in prothrombin activity.[28] More than a decade ago, TIC was identified based on the traditional transfusion triggers recommended by massive transfusion guidelines,[28] a 50% increment of the conventional coagulation assays namely PT, aPTT, or international normalized ratio (INR).[39,73] However, subsequent experimental studies confirmed that TIC defined by standard clotting times of PT ratio >1.2 is associated with increased mortality and transfusion requirements in a dose dependent manner.[40] In 2003 Brohi *et al.*[38] characterized TIC as PT >18s, aPTT >60s or INR >1.5 and MacLeod *et al.* identified TIC as a PT >14s and aPTT >34s.[39] Conventional coagulation assays continued to be the primary investigation for identification of TIC for a decade, being ubiquitous and established to predict unfavourable outcome and need of transfusion in trauma patients. Lately, Van Zyl and colleagues reported INR >1.2 as a clinically significant threshold for increased mortality and blood product requirements.[74] Other markers, such as low initial haemoglobin level, have also been reported to be an indicator for severe bleeding and coagulopathy.[73] Similarly, fibrinogen is increasingly being recognized as playing a vital role in trauma-related bleeding and is not only the precursor of fibrin, but also an important mediator of platelet aggregation.[75] Fibrinogen levels of >2.0 g/L have been reported as a risk factor for the development of progressive haemorrhagic injury.[76] Viscoelastic tests such as thromboelastography (TEG) and rotational thromboelastometry (ROTEM) have emerged as point-of-care tools to assess coagulation function in real time. These tests offer a more comprehensive evaluation of clot formation, strength, and stability than conventional assays. A Cochrane review (2015) concluded that TEG and ROTEM may help detect TIC in adult trauma patients, but the evidence is limited and of low certainty.[77] While they offer rapid, dynamic assessment of clotting abnormalities, their use is still largely guided by local protocols and availability, and they have not replaced standard coagulation tests in most centres.

PATHOPHYSIOLOGICAL MECHANISM OF TIC

It originates from severe tissue damage and haemorrhagic shock, resulting in an inability of the body to form and maintain clot strength leading to excessive bleeding and worsening shock, thus cascading into a vicious cycle.[78] In TIC, the cell-mediated regulation of haemostasis is impaired. The endogenous TIC differs from the iatrogenic exogenous resuscitation-induced coagulopathy caused by dilution of coagulation factors. However, it may be present concomitantly. Extensive tissue and endothelial cell damage results in loss of endothelial glycocalyx and increased TF expression, both of which activate coagulation. Dying cells release intracellular components, such as cell-free DNA, histones, and high-mobility group box protein 1 (HMGB-1), that signal tissue injury and are therefore termed "damage-associated molecular patterns" (DAMPs). In about half of patients with TIC, platelets are dysfunctional in their adhesion and aggregation capabilities. This platelet dysfunction, is often not revealed by the normal platelet count, and impairs the haemostasis even if the blood levels of coagulation factors are normalized. Exhaustion has been attributed to platelet overactivation from TF, von Willebrand factor, and DAMPs. Platelets interact bidirectionally with circulating leukocytes by forming platelet-leukocyte aggregates (PLAs). PLAs are potent activators of the immune response, stimulating leukocyte migration towards the injury site. On the other hand, extracellular traps from activated neutrophils and macrophages are released, promoting platelet aggregation and thrombin formation.[79-82] Coagulation factors are usually depleted in TIC due to systemic consumption, dilution, and degradation by overproduction of several proteins of the anticoagulation and fibrinolytic systems, mainly APC and plasmin. APC degrades coagulation factor Va and factor VIIIa and promotes the activity of tissue plasminogen activator, which converts plasminogen to plasmin. High plasmin production degrades fibrin and fibrinogen, leading to hyperfibrinolysis. Moreover, reduced thrombin formation alters clot formation, resulting in a thick loose fibrin network that is more prone to lysis. Resultant breakdown of newly formed clots further amplifies bleeding. Ionized calcium is required as a co-factor for various coagulation reactions. Calcium consumption in TIC during coagulation and inactivation by citrate-containing blood products, further worsens the coagulation disturbances.[83,84] When patients survive their initial traumatic bleeding and injuries, TIC shifts from a hypocoagulable to a hypercoagulable profile, with a consequent increased risk of thromboembolic events and organ dysfunction. This shift can occur within minutes to hours following injury. The persistence of endothelial damage, activated immune cells and platelets, and circulating DAMPs that create a procoagulant environment may all be responsible for the shift.[85]

The mechanisms associated with the hypocoagulable and hypercoagulable state of TIC are depicted in Figure 1.6. Thus, it can be concluded that TIC consists of three important variables a pathophysiological process linked to trauma (acute traumatic coagulopathy), iatrogenic factors (coagulopathy induced by resuscitation) and detrimental factors (both iatrogenic and pathophysiological). This is represented schematically in Figure 1.7.

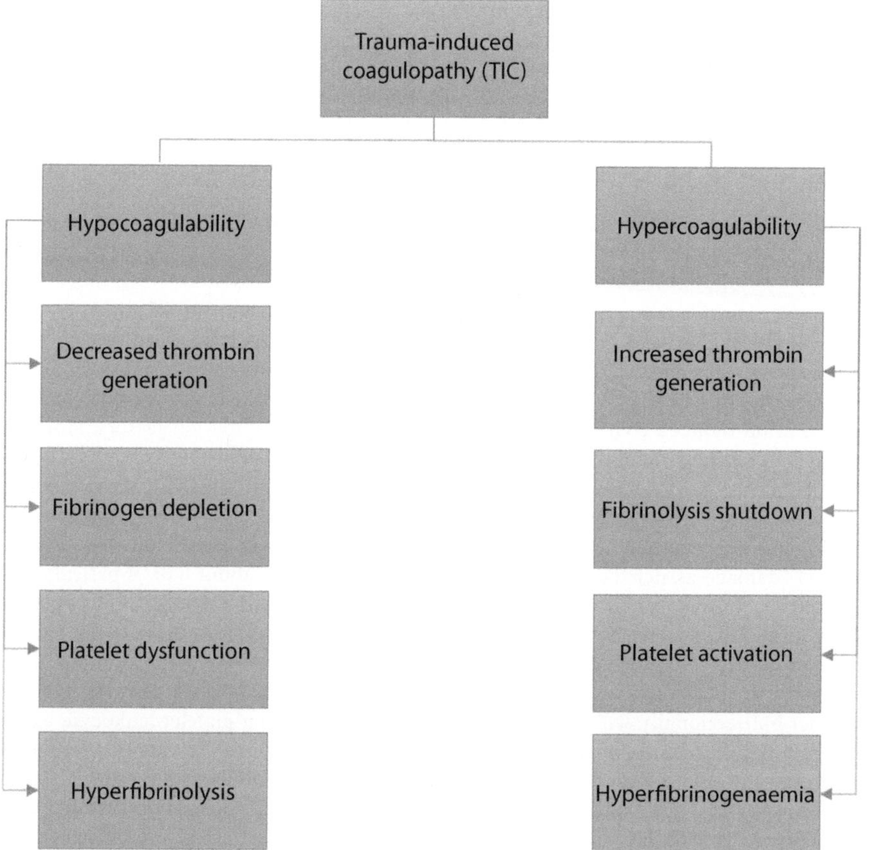

Figure 1.6 The mechanism associated with hypocoagulable and hypercoagulable states of trauma-induced coagulopathy (TIC).

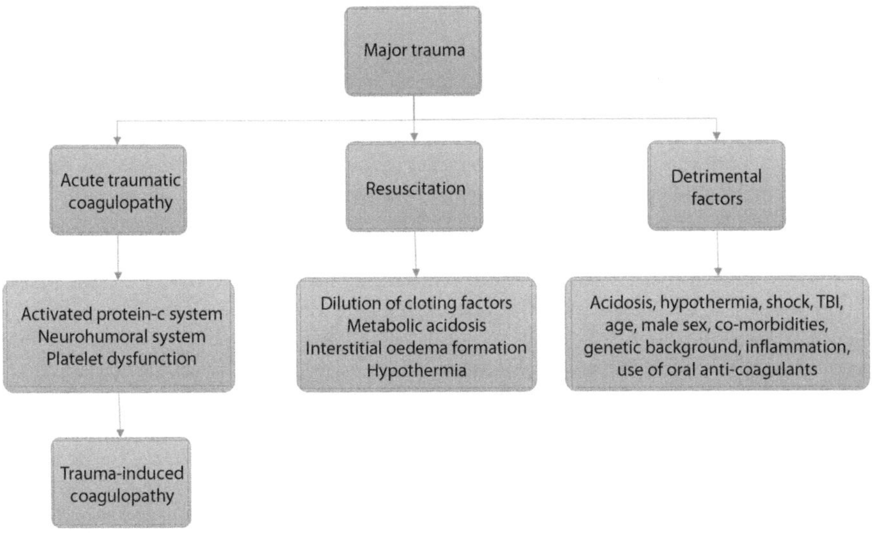

Figure 1.7 Mechanism of TIC.

CLINICAL FEATURES

Although blood loss is usually noticeable, neither visual evaluation nor physiological parameters are effective guides for understanding the degree of haemorrhage. Trauma dynamics, *i.e.*, the mechanism of injury works as an excellent guide for identifying patients at risk of significant bleeding. For instance, patients who have suffered trauma due to injury, are more likely to receive massive transfusion and are thus more likely to develop TIC. TIC is a complex process that involves the endothelium, platelets, circulating coagulation factors and the immune system and no single assay or set of assays available to date can effectively integrate the measurements of the crucial coordinated events involved in vascular homeostasis to provide a comprehensive evaluation.

Early TIC – Massively bleeding patients are at increased risk of developing TIC. Shock is a predominant feature seen in these patients. Identification of patients with TIC amongst a cohort of massively bleeding patients is augmented by the use of laboratory tests. The problem in early TIC is that of hyperfibrinolysis, and the conventional laboratory tests fail to identify this. However, studies have shown that mortality is higher amongst similarly injured patients who have prolonged PT/international normalized ratio (INR), suggesting the role of conventional tests,[85]

Late TIC – Tissue injury is the predominant pathophysiology in late TIC. Hypercoagulability is often the core problem with late TIC. The patients at great risk of late TIC are those that developed early TIC. Management of shock with resuscitation, administration of fluids, blood products and haemostatic agents results in potential secondary coagulopathies as well as haemodilution, acidosis and hypothermia. Coagulopathy is exacerbated in the event of ongoing blood loss due to lack of mechanical control. The majority of the patients shift from a hypocoagulable to a hypercoagulable state within 24 hours, following correction of haemorrhage and hypoperfusion. Patients with spine, pelvic and femur fractures, which limit post-injury mobilization, are particularly at high risk of late thrombotic complications.[26]

CONCLUSION

TIC is a critical and complex physiological response to severe injury that significantly increases morbidity and mortality. Unlike classical coagulopathy, TIC develops rapidly, often within minutes of trauma, and is not solely due to dilution, hypothermia, or acidosis. Instead, it reflects a dysregulated haemostatic response involving the coagulation cascade, anticoagulant pathways, and fibrinolysis. Understanding these mechanisms is vital for early recognition and timely intervention. The pathophysiology of TIC underscores the need for a shift from traditional volume-based resuscitation to targeted, damage-control strategies. Diagnostic tools such as viscoelastic assays can support rapid detection, while protocol-driven use of blood products and adjunct therapies can limit further bleeding and prevent complications such as thrombosis. Despite advances in high-income settings, significant challenges remain in low- and middle-income countries, where limited resources hinder early diagnosis and treatment. Addressing these gaps through training, standardized protocols, and access to diagnostics is essential. A robust understanding of TIC, from its biological basis to its clinical manifestations, can improve trauma care outcomes globally. Continued research, especially in diverse populations, and integration of TIC focused practices into trauma systems will help reduce preventable deaths and advance precision care in trauma settings.

TAKE-HOME MESSAGE

TIC is an early, dynamic, and multifactorial condition distinct from traditional coagulopathies. Recognizing its complex interplay of vascular, cellular, and biochemical disruptions is essential for timely diagnosis and management. A solid foundation in its principles is key to improving trauma outcomes.

REFERENCES

1. O'Donovan S, van den Heuvel C, Baldock M, Byard RW. Causes of fatalities in motor vehicle occupants: An overview. Forensic Sci Med Pathol. 2022;18(4):511–5.

2. Pfeifer R, Tarkin IS, Rocos B, Pape H-C. Patterns of mortality and causes of death in polytrauma patients—Has anything changed? Injury. 2009;40(9):907–11.

3. Theusinger OM, Baulig W, Levy JH. Coagulation in trauma. Trends in Anaesthesia and Critical Care. 2015;5(1):23–7.

4. Kushimoto S, Kudo D, Kawazoe Y. Acute traumatic coagulopathy and trauma-induced coagulopathy: An overview. J Intensive Care. 2017;5(1):6.

5. Seidu AS, Alhassan AR, Buunaaim ADB. Epidemiology of polytrauma at a teaching hospital in Northern Ghana: A cross-sectional study. Int J Clin Pract. 2024;2024(1):4131822.

6. Park JH, Song KJ, Shin SD, Hong KJ, Ro YS, Jeong J, et al. Epidemiology and outcomes of severe injury patients: Nationwide community-based study in Korea. Injury. 2022;53(6):1935–46.

7. Hayakawa M, Sawamura A, Gando S, Kubota N, Uegaki S, Shimojima H, et al. Disseminated intravascular coagulation at an early phase of trauma is associated with consumption coagulopathy and excessive fibrinolysis both by plasmin and neutrophil elastase. Surgery. 2011;149(2):221–30.

8. Hayakawa M. Pathophysiology of trauma-induced coagulopathy: Disseminated intravascular coagulation with the fibrinolytic phenotype. J Intensive Care. 2017;5:14.

9. Thornton P, Douglas J. Coagulation in pregnancy. Best Pract Res Clin Obstet Gynaecol. 2010;24:339–52.

10. Green D. Coagulation cascade. Hemodial Int. 2006;10(Suppl 2):S2–4.

11. Chaturvedi S, Brodsky RA, McCrae KR. Complement in the pathophysiology of the antiphospholipid syndrome. Front Immunol. 2019;10:449.

12. Franchi T, Eaton S, De Coppi P, Giuliani S. The emerging role of immunothrombosis in paediatric conditions. Pediatr Res. 2019;86(1):19–27.

13. Habib A, Petrucci G, Rocca B. Pathophysiology of thrombosis in peripheral artery disease. Curr Vasc Pharmacol. 2020;18(3):204–14.

14. Achneck HE, Sileshi B, Parikh A, Milano CA, Welsby IJ, Lawson JH. Pathophysiology of bleeding and clotting in the cardiac surgery patient: From vascular endothelium to circulatory assist device surface. Circulation. 2010;122:2068–77.

15. Previtali E, Bucciarelli P, Passamonti SM, Martinelli I. Risk factors for venous and arterial thrombosis. Blood Transfus. 2011;9:120–38.

16. Bombeli T, Spahn DR. Updates in perioperative coagulation: Physiology and management of thromboembolism and haemorrhage. Br J Anaesth. 2004;93:275–87.

17. Hall JE. Guyton and Hall Textbook of Medical Physiology: Enhanced E-Book. 11th ed. Philadelphia: Elsevier Health Sciences; 2010. Hemostasis and blood coagulation; pp. 457–9.

18. Kumar V, Abbas AK, Fausto N, Aster JC. Robbins and Cotran Pathologic Basis of Disease. 8th ed. Philadelphia, PA: Saunders Elsevier; 2010. Hemodynamic disorders, thromboembolic disease and shock; pp. 118–20.

19. Lasne D, Jude B, Susen S. From normal to pathological hemostasis. Can J Anesth. 2006;53:S2–11.

20. Owens AP, 3rd, Mackman N. Tissue factor and thrombosis: The clot starts here. Thromb Haemost. 2010;104:432–9.

21. Chaudhry R, Usama SM, Babiker HM. Physiology, Coagulation Pathways. [Updated 2025 Jun 2]. In: StatPearls [Internet]. Treasure Island (FL): StatPearls Publishing; 2026.

22. Palta S, Saroa R, Palta A. Overview of the coagulation system. Indian J Anaesth. 2014;58(5):515–23.

23. Rawala-Sheikh R, Ahmad SS, Monroe DM, Roberts HR, Walsh PN. Role of gamma-carboxyglutamic acid residues in the binding of factor IXa to platelets and in factor-X activation. Blood. 1992;79(2):398–405.

24. Colvin BT. Physiology of haemostasis. Vox Sang. 2004;87(Suppl 1):43–6.

25. Dobson GP, Letson HL, Sharma R, Sheppard FR, Cap AP. Mechanisms of early trauma-induced coagulopathy: The clot thickens or not? J Trauma Acute Care Surg. 2015;79(2):301–9.

26. Moore EE, Moore HB, Kornblith LZ, Neal MD, Hoffman M, Mutch NJ, et al. Trauma-induced coagulopathy. Nat Rev Dis Primers. 2021;7(1):30. Erratum in: Nat Rev Dis Primers. 2022 Apr 22;8(1):25.

27. Buzzard L, Schreiber M. Trauma-induced coagulopathy: What you need to know. J Trauma Acute Care Surg. 2024;96(2):179–85.

28. Simmons RL, Collins JA, Heisterkamp CA, Mills DE, Andren R, Phillips L. Coagulation disorders in combat casualties. I. Acute changes after wounding. II. Effects of massive transfusion. 3. Post-resuscitative changes. Ann Surg. 1969;169(4):455–82.

29. Kashuk JL, Moore EE, Millikan JS, Moore JB. Major abdominal vascular trauma–a unified approach. J Trauma. 1982;22(8):672–9.

30. Tieu BH, Holcomb JB, Schreiber MA. Coagulopathy: Its pathophysiology and treatment in the injured patient. World J Surg. 2007;31(5):1055–64.

31. Cohen MJ, West M. Acute traumatic coagulopathy: From endogenous acute coagulopathy to systemic acquired coagulopathy and back. J Trauma. 2011;70(5 Suppl):S47–9.

32. McMullin NR, Kauvar DS, Currier HM, Baskin TW, Pusateri AE, Holcomb JB. The clinical and laboratory response to recombinant factor VIIA in trauma and surgical patients with acquired coagulopathy. Curr Surg. 2006;63(4):246–51.

33. Gando S, Tedo I, Hanaoka Y, Makise N, Tsujinaga H, Kubota M. Masui. Blood coagulation and fibrinolysis in trauma patients with special reference to FPA and FPBbeta 15-42. [Jpn]J Acute Med. 1988;37(4):451–6.

34. Gando S, Tedo I, Kubota M. Posttrauma coagulation and fibrinolysis. Crit Care Med. 1992;20:594–600.

35. Engelman DT, Gabram SG, Allen L, Ens GE, Jacobs LM. Hypercoagulability following multiple trauma. World J Surg. 1996;20(1):5–10.

36. Guay J, Ozier Y, de Moerloose P, Samana CM, Bélisle S, Hardy JF. Le polytraumatisé et les anomalies de l'hémostase [Polytrauma and hemostatic anomalies]. Can J Anaesth. 1998;45(7):683–91.

37. Ordog GJ, Wasserbergaer J. Coagulation abnormalities in traumatic shock. Crit Care Med. 1986;14:519.

38. Brohi K, Singh J, Heron M, Coats T. Acute traumatic coagulopathy. J Trauma. 2003;54(6):1127–30.

39. MacLeod J, Lynn M, McKenney M, Cohn S, Murtha M. Early coagulopathy predicts mortality in trauma. J Trauma. 2003;55(1):39–44.

40. Peng N, Su L. Progresses in understanding trauma-induced coagulopathy and the underlying mechanism. Chin J Traumatol. 2017;20(3):133–6.

41. Brohi K, Cohen MJ, Davenport RA. Acute coagulopathy of trauma: Mechanism, identification and effect. Curr Opin Crit Care. 2007;13(6):680–5.

42. Rani P, Panda NB, Hazarika A, Ahluwalia J, Chhabra R. Trauma-induced coagulopathy: Incidence and outcome in patients with isolated traumatic brain injury in a level I trauma care center in India. Asian J Neurosurg. 2019;14(4):1175–80.

43. Albert V, Arulselvi S, Agrawal D, Pati HP, Pandey RM. Early posttraumatic changes in coagulation and fibrinolysis systems in isolated severe traumatic brain injury patients and its influence on immediate outcome. Hematol Oncol Stem Cell Ther. 2019;12(1):32–43.

44. Chong SL, Dang H, Ming M, Mahmood M, Zheng CQS, Gan CS, *et al.* Pediatric acute & critical care medicine Asian network (PACCMAN). Traumatic brain injury outcomes in 10 Asian pediatric ICUs: A pediatric acute and critical care medicine Asian network retrospective study. Pediatr Crit Care Med. 2021;22(4):401–11.

45. Strumwasser A, Speer AL, Inaba K, Branco BC, Upperman JS, Ford HR, *et al.* The impact of acute coagulopathy on mortality in pediatric trauma patients. J Trauma Acute Care Surg. 2016;81(2):312–8.

46. Rugeri L, Levrat A, David JS, Delecroix E, Floccard B, Gros A, *et al.* Diagnosis of early coagulation abnormalities in trauma patients by rotation thrombelastography. J Thromb Haemost. 2007;5(2):289–95.

47. Cohen MJ, Brohi K, Ganter MT, Manley GT, Mackersie RC, Pittet JF. Early coagulopathy after traumatic brain injury: The role of hypoperfusion and the protein C pathway. J Trauma. 2007;63(6):1254–62.

48. Zehtabchi S, Soghoian S, Liu Y, Carmody K, Shah L, Whittaker B, *et al.* The association of coagulopathy and traumatic brain injury in patients with isolated head injury. Resuscitation. 2008;76(1):52–6.

49. Talving P, Benfield R, Hadjizacharia P, Inaba K, Chan LS, Demetriades D. Coagulopathy in severe traumatic brain injury: A prospective study. J Trauma. 2009;66(1):55–61; discussion 61-2

50. Allard CB, Scarpelini S, Rhind SG, Baker AJ, Shek PN, Tien H, *et al.* Abnormal coagulation tests are associated with progression of traumatic intracranial hemorrhage. J Trauma. 2009;67(5):959–67.

51. Lustenberger T, Talving P, Kobayashi L, Inaba K, Lam L, Plurad D, *et al.* Time course of coagulopathy in isolated severe traumatic brain injury. Injury. 2010;41(9):924–8.

52. Lustenberger T, Talving P, Kobayashi L, Barmparas G, Inaba K, Lam L, *et al.* Early coagulopathy after isolated severe traumatic brain injury: Relationship with hypoperfusion challenged. J Trauma. 2010;69(6):1410–4.

53. Wafaisade A, Lefering R, Tjardes T, Wutzler S, Simanski C, Paffrath T; Trauma Registry of DGU, *et al.* Acute coagulopathy in isolated blunt traumatic brain injury. Neurocrit Care. 2010;12(2):211–9.

54. Wu X, Du Z, Yu J, Sun Y, Pei B, Lu X, *et al.* Activity of factor VII in patients with isolated blunt traumatic brain injury: Association with coagulopathy and progressive hemorrhagic injury. J Trauma Acute Care Surg. 2014;76(1):114–20.

55. Chhabra G, Sharma S, Subramanian A, Agrawal D, Sinha S, Mukhopadhyay AK. Coagulopathy as prognostic marker in acute traumatic brain injury. J Emerg Trauma Shock. 2013;6(3):180–5.

56. Greuters S, van den Berg A, Franschman G, Viersen VA, Beishuizen A, Peerdeman SM; ALARM-BLEEDING investigators, *et al.* Acute and delayed mild coagulopathy are related to outcome in patients with isolated traumatic brain injury. Crit Care. 2011;15(1):R2.

57. Franschman G, Boer C, Andriessen TM, van der Naalt J, Horn J, Haitsma I, *et al.* Multicenter evaluation of the course of coagulopathy in patients with isolated traumatic brain injury: Relation to CT characteristics and outcome. J Neurotrauma. 2012;29(1):128–36.

58. Genét GF, Johansson PI, Meyer MA, Sølbeck S, Sørensen AM, Larsen CF, *et al.* Trauma-induced coagulopathy: Standard coagulation tests, biomarkers of coagulopathy, and endothelial damage in patients with traumatic brain injury. J Neurotrauma. 2013;30(4):301–6.

59. Epstein DS, Mitra B, O'Reilly G, Rosenfeld JV, Cameron PA. Acute traumatic coagulopathy in the setting of isolated traumatic brain injury: A systematic review and meta-analysis. Injury. 2014;45(5):819–24.

60. Shaz BH, Winkler AM, James AB, Hillyer CD, MacLeod JB. Pathophysiology of early trauma-induced coagulopathy: Emerging evidence for hemodilution and coagulation factor depletion. J Trauma. 2011;70(6):1401–7.

61. de Oliveira Manoel AL, Neto AC, Veigas PV, Rizoli S. Traumatic brain injury associated coagulopathy. Neurocrit Care. 2015;22(1):34–44.

62. Dekker SE, Duvekot A, de Vries HM, Geeraedts LMG, Peerdeman SM, de Waard MC, *et al.* Relationship between tissue perfusion and coagulopathy in traumatic brain injury. J. Surg. Res. 2016;205:147–54.

63. Böhm JK, Schaeben V, Schäfer N, Güting H, Lefering R, Thorn S, *et al.* CENTER-TBI participants and investigators. Extended coagulation profiling in isolated traumatic brain injury: A CENTER-TBI analysis. Neurocrit Care. 2022;36(3):927–41.

64. Du X, Wang W, Xu B, Zheng J, Xia VW, Guo Y, *et al.* Predicting postoperative trauma-induced coagulopathy in patients with severe injuries by machine learning. Sci Rep. 2025;15(1):27072.

65. Sun Y, Wang J, Wu X, Xi C, Gai Y, Liu H, *et al.* Validating the incidence of coagulopathy and disseminated intravascular coagulation in patients with traumatic brain injury–analysis of 242 cases. Br J Neurosurg. 2011;25(3):363–8.

66. Folkerson LE, Sloan D, Davis E, Kitagawa RS, Cotton BA, Holcomb JB, *et al.* Coagulopathy as a predictor of mortality after penetrating traumatic brain injury. Am J Emerg Med. 2018;36(1):38–42.

67. Brown JB, Cohen MJ, Minei JP, Maier RV, West MA, Billiar TR; Inflammation and the Host Response to Injury Investigators, *et al.* Characterization of acute coagulopathy and sexual dimorphism after Injury: Females and coagulopathy just do not mix. J Trauma Acute Care Surg. 2012;73(6):1395–400.

68. Xu SX, Wang L, Zhou GJ, Zhang M, Gan JX. Risk factors and clinical significance of trauma-induced coagulopathy in ICU patients with severe trauma. Eur J Emerg Med. 2013;20(4):286–90.

69. Global status report on road safety [Internet]; 2018 June 17 [Accessed 16 November 2025]. Available from https://www.who.int/publications/i/item/9789241565684

70. Kauvar DS, Lefering R, Wade CE. Impact of hemorrhage on trauma outcome: An overview of epidemiology, clinical presentations, and therapeutic considerations. J Trauma. 2006;60(6 Suppl):S3–S11.

71. Holcomb JB, Tilley BC, Baraniuk S, Fox EE, Wade CE, Podbielski JM; PROPPR Study Group, *et al.* Transfusion of plasma, platelets, and red blood cells in a 1:1:1 vs a 1:1:2 ratio and mortality in patients with severe trauma: The PROPPR randomized clinical trial. JAMA. 2015;313(5):471–82.

72. Baranwal AK, Kumar MP, Gupta PK. Comparison of ventilator-free days at 14 and 28 days as a clinical trial outcome in low- and middle-income countries. Indian J Crit Care Med. 2020;24(10):960–6.

73. van Zyl N, Reade MC, Fraser JF. Experimental animal models of traumatic coagulopathy: A systematic review. Shock. 2015;44(1):16–24.

74. Practice guidelines for perioperative blood transfusion and adjuvant therapies: An updated report by the American society of anesthesiologists task force on perioperative blood transfusion and adjuvant therapies. Anesthesiology. 2006;105(1): 198–208.

75. Rossaint R, Bouillon B, Cerny V, Coats TJ, Duranteau J, Fernández-Mondéjar E, *et al.* The European guideline on management of major bleeding and coagulopathy following trauma: Fourth edition. Crit Care. 2016;20:100.

76. Schlimp CJ, Schöchl H. The role of fibrinogen in trauma-induced coagulopathy. Hamostaseologie. 2014;34:29–39.

77. Hunt H, Stanworth S, Curry N, Woolley T, Cooper C, Ukoumunne O, *et al.* Thromboelastography (TEG) and rotational thromboelastometry (ROTEM) for trauma induced coagulopathy in adult trauma patients with bleeding. Cochrane Database Syst Rev. 2015;2015(2):CD010438.

78. Gando S, Kameue T, Matsuda N, Hayakawa M, Ishitani T, Morimoto Y, *et al.* Combined activation of coagulation and inflammation has an important role in multiple organ dysfunction and poor outcome after severe trauma. Thromb Haemost. 2002;88(6):943–9.

79. Ostrowski SR, Henriksen HH, Stensballe J, Gybel-Brask M, Cardenas JC, Baer LA, *et al.* Sympathoadrenal activation and endotheliopathy are drivers of hypocoagulability and

hyperfibrinolysis in trauma: A prospective observational study of 404 severely injured patients. J Trauma Acute Care Surg. 2017;82(2):293–301.

80. Vulliamy P, Kornblith LZ, Kutcher ME, Cohen MJ, Brohi K, Neal MD. Alterations in platelet behavior after major trauma: Adaptive or maladaptive? Platelets. 2021; 32(3):295–304.

81. Zhang Q, Raoof M, Chen Y, Sumi Y, Sursal T, Junger W, *et al.* Circulating mitochondrial DAMPs cause inflammatory responses to injury. Nature. 2010;464(7285):104–7.

82. Kleinveld DJB, Hamada SR, Sandroni C. Trauma - induced coagulopathy. Intensive Care Med. 2022;48(11):1642–5.

83. Davenport RA, Guerreiro M, Frith D, Rourke C, Platton S, Cohen M, *et al.* Activated protein C drives the hyperfibrinolysis of acute traumatic coagulopathy. Anesthesiology. 2017;126(1):115–27.

84. Wolberg AS. Thrombin generation and fibrin clot structure. Blood Rev. 2007;21(3): 131–42.

85. Shepherd JM, Cole E, Brohi K. Contemporary patterns of multiple organ dysfunction in trauma. Shock. 2017;47(4):429–35.

Chapter 2

MECHANISM AND PATHOPHYSIOLOGY OF TRAUMA-INDUCED COAGULOPATHY

Abhishek Satapathy, Babita Gupta, Venencia Albert,
Nitin Tiwari, and Arulselvi Subramanian

DOI: 10.1201/9781003711070-2

INTRODUCTION

Trauma-induced coagulopathy (TIC) is a spectrum of hemostatic disorders caused by severe mechanical trauma. The clinical presentation of TIC can vary widely, ranging from uncontrolled hemorrhage to thrombotic complications such as deep vein thrombosis (DVT) and pulmonary embolism (PE). Early hypocoagulability is often characterized by diffuse bleeding from multiple sites, while later stages may present with hypercoagulability and thrombotic events. The pathophysiology of TIC is intricate, involving a multitude of factors, such as hypovolemic shock, tissue injury, endothelial damage, and dysregulated fibrinolysis. This chapter delves into the elaborate pathogenetic processes underlying TIC. A comprehensive understanding of the mechanism is essential for strategizing diagnostic and therapeutic approaches.

The classical concept of TIC is based on the foundation of the lethal triad framework.[1] The components are hypothermia, acidosis, and hemodilution. They are believed to arise because of significant hemorrhage and insufficient resuscitation. These events result in atypical enzymatic activity, depletion of clotting factors, and ineffective clot formation. The traditional notion posits that coagulopathy arising in the later stages of clinical progression is predominantly iatrogenic, induced by fluid replacement strategies that lead to hypothermia and the dilution of coagulation factors.[1]

Nonetheless, this traditional concept has faced criticism due to clinical observations of coagulopathy present upon admission to the emergency department, before the commencement of fluid replacement strategies. The new concept identifies this initial phase as characterized by hypoperfusion-induced endogenous coagulopathy, referred to as acute coagulopathy of trauma shock.[2] Unlike the classical model, this modern understanding emphasizes that TIC is largely an intrinsic response to tissue injury, augmented by systemic hypoperfusion.[3] It acknowledges that intricate biological cascades are implicated in this process, including the activation of the protein C pathway, disruption of the endothelial glycocalyx, release of tissue factor-bearing microparticles, systemic inflammation, and dysregulation of fibrinolysis. These processes exhibit a dynamic interaction, leading to an unstable equilibrium between procoagulant and anticoagulant forces. Additional modulation occurs based on the degree of shock, injury burden, and host response (Figure 2.1). A comparison of the classical post-trauma coagulopathy concept and the modern view of TIC is shown in Table 2.1.

Modern trauma protocols emphasize personalized hemostatic resuscitation based on real-time assessments of patients' coagulation profiles, due to the temporal variations in their clinical courses.[4]

Table 2.1   Classical post-trauma coagulopathy concept vs. the modern view of TIC

Dimension	Classical post-trauma coagulopathy concept	TIC (modern view)
Onset/Cause/Driver	Secondary, after resuscitation: Dilution, hypothermia, acidosis	Primary, on arrival: Shock, tissue injury leading to endotheliopathy
Core mechanisms	Factor depletion and thrombocytopenia, impaired thrombin generation	PC activation, glycocalyx loss, platelet dysfunction, sympathetic stimulation
Phenotype	PT/aPTT increased, decreased fibrinogen, thrombocytopenia	Variable phenotype according to fibrinolysis status, platelet hypofunction with or without thrombocytopenia
Management	Balanced replacement to address dilution	Mechanism guided- hemorrhage control to protect endothelium, early TXA in hyperfibrinolysis, no reflex TXA in fibrinolytic shutdown

Abbreviations: *PT: prothrombin time; aPTT: activated partial thromboplastin time; TXA: tranexamic acid.*

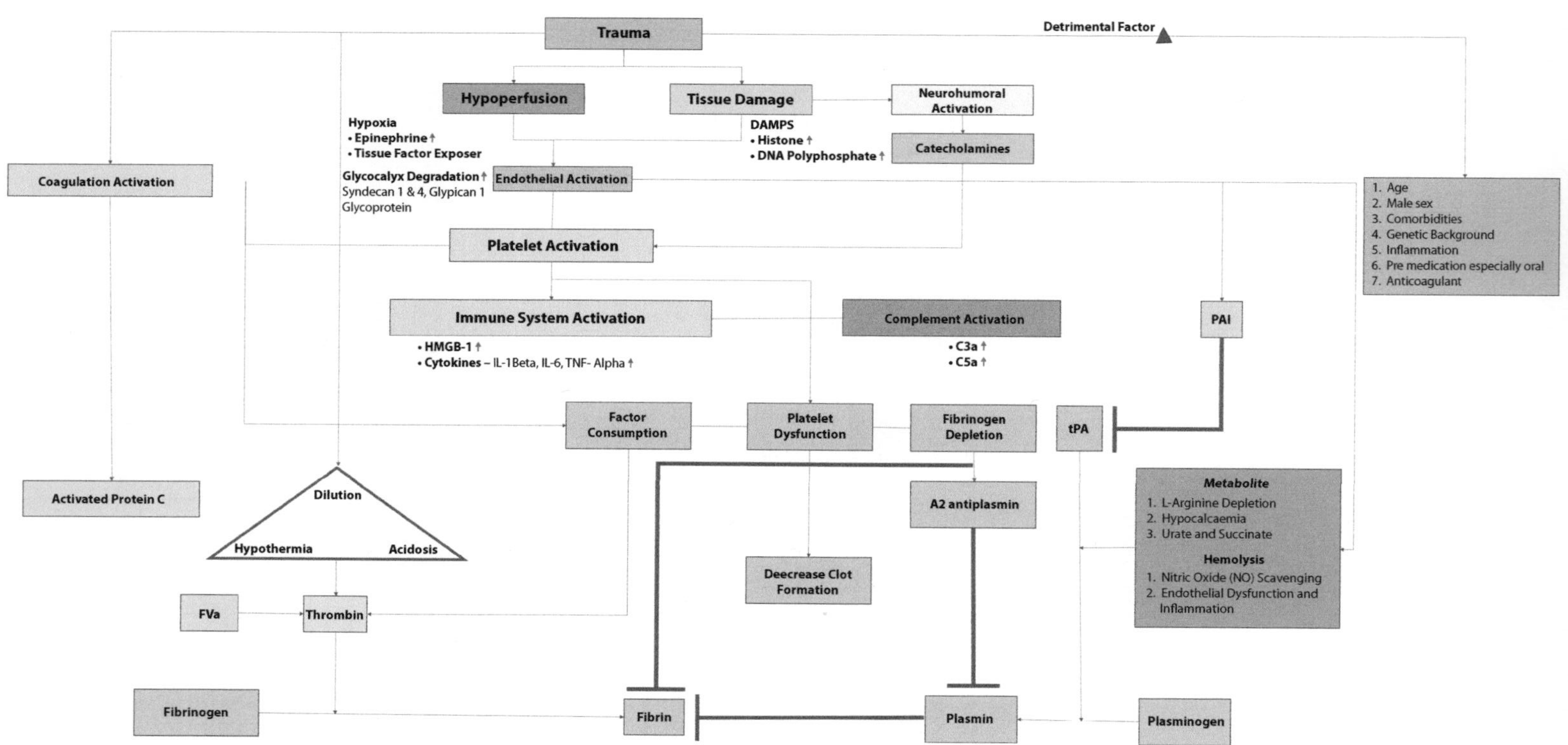

Trauma
Detrimental Factor
Hypoperfusion
Tissue Damage
Neurohumoral Activation
Hypoxia
• Epinephrine ↑
• Tissue Factor Exposer
DAMPS
• Histone ↑
• DNA Polyphosphate ↑
Catecholamines
Coagulation Activation
Glycocalyx Degradation ↑
Syndecan 1 & 4, Glypican 1
Glycoprotein
Endothelial Activation
1. Age
2. Male sex
3. Comorbidities
4. Genetic Background
5. Inflammation
6. Pre medication especially oral
7. Anticoagulant
Platelet Activation
Immune System Activation
• HMGB-1 ↑
• Cytokines – IL-1Beta, IL-6, TNF- Alpha ↑
Complement Activation
• C3a ↑
• C5a ↑
PAI
Factor Consumption
Platelet Dysfunction
Fibrinogen Depletion
tPA
Activated Protein C
Dilution
Hypothermia
Acidosis
A2 antiplasmin
Metabolite
1. L-Arginine Depletion
2. Hypocalcaemia
3. Urate and Succinate
Hemolysis
1. Nitric Oxide (NO) Scavenging
2. Endothelial Dysfunction and Inflammation
Deecrease Clot Formation
FVa
Thrombin
Fibrinogen
Fibrin
Plasmin
Plasminogen

Figure 2.1   Pathophysiological pathway of trauma-induced coagulopathy (TIC).

This diagram shows the interconnected pathways causing trauma-induced coagulopathy (TIC). Traumatic injury sets off a chain reaction of hypoperfusion, tissue destruction, and neurohumoral activation, which results in the release of catecholamines and endothelial activation. Activated endothelium causes coagulation, platelet, immune, and complement system activation, all of which contribute to dysregulated hemostasis. Coagulation activation causes clotting factor consumption, platelet dysfunction, and fibrinogen depletion, all of which result in impaired thrombin and fibrin production and clot formation. The protein C pathway becomes overactive, encouraging fibrinolysis and fibrinogen destruction, whereas tissue-type plasminogen activator (tPA) increases the conversion of plasminogen to plasmin, increasing fibrinolytic activity. Plasminogen activator inhibitor (PAI) and α2-antiplasmin can reduce fibrinolysis; however, they can become overly effective. Trauma-induced hypoperfusion and tissue injury generate metabolic abnormalities such as L-arginine depletion, acidosis (caused by lactate and carboxylic acid buildup), hypocalcemia, and elevated urate and succinate levels. These modifications decrease endothelial function, limit nitric oxide (NO) availability, and inhibit coagulation enzyme activity, exacerbating coagulopathy and tissue hypoxia. Hemolysis generates free hemoglobin, which scavenges nitric oxide, causing vasoconstriction, endothelial dysfunction, and inflammation. It also causes platelet activation and fibrinolysis dysregulation, exacerbating both thrombotic and bleeding tendencies in TIC patients. Multiple detrimental factors influence the severity and expression of these processes, including acidosis, shock, hypothermia, traumatic brain injury, age, sex, comorbidities, genetic predisposition, inflammation, pre-injury medication, and anticoagulant use.

MECHANISMS OF TRAUMA-INDUCED COAGULOPATHY

The early development of TIC is primarily driven by systemic hypoperfusion and endothelial injury, which together initiate a series of maladaptive responses within the coagulation system. These responses are interconnected processes that swiftly develop within minutes of significant trauma.[5]

The endothelium is crucial for sustaining hemostatic balance, rather than a mere passive vascular lining. In reaction to trauma and hypoperfusion, the endothelium experiences significant structural and functional modifications. The shedding of the endothelial glycocalyx, a carbohydrate-dense network crucial for regulating vascular permeability, leukocyte adhesion, and coagulation, is among the earliest and most significant occurrences.[6]

Degradation of the glycocalyx is initiated by ischemia-reperfusion injury, surges in catecholamines, and inflammatory mediators. This process reveals the subendothelial surface, facilitates platelet adhesion, and results in the systemic release of syndecan-1, a biomarker indicative of endothelial injury. The loss of the glycocalyx undermines the endothelial anticoagulant interface, promoting thrombin generation and exacerbating coagulopathy.[7]

Furthermore, damaged endothelium upregulates expression of thrombomodulin, which binds thrombin and alters its activity from procoagulant to anticoagulant, resulting in activation of the protein C pathway. The net result is a state of paradoxical hypocoagulability, wherein, despite ongoing thrombin generation, clot stabilization is impaired.[7]

The initial trauma activates the sympathetic nervous system. This activation results in a surge of catecholamines, which elevates heart rate and blood pressure, enhances cardiac output, and induces peripheral vasoconstriction, all of which are critical for sustaining the perfusion of vital organs. It also induces glycogenolysis and lipolysis to provide rapid energy for heightened metabolic demands. Catecholamines modify immunological responses, which may affect inflammation and healing processes.

The shock index (SI) is a basic measure calculated by dividing the heart rate by systolic blood pressure. This score is crucial for diagnosing the initial stages of hemorrhagic shock, a crucial component of TIC. Prompt recognition of shock ahead of the onset of overt symptoms is crucial for guiding rapid resuscitation efforts. An increased SI, above 0.9, is correlated with an increased probability of mortality. A higher SI reflects an excessive increase in heart rate compared to systolic blood pressure, suggesting that the body's compensatory mechanisms are being overloaded.

HYPOPERFUSION AND ENDOGENOUS ANTICOAGULATION THROUGH THE PROTEIN C PATHWAY

Severe trauma leads to systemic hypoperfusion and causes hypoxia, which redirects metabolism toward anaerobic glycolysis, causing lactic acidosis.[8] Hypoxia and acidosis both impact the endothelium's normal function and coagulation enzymes. Severe acidosis is associated with significantly increased mortality in trauma patients.[9]

The injured endothelium expresses higher levels of thrombomodulin, which promotes the conversion of protein C into activated protein C (aPC). Activated PC is a potent anticoagulant and profibrinolytic agent. It inhibits factors Va and VIIIa, reducing thrombin generation. Fibrinolytic activity is increased by its suppression of plasminogen activator inhibitor-1 (PAI-1), enhancing tissue-type plasminogen activator (tPA) activity. It also modulates the action of nuclear factor kappa B (NF-κB) signaling and leukocyte-endothelium interactions.[10,11]

Table 2.2 Activated protein C (aPC) state and fibrinolysis phenotype in TIC

Activated protein C (APC) state	Effect on coagulation	Effect on fibrinolysis	Diagnostic findings	Management
Increased (early hypoperfusion)	Decreased thrombin, decreased FVa/ VIIIa activity	Hyperfibrinolysis	LY30 >3%, Low/Normal Fibrinogen	Strong predictor of mortality, time-sensitive TXA
Decreased	Increased thrombin, dense cross-linked fibrin	Fibrinolysis shutdown	LY30 ≤ 0.8%,	Avoiding TXA, prioritizing endothelial protection
Normal/physiologic level	Adequate thrombin generation	Physiologic lysis	LY30 0.8–3%	No fibrinolysis directed therapy, correct substrates as needed

Abbreviations: *APC: activated protein C; LY30: lysis at 30 minutes; TXA: tranexamic acid.*

The aPC-mediated pathway is crucial to the initial hypocoagulable phenotype of TIC and signifies an intrinsic effort to mitigate extensive microvascular thrombosis and organ failure. Nonetheless, when excessive or dysregulated, it facilitates uncontrolled hemorrhage.[5] The activated protein C (aPC) state and fibrinolysis phenotypes in TIC are summarized in Table 2.2.

COAGULATION SYSTEM DYSFUNCTION

The inadequate regulation of the coagulation cascade in TIC is characterized by a paradoxical phenomenon: The simultaneous activation and depletion of clotting factors. This leads to either a hemorrhagic or thrombotic phenotype, contingent upon the balance of the implicated variables. This dysfunction encompasses increased thrombin synthesis, factor depletion, and platelet irregularities, all of which are initiated early in the trauma phase.

ACTIVATION OF THE COAGULATION CASCADE

The tissue factor (TF) is situated on the subendothelial surfaces. Significant tissue damage exposes this TF and microparticles released from activated monocytes, platelets, and injured tissues. It forms a complex with factor VIIa, initiating the extrinsic pathway of coagulation leading to a sudden surge in thrombin generation.[12] Moreover, trauma triggers the production of damage-associated molecular patterns (DAMPs), such as high-mobility group box 1 (HMGB1), extracellular histones, and mitochondrial DNA. These compounds act as procoagulant and proinflammatory agents by activating Toll-like receptors (TLRs) and inflammasomes, therefore augmenting coagulation and endothelial activation.[13]

Although thrombin generation is initially advantageous for hemostasis, its uncontrolled and systemic activation leads to microvascular thrombosis, organ ischemia, and consumptive coagulopathy. This thrombo-inflammatory disease embodies the core of immunothrombosis, an erroneous host defensive mechanism.[14]

COAGULATION FACTOR DEPLETION

The coagulation system hyperactivity results in a rapid depletion of clotting factors. Fibrinogen levels show more vulnerability than other parameters, indicating a robust association with injury severity and mortality.[15] The depletion of factors V, VIII, and XIII exacerbates the impairment of clot structural integrity. Contrary to inherited coagulopathies characterized by isolated factor deficiencies, TIC exhibits extensive factor consumption, augmented by dilution from fluid resuscitation and blood products.[1] This consumption results in hypocoagulability.[16]

PLATELET DYSFUNCTION

Platelets are essential for primary hemostasis and play an important role in coagulation. Their functionality is markedly impaired in TIC, even with a normal platelet count.[17] This qualitative platelet dysfunction signifies early coagulopathy.[18]

Trauma disrupts platelet intracellular signaling pathways critical for adhesion and aggregation, including glycoprotein VI (GPVI) mediated collagen response and ADP activated P2Y12 receptor signaling, affects cytoskeletal rearrangement, and reduces surface expression of P selectin and GPIIb/IIIa.[19]

Endothelial activity facilitates the release of NO and prostacyclin (PGI2), which inhibit platelet activation. Trauma-induced shear stress and oxidative stress further impede platelet activity. Recent results indicate that defective platelets in TIC exhibit diminished responsiveness to thrombin and may be unable to facilitate procoagulant membrane flipping, a critical mechanism for thrombin burst and fibrin production.

FIBRINOLYTIC DYSREGULATION

Fibrinolysis, the process by which fibrin clots are dissolved, is a well-regulated component of hemostasis. Trauma causes dysregulation of fibrinolysis, contributing to the coagulopathic phenotype. Patients may exhibit hyperfibrinolysis, leading to uncontrolled hemorrhage, or fibrinolytic shutdown, heightening the risk of thrombotic events and organ failure. This bimodal dysregulation signifies an inappropriate response due to trauma and shock.[20]

EARLY HYPERFIBRINOLYSIS

Hyperfibrinolysis is a characteristic feature of early TIC and is strongly correlated with extensive transfusion needs and mortality rates. Primary drivers are as follows:

i. Release of tPA in response to hypoperfusion and catecholamine elevation.[21]

ii. Inhibition of PAI-1 by activated protein C, promoting unopposed tPA activity.[22]

iii. Expedited conversion of plasminogen into plasmin, resulting in the swift degradation of fibrin and fibrinogen.[23]

The outcome is the creation of fragile, unstable clots that are swiftly dissolved. Fibrin degradation products (FDPs), particularly D-dimer, exhibit a surge during this phase and correlate with poor prognosis. This condition is difficult to recognize by standard coagulation assays but can be easily diagnosed by viscoelastic testing (e.g., thromboelastography [TEG] or rotational thromboelastometry [ROTEM]), which shows early lysis patterns.

FIBRINOLYTIC SHUTDOWN: A PARADOXICAL RISK

In contrast, some trauma patients exhibit fibrinolytic shutdown, marked by diminished tPA activity and elevated PAI-1 levels.[24] This phenotype is associated with:

i. Microvascular thrombosis and multiple organ dysfunction syndrome (MODS).

ii. Elevated risk of venous thromboembolism (VTE) despite the risk of hemorrhage.

This shutdown is presumed to be a compensatory phase succeeding early hyperfibrinolysis. The change is driven by significant endothelial injury, inflammation, and elevated thrombin levels, which strengthen fibrin clots and resist fibrinolysis.[25]

INFLAMMATION COAGULATION CROSSTALK

The intersection of inflammation and coagulation is a key characteristic of TIC. Severe trauma triggers an immunothrombotic response that links the innate immune system with the coagulation cascade. This integration plays a key role in limiting microbial invasion and closure of vascular injuries. In cases of systemic trauma, it frequently loses regulatory control and self-propagates, leading to tissue destruction, microvascular thrombosis, and organ failure.[26]

DAMAGE-ASSOCIATED MOLECULAR PATTERNS (DAMPS) AND PATTERN RECOGNITION RECEPTORS (PRRS)

Tissue injury leads to cellular release of DAMPs, including intracellular compounds including HMGB1, histones, ATP, and mitochondrial DNA. DAMPs activate pattern recognition receptors (PRRs), namely TLRs and NOD-like receptors on endothelial cells, leukocytes, and platelets. This causes the following:

i. Initiation of pro-inflammatory signaling pathways (e.g., NF-κB)

ii. Augmentation the expression of TF on monocytes and endothelium

iii. Activation of the inflammasome pathway, leading to interleukin(IL)-1β and IL-18 release

iv. Neutrophil extracellular trap (NET) formation

These responses transform trauma into a systemic inflammatory state with disruption of hemostatic balance.

IMMUNOTHROMBOSIS AND MICROVASCULAR INJURY

Immunothrombosis is a mechanism of defense by which neutrophils and monocytes coordinate with platelets and the coagulation system to form fibrin-rich microthrombi to entrap pathogens and cellular debris. In TIC, this defensive system becomes maladaptive: NETs, consisting of DNA, histones, and proteases, not only capture pathogens but also create a procoagulant surface. Extracellular histones activate platelets and damage the endothelium, promoting thrombosis.[27] Thus, NETs are complex players involved in pathogen clearance and tissue repair but can also lead to the development of severe inflammatory conditions if unchecked. Activated monocytes also release pro-inflammatory cytokines, as discussed subsequently. Activated complement components, including C5a, recruit inflammatory cells and enhance coagulation. The outcome is extensive microvascular thrombosis and disruption of the endothelial barrier.[28]

CYTOKINES, ENDOTHELIOPATHY, AND DISSEMINATED COAGULOPATHY

Trauma triggers a cytokine storm marked by increased release of tumor necrosis factor-alpha (TNF-α), IL-6, IL-1β, and Interferon-gamma (IFN-γ) from activated immune cells. These cytokines cause tissue edema by increasing endothelial permeability and upregulating the expression of adhesion molecules (Intercellular Adhesion Molecule-1 (ICAM-1) and Vascular Cell Adhesion Molecule-1 (VCAM-1)), promoting leukocyte-endothelial interactions. They also promote a procoagulant state by downregulating anticoagulant pathways (e.g., thrombomodulin, antithrombin) and upregulating TF expression. A fundamental characteristic of TIC is trauma-associated endotheliopathy, a cytokine-mediated endothelial dysfunction. This promotes the progression from localized coagulopathy to full-blown disseminated intravascular coagulation (DIC). In summary, trauma causes endotheliopathy, which contributes to the development of DIC.[6]

ROLE OF THE ENDOTHELIUM AND GLYCOCALYX IN TIC

The endothelium functions not just as a physical barrier but also as a critical regulator of vascular tone, permeability, leukocyte trafficking, and hemostasis. Trauma-associated hypoperfusion, inflammation, and mechanical damage significantly impair the structural and functional integrity of the endothelial glycocalyx, a critical factor in the onset and sustaining of TIC.[29]

STRUCTURE AND FUNCTION OF THE GLYCOCALYX

The glycocalyx is a gel-like layer on the surface of endothelial cells made up of proteoglycans (e.g., syndecans, glypicans) and glycosaminoglycans (e.g., heparan sulfate, chondroitin sulfate). It functions as a mechanotransducer for shear stress, a selective barrier that regulates vascular permeability, and a reservoir for anticoagulant and anti-inflammatory mediators such as antithrombin, tissue factor pathway inhibitor (TFPI), and extracellular superoxide dismutase.[30]

GLYCOCALYX SHEDDING IN TRAUMA

Trauma-induced hypoperfusion and oxidative stress promote enzymatic degradation of the glycocalyx through matrix metalloproteinases (MMPs), heparinase, hyaluronidase, and proinflammatory cytokines. This leads to the release of syndecan-1, which serves as a quantifiable marker of endothelial injury. Syndecan-1 levels are proportional to the severity of damage, coagulopathy and translate to increased mortality. The loss of the glycocalyx exposes the adhesion molecules such as endothelial (E)-selectin and ICAM-1, promoting leukocyte and platelet attachment. Concurrently, the loss of this anticoagulant barrier promotes a shift towards procoagulant activity.[31]

ENDOTHELIAL SIGNALING AND COAGULOPATHY

Glycocalyx shedding also disrupts thrombomodulin-thrombin interactions, leading to excess thrombin activity, promotion of platelet activation, and fibrin generation. Excessive activation of protein C results in anticoagulation and fibrinolysis in the initial stages of TIC. Elevated vascular permeability, leading to edema and systemic inflammation. Malfunction of endothelial nitric oxide synthase (eNOS) due to glycocalyx degradation and oxidative stress reduces NO bioavailability, facilitating vasoconstriction, platelet aggregation, and endothelial damage. These processes cause significant endotheliopathy, marked by coagulopathy, inflammation, capillary leakage, and organ failure. The integrated endothelial response is a primary factor in TIC, making the glycocalyx a candidate for a potential therapeutic target for endothelium-protective nterventions (Figure 2.2).[31]

METABOLIC DYSREGULATION

Trauma induces profound changes in the metabolic profile of endothelial cells, notably disturbing glucose uptake and fatty acid metabolism. These metabolic shifts impair mitochondrial function, increase reactive oxygen species, and favor the accumulation of lipid droplets.[32] High glucose states seen in acute stress promote mitochondrial fragmentation and decrease fatty acid β-oxidation, leading to an overload of triglyceride-derived fatty acids stored as lipid droplets, which is both an adaptive and maladaptive response to metabolic stress.[33] Disordered glucose and fatty acid handling impair endothelial ATP production, reducing NO synthesis, and fostering oxidative stress, which together drive endothelial dysfunction, a core feature of endotheliopathy of trauma (EoT).[34] Understanding these intricate metabolic mechanisms is critical for the development of targeted therapies that aim to restore endothelial homeostasis and minimize the sequelae of trauma-induced endothelial dysfunction.[35] Ongoing research continues to unravel how metabolic derangements interact with inflammatory and coagulation pathways in the pathogenesis and progression of EoT, with the ultimate goal of designing interventions that enhance outcomes in trauma patients.

IATROGENIC CONTRIBUTORS TO TRAUMA-INDUCED COAGULOPATHY

Iatrogenic TIC refers to coagulopathy generated or worsened by medical interventions during trauma care, distinct from the endogenous mechanisms triggered by injury itself. These interventions historically include large-volume crystalloid and red cell transfusions, aggressive resuscitation, and surgical procedures, which disrupt the balance of coagulation homeostasis. Impaired coagulation after trauma was previously attributed mainly to such iatrogenic factors, including dilutional coagulopathy, hypothermia, and metabolic acidosis

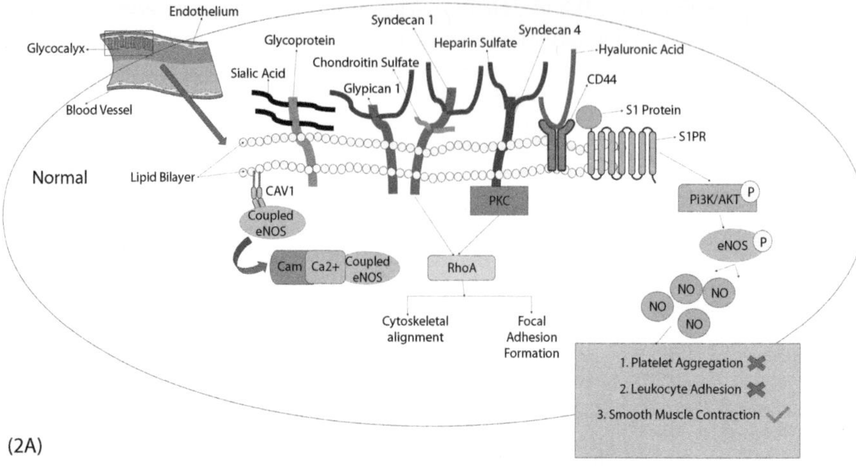

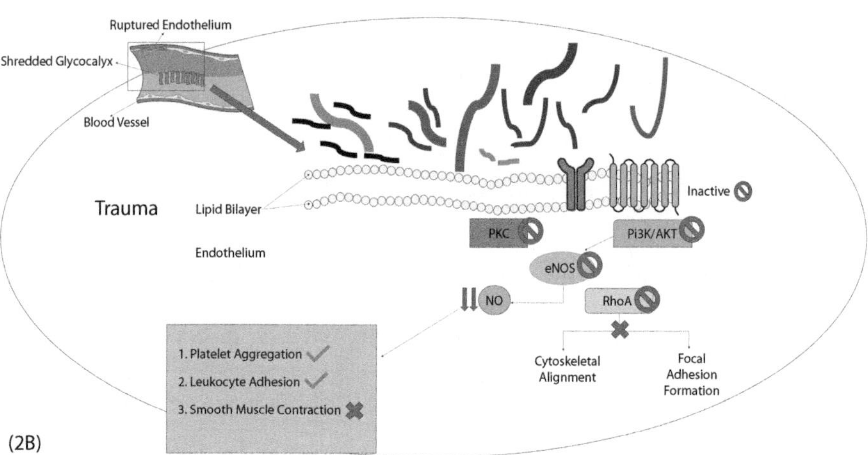

Figure 2.2 Schematic illustration of endothelial glycocalyx mediated signaling under normal (2A) and trauma conditions (2B). Selected elements were sourced from the National Institute of Allergy and Infectious Diseases (NIAID) of the National Institutes of Health (NIH) BioArt Source (bioart. niaid.nih.gov).

The image depicts the molecular pathways that regulate eNOS activation and nitric oxide (NO) generation in the presence and absence of the endothelial glycocalyx. (Left) Under normal physiological settings, laminar shear stress works as a mechanical ligand, passing through the intact glycocalyx and transmembrane receptors to activate intracellular signaling via protein kinase C (PKC) and the PI3K/AKT pathway. This enhances Ca^{2+}/calmodulin (CaM)-dependent coupling and phosphorylation of eNOS, leading to increased production of NO. Released NO diffuses into vascular smooth muscle cells, causing vasodilation, inhibiting platelet aggregation, and suppressing leukocyte adhesion, so preserving vascular homeostasis. (Right) After trauma or endothelial injury, glycocalyx shedding affects mechanotransduction and suppresses PKC, PI3K/AKT, and Ca^{2+}/CaM-eNOS signaling. The resulting decrease in eNOS activation and NO bioavailability promotes platelet aggregation and leukocyte adhesion, contributing to endothelial dysfunction and vascular inflammation.

induced by resuscitation practices. The "lethal triad" of dilution, hypothermia, and acidosis impairs thrombin production, fibrinogen concentration, and platelet function.[1] Modern understanding distinguishes iatrogenic TIC from the endogenous acute coagulopathy that occurs within minutes of injury. While iatrogenic mechanisms can coexist with endogenous TIC, they involve separate biology and are now less common due to goal-directed resuscitation and hemostatic techniques.

KEY IATROGENIC CONTRIBUTORS

i. Dilutional coagulopathy: Excessive crystalloid or colloid resuscitation dilutes clotting factors and platelets, diminishing the ability to form a blood clot effectively.[36]

ii. Anticoagulant and antiplatelet medications: Prior use of low-molecular-weight heparin (LMWH), direct oral anticoagulants (DOACs), or agents like aspirin can heighten bleeding risk after trauma. The timing of the last dose and reversal strategies becomes critical in management.

iii. Surgical and procedural factors: Large tissue dissection, massive transfusion protocols, and bypass techniques can further deplete coagulation factors and platelets; operative hypothermia hampers enzymatic clotting function.[37]

iv. Acidosis-induced coagulopathy: Trauma resuscitation practices sometimes result in metabolic acidosis, disturbing coagulation by preventing normal thrombin generation and impairing clot formation.

Contemporary protocols focus on minimizing iatrogenic harm through goal-directed, hemostatic resuscitation, temperature management, judicious fluid use, and early identification of patients at risk for coagulopathy. Understanding both endogenous and iatrogenic contributors is vital for optimizing trauma outcomes.[36]

SYMPATHETIC SYSTEM DYSFUNCTION

In TIC, the sympathoadrenal surge is not only a hemodynamic response, but also a driver of hemostasis. There is a strong correlation between high circulating catecholamine levels and glycocalyx shedding, protein C activation, and fibrinolysis. Mechanisms include direct endothelial injury, increased permeability, and proinflammatory signaling activation. Therefore, the state of hemodynamic shock has devastating results for the endothelium. This fact is supported by the study showing the potential benefit of prehospital plasma transfusion during long transport time, minimizing the endothelial exposure to shock.[23,24]

SEX-BASED DIFFERENCES IN TIC

Research strongly supports that coagulation demonstrates a powerful sex-dependent effect, resulting in significant sex-based differences in TIC pathophysiology, mechanism, and impact on clinical outcomes. Sex dimorphisms influence thrombin formation, fibrinogen activity, platelet function, and fibrinolysis.

Females exhibit a relative state of hypercoagulability compared to males, a status that persists following injury.[38] Hormonally active females display a better physiological response to trauma and shock than their male counterparts. Females typically have higher levels of coagulation factors (II, VII, VIII, IX, X, XI, and XII), Factor V, TF, and a aPTT compared to males.[39,40] These differences result in a net increased thrombin generation in females,[41] which is relevant because thrombin generation is impaired in TIC and is predictive of the need for massive transfusion and mortality. The mechanisms are not fully elucidated, but circulating sex hormones,[42] particularly estrogen, are suspected to play a significant role.[43,44] Estradiol levels are increased in circulation in correlation with injury severity. Estradiol provokes a hypercoagulable phenotype in both males and females, evidenced by a shorter time to clot formation, greater thrombin generation, a greater rate of clot propagation and functional fibrinogen, and higher clot strength.

Similar changes are observed *in vivo* during the peak estrus phase of the menstrual cycle.[43] Estradiol affects fibrin biology, increasing the abundance of several factor XIII (FXIII) crosslinks within the fibrinogen alpha chain, suggesting alterations in clot structure. The estradiol-to-progesterone ratio also positively correlates with fibrin cross-linking and overall clot strength.[45,46] Sex-based differences in platelet biology are well established, with women showing higher platelet reactivity at baseline than men. Female platelets demonstrate stronger fibrinogen binding and greater spontaneous aggregation.[47] When stimulated with agonists such as ADP or epinephrine, they exhibit enhanced aggregation and activation responses. Women also tend to respond less effectively to antiplatelet therapy; younger females, in particular, show reduced sensitivity to clopidogrel and higher residual platelet reactivity while on dual therapy with aspirin and clopidogrel.[48] These differences appear to be influenced by estrogen, as platelets express estradiol beta receptors.[49] Experimental studies have shown that exposure of male platelets to physiological levels of estradiol induces a phenotype similar to that of female platelets, underscoring the hormonal regulation of platelet function.[50]

Sex dimorphism extends to fibrinogen and fibrinolysis pathways as well.[51] Women generally display higher circulating and functional fibrinogen levels, contributing to stronger and more stable clots.[52] Female clots exhibit greater resistance to fibrinolysis, likely due to elevated levels of PAI-1.[53,54] Consequently, following trauma, women tend to have a more antifibrinolytic profile and show reduced fibrinolytic activity compared with men.[55]

CONCLUSION AND FUTURE PERSPECTIVES

TIC is a multifaceted disorder that encompasses hemostasis, inflammation, immunology, and endothelial biology. TIC is not merely a frank dilutional or consumptive disorder; rather, it incorporates a systemic host response to injury, shaped by shock, tissue disruption, and cellular stress signals that compromise vascular integrity, trigger immunothrombosis, and modify hemostasis. The recognition of distinct phenotypes, hyperfibrinolysis, fibrinolytic shutdown, and hypocoagulability has significantly transformed our diagnostic and treatment strategies. Viscoelastic assays provide real-time, actionable data, enabling tailored therapy that aligns with each patient's unique presentation. The interdependence of trauma, immunity, and coagulation is evidenced by the pivotal roles played by the endothelium and glycocalyx, the influence of DAMPs and NETs, and the dysregulation of anticoagulant pathways. These mechanistic findings influence transfusion protocols, resuscitation techniques, and new treatment approaches.

TAKE-HOME MESSAGE

TIC starts early after injury and is driven by shock and tissue damage, not only by dilution or hypothermia from resuscitation. The condition moves between bleeding and clotting tendencies because of changes in coagulation factors, platelets, endothelial injury and fibrinolysis. Understanding these pathways helps guide targeted treatment, including early control of bleeding, protection of the endothelium and careful use of antifibrinolytics based on the patient's real-time coagulation status.

REFERENCES

1. Savioli G, Ceresa IF, Caneva L, Gerosa S, Ricevuti G. Trauma-induced coagulopathy: Overview of an emerging medical problem from pathophysiology to outcomes. *Medicines.* 2021;8(4):16.

2. Frith D, Brohi K. The acute coagulopathy of trauma shock: Clinical relevance. *Surgeon.* 2010;8(3):159–163.

3. Moore EE, Moore HB, Kornblith LZ, *et al.* Trauma-induced coagulopathy. *Nat Rev Dis Primers.* 2021;7(1):30.

4. Moore EE, Moore HB, Chapman MP, Gonzalez E, Sauaia A. Goal-directed hemostatic resuscitation for trauma induced coagulopathy: Maintaining homeostasis. *J Trauma Acute Care Surg.* 2018;84:S35–S40.

5. Zanza C, Romenskaya T, Racca F, Rocca E, Piccolella F, Piccioni A, *et al.* Severe trauma-induced coagulopathy: Molecular mechanisms underlying critical illness. *Int J Mol Sci.* 2023;24(8):7118.

6. Matsumoto H, Annen S, Mukai N, Ohshita M, Ogawa S, Okita M, *et al.* Association of endotheliopathy with coagulofibrinolytic reactions and disseminated intravascular coagulation after trauma: A retrospective observational study. *Sci Rep.* 2024;14(1):29630.

7. Abassi Z, Armaly Z, Heyman SN. Glycocalyx degradation in ischemia-reperfusion injury. *Am J Pathol.* 2020;190(4):752–767.

8. Corwin GS, Sexton KW, Beck WC, Taylor JR, Bhavaraju A, Davis B, *et al.* Characterization of acidosis in trauma patient. *J Emerg Trauma Shock.* 2020;13(3):213–218.

9. Ross SW, Thomas BW, Christmas AB, Cunningham KW, Sing RF. Returning from the acidotic abyss: Mortality in trauma patients with a pH < 7.0. *Am J Surg.* 2017;214(6):1067–1072.

10. Komarova YA, Kruse K, Mehta D, Malik AB. Protein interactions at endothelial junctions and signaling mechanisms regulating endothelial permeability. *Circ Res.* 2017;120(1):179–206.

11. Cohen MJ, Call M, Nelson M, Calfee CS, Esmon CT, Brohi K, *et al.* Critical role of activated protein c in early coagulopathy and later organ failure, infection and death in trauma patients. *Ann Surg.* 2012;255(2):379–385.

12. Duque P, Mora L, Levy JH, Schöchl H. Pathophysiological response to trauma-induced coagulopathy: A comprehensive review. *Anesth Analg.* 2020;130(3):654–664.

13. Relja B, Land WG. Damage-associated molecular patterns in trauma. *Eur J Trauma Emerg Surg.* 2020;46(4):751–775.

14. Mitrophanov AY, Vandyck K, Tanaka KA. Thrombin generation in trauma patients: How do we navigate through scylla and Charybdis? *Curr Anesthesiol Rep.* 2022;12(2):308–319.

15. Schlimp CJ, Schöchl H. The role of fibrinogen in trauma-induced coagulopathy. *Hamostaseologie*. 2014;34(1):29–39.

16. Brenni M, Worn M, Brüesch M, Spahn DR, Ganter MT. Successful rotational thromboelastometry-guided treatment of traumatic haemorrhage, hyperfibrinolysis and coagulopathy. *Acta Anaesthesiol Scand*. 2010;54(1):111–117.

17. Kutcher ME, Redick BJ, McCreery RC, Crane IM, Greenberg MD, Cachola LM, et al. Characterization of platelet dysfunction after trauma. *J Trauma Acute Care Surg*. 2012;73(1):13–19.

18. Sloos PH, Vulliamy P, van 't Veer C, Gupta AS, Neal MD, Brohi K, et al. Platelet dysfunction after trauma: From mechanisms to targeted treatment. *Transfusion*. 2022;62:S281–S300.

19. Vulliamy P, Kornblith LZ, Kutcher ME, Cohen MJ, Brohi K, Neal MD. Alterations in platelet behavior after major trauma: Adaptive or maladaptive? *Platelets*. 2021;32(3):295–304.

20. Madurska MJ, Sachse KA, Jansen JO, Rasmussen TE, Morrison JJ. Fibrinolysis in trauma: A review. *Eur J Trauma Emerg Surg*. 2018;44(1):35–44.

21. Bunch CM, Chang E, Moore EE, Moore HB, Kwaan HC, Miller JB, et al. SHock-INduced Endotheliopathy (SHINE): A mechanistic justification for viscoelastography-guided resuscitation of traumatic and non-traumatic shock. *Front Physiol*. 2023;14:1094845.

22. Reda S, Winterhagen FI, Berens C, Müller J, Oldenburg J, Pötzsch B, et al. Circulating plasminogen activator inhibitor-1 (PAI-1) is reduced by in vivo thrombin generation and subsequent formation of activated protein C (APC). *Blood*. 2019;134:2389–2389.

23. Gibson BHY, Duvernay MT, Moore-Lotridge SN, Flick MJ, Schoenecker JG. Plasminogen activation in the musculoskeletal acute phase response: Injury, repair, and disease. *Res Pract Thromb Haemost*. 2020;4(4):469–480.

24. Favors L, Harrell K, Miles V, Hicks RC, Rippy M, Parmer H, et al. Analysis of fibrinolytic shutdown in trauma patients with traumatic brain injury. *Am J Surg*. 2024;227:72–76.

25. Moore HB, Moore EE, Neal MD, Sheppard FR, Kornblith LZ, Draxler DF, et al. Fibrinolysis shutdown in trauma: Historical review and clinical implications. *Anesth Analg*. 2019;129(3):762–773.

26. Costantini TW, Kornblith LZ, Pritts T, Coimbra R. The intersection of coagulation activation and inflammation after injury: What you need to know. *J Trauma Acute Care Surg*. 2024;96(3):347–356.

27. Keulen GM, Huckriede J, Wichapong K, Nicolaes GAF. Histon activities in the extracellular environment: regulation and prothrombotic implications. *Curr Opin Hematol*. 2024;31(5):230–237.

28. Rawish E, Sauter M, Sauter R, Nording H, Langer HF. Complement, inflammation and thrombosis. *Br J Pharmacol*. 2021;178(14):2892–2904.

29. Patterson EK, Cepinskas G, Fraser DD. Endothelial glycocalyx degradation in critical illness and injury. *Front Med*. 2022;9:898592.

30. Ostrowski SR, Johansson PI. Endothelial glycocalyx degradation induces endogenous heparinization in patients with severe injury and early traumatic coagulopathy. *J Trauma Acute Care Surg*. 2012;73(1):60–66.

31. Rahbar E, Cardenas JC, Baimukanova G, Usadi B, Bruhn R, Pati S, et al. Endothelial glycocalyx shedding and vascular permeability in severely injured trauma patients. *J Transl Med*. 2015;13:117.

32. Clyne AM. Endothelial response to glucose: dysfunction, metabolism, and transport. *Biochem Soc Trans*. 2021;49(1):313–325.

33. Scrimieri R, Locatelli L, Cazzaniga A, Cazzola R, Malucelli E, Sorrentino A, *et al.* Ultrastructural features mirror metabolic derangement in human endothelial cells exposed to high glucose. *Sci Rep.* 2023;13(1):15133.

34. Capponi A, Rostagno C. Trauma-induced coagulopathy: A review of specific molecular mechanisms. *Diagnostics.* 2025;15(11):1435.

35. Oft HC, Simon DW, Sun D. New insights into metabolism dysregulation after TBI. *J Neuroinflammation.* 2024;21(1):184.

36. Kornblith LZ, Moore HB, Cohen MJ. Trauma-induced coagulopathy: The past, present, and future. *J Thromb Haemost.* 2019;17(6):852–862.

37. Rajagopalan S, Mascha E, Na J, Sessler DI. The effects of mild perioperative hypothermia on blood loss and transfusion requirement. *Anesthesiology.* 2008;108(1):71–77.

38. Coleman JR, Gumina R, Hund T, Cohen M, Neal MD, Townsend K, *et al.* Sex dimorphisms in coagulation: Implications in trauma-induced coagulopathy and trauma resuscitation. *Am J Hematol.* 2024;99:S28–S35.

39 Favaloro EJ, Soltani S, McDonald J, Grezchnik E, Easton L. Cross-laboratory audit of normal reference ranges and assessment of ABO blood group, gender and age on detected levels of plasma coagulation factors. *Blood Coagul Fibrinolysis.* 2005;16(8):597–605.

40. Lindmark E, Wallentin L, Siegbahn A. Blood cell activation, coagulation, and inflammation in men and women with coronary artery disease. *Thromb Res.* 2001;103(3): 249–259.

41. Krarup A, Wallis R, Presanis JS, Gál P, Sim RB. Simultaneous activation of complement and coagulation by MBL-associated serine protease 2. *PLoS One.* 2007;2(7):e623.

42. Brown JB, Cohen MJ, Minei JP, Maier RV, West MA, Billiar TR, Peitzman AB, Moore EE, Cuschieri J, Sperry JL Inflammation and the Host Response to Injury Investigators. Characterization of acute coagulopathy and sexual dimorphism after injury: Females and coagulopathy just do not mix. *J Trauma Acute Care Surg.* 2012;73(6):1395–400.

43. Coleman JR, Moore EE, Schmitt L, Hansen K, Dow N, Freeman K, *et al.* Estradiol provokes hypercoagulability and affects fibrin biology: A mechanistic exploration of sex dimorphisms in coagulation. *J Trauma Acute Care Surg.* 2023;94(2):179–186.

44. Orbach-Zinger S, Eidelman LA, Lutsker A, Oron G, Fisch B, Ben-Haroush A. The effect of in vitro fertilization on coagulation parameters as measured by thromboelastogram. *Eur J Obstet Gynecol Reprod Biol.* 2016;201:118–120.

45. Gee AC, Sawai RS, Differding J, Muller P, Underwood S, Schreiber MA. The influence of sex hormones on coagulation and inflammation in the trauma patient. *Shock.* 2008;29(3):334–341.

46. Gang W, Limin X, Yang W, Zhanzhi W, Lijun X. The effects of craniocerebral and extracranial trauma on the changes in serum testosterone and estradiol in the early stage and their clinical significance. *J Trauma Acute Care Surg.* 2013;74(1):254–258.

47. Coleman JR, Moore EE, Kelher MR, Samuels JM, Cohen MJ, *et al.* Female platelets have distinct functional activity compared with male platelets: Implications in transfusion practice and treatment of trauma-induced coagulopathy. *J Trauma Acute Care Surg.* 2019;87(5):1052–1060.

48. Hobson AR, Qureshi Z, Banks P, Curzen N. Gender and responses to aspirin and clopidogrel: Insights using short thrombelastography. *Cardiovasc Ther.* 2009;27(4): 246–252.

49. Hadley JB, Kelher MR, Coleman JR, Kelly KK, Dumont LJ, Esparza O, Banerjee A, Cohen MJ, Jones K, Silliman CC. Hormones, age, and sex affect platelet responsiveness in vitro. *Transfusion.* 2022;62(9):1882–1893.

50. Farkas S, Szabó A, Hegyi AE, Török B, Fazekas CL, Ernszt D, *et al*. Estradiol and estrogen-like alternative therapies in use: The importance of the selective and non-classical actions. *Biomedicines*. 2022;10(4):861.

51. Coleman JR, Moore EE, Sauaia A, Samuels JM, Moore HB, Ghasabyan A, *et al*. Untangling sex dimorphisms in coagulation: Initial steps toward precision medicine for trauma resuscitation. *Ann Surg*. 2020;271(6):e128–e130.

52. Gorton HJ, Warren ER, Simpson NA, Lyons GR, Columb MO. Thromboelastography identifies sex-related differences in coagulation. *Anesth Analg*. 2000;91(5):1279–1281.

53. DiMusto PD, Lu G, Ghosh A, Roelofs KJ, Su G, Zhao Y, *et al*. Increased PAI-1 in females compared with males is protective for abdominal aortic aneurysm formation in a rodent model. *Am J Physiol Heart Circ Physiol*. 2012;302(7):H1378–H1386.

54. Asselbergs FW, Williams SM, Hebert PR, Coffey CS, Hillege HL, Navis G, *et al*. The gender-specific role of polymorphisms from the fibrinolytic, renin-angiotensin, and bradykinin systems in determining plasma t-PA and PAI-1 levels. *Thromb Haemost*. 2006;96(4):471–477.

55. Piróg M, Piwowarczyk S, Undas A. Plasma fibrin clot properties are unfavorably altered in women following venous thromboembolism associated with combined hormonal contraception. *Dis Markers*. 2019:4923535.

Chapter 3

RISK FACTORS AND CONTRIBUTING ELEMENTS TO TRAUMA-INDUCED COAGULOPATHY

Vineeth Chandran K P and Ajay Ambalakkatte

DOI: 10.1201/9781003711070-3

INTRODUCTION

This chapter focuses on the various factors that contribute to the development of trauma-induced coagulopathy (TIC). These include patient factors, characteristics of trauma, and the role of initial resuscitation in the development of TIC. It is important to understand these factors as they will directly affect the management and prognosis of the patient. Elderly trauma patients often face worse prognoses due to baseline comorbidities and medications, unlike younger patients with fewer physiological stressors. We therefore try to ascertain the relationship between these various factors and identify how they will affect the development of TIC. The Venn diagram in Figure 3.1 illustrates how different categories of health-related risk factors, physiological, comorbidities, and injury- and treatment-related risks, interact and overlap to influence a patient's overall risk profile.

CLINICAL AND PHYSIOLOGICAL INFLUENCES

AGE AND GENDER

Age is an independent risk factor for worse outcomes following major trauma.[1] Reduction of the physiological reserve, presence of comorbidities and use of regular medications play major roles in the increased risk. Declining cellular function eventually leading to organ failure happens with aging. They have an impaired adaptive and homeostatic mechanism to the stress of trauma. Insults commonly tolerated by young people can have serious effects on the elderly.[1] Observational studies claim the possibility of a higher incidence of TIC in the elderly after

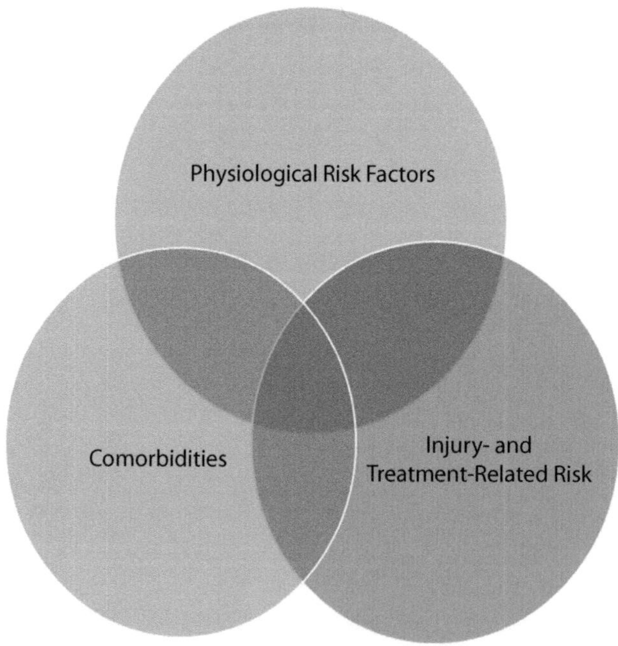

Figure 3.1 Venn diagram of overlapping risk categories.

examining various coagulation parameters in this group.[2-5] Platelets and endothelial cells play a major role in haemostasis following trauma. Progressive disruption and dysfunction of the endothelium and declining platelet number with old age result in deranged haemostasis.[2,3] Adding to this, it should be noted that the coagulation proteins alter with age.[6-8] Endogenous thrombin potential reduces after trauma, and there is a higher probability of exsanguination due to early depletion of coagulation factors.[9,10] Conversely, there is an increase in fibrinogen, factor VIII, and von Willebrand factor (vWF) levels with age and hence there is a shift towards inhibition of fibrinolysis. These factors contribute to an increased chance of dysregulated coagulation in older individuals when compared to the young, as seen in TIC.[11,12] Like age, gender also plays a role in the development of TIC. It may be the physiological process of bleeding every month after menarche and the preparation for massive bleeding following pregnancy, would have possibly rendered females more resilient against TIC.

GENDER

The female gender is supposed to have protection against TIC after severe trauma. Females show a relative hypercoagulability status compared to males, as evidenced by the shorter time for clot formation, increased rate of clot propagation, increased platelet activity and clot strength, and decreased fibrinolysis.[13] It was evidenced by the Pragmatic Randomized Optimal Platelet and Plasma Ratios (PROPPR) trial that females received lower volumes of all blood products in trauma after attaining haemostasis, although this did not translate to mortality benefits.[14] The following are the proposed mechanisms associated with increased hypercoagulability in females:

i. Hypoxia and tissue injury secondary to trauma lead to dysfunction of the neuroendocrine system, resulting in increased circulating levels of estradiol.[15,16] This is associated with hypercoagulability. Estradiol has been shown to be positively correlated with the rate of fibrin deposition, crosslinking, and overall clot strength. Also, they have higher circulating levels of fibrinogen and higher levels of functional fibrinogen.

ii. Females have higher levels of factors II, VII, VIII, IX, X, XI, and XII and shorter activated partial thromboplastin time (aPTT).[17] Females also have demonstrated higher levels of proteins that propagate thrombin generation, like complement factor H and C4b-binding protein (C4BP), and also decreased levels of antithrombin.[18,19]

iii. Gender difference in the platelet response secondary to trauma due to the presence of sex hormone receptors on megakaryocytes and platelets.[20] Female platelets have an increased activation with adenosine diphosphate (ADP), whereas male platelets have increased activation with platelet activating factor (PAF). This difference in activation results in different responses in the downstream intracellular cascades.[20]

iv. Female clots are found to have increased fibrinolytic resistance when compared to male. Following ischaemic insults, they also are seen to have higher levels of plasminogen activator inhibitor-1 (PAI-1). This contributes to increased tissue-type plasminogen activator (tPA) resistance and thereby decreased fibrinolysis.[21] Also, in the presence of estradiol, factor XIII and fibrinogen form increased crosslinks.[22] Females tolerate depressed clot strength better than males and therefore have a survival benefit.

All these factors suggest a higher protection for females when compared to males in the development of TIC following trauma. However, what happens when an obese female presents with trauma? How the body habitus will affect the development of TIC is an interesting take.

OBESITY

Overweight and obesity are pressing problems worldwide. According to the World Health Organization (WHO), 43% of adults aged 18 years and over were overweight and 16% were living with obesity during the time period involved.[23] Obesity is an independent risk factor for morbidity and mortality following trauma.[24] However, since obesity is a state of chronic inflammation, patients are more prone to hypercoagulable states than bleeding.[25] Various proposed mechanisms of obesity in the coagulation pathway are as follows:

i. Increased circulating levels of cytokines like Interleukin-6 (IL-6) and tumour necrosis factor-alpha (TNF-α) and leptin upregulate procoagulant factors in vascular endothelium and increase platelet activity and thrombin generation[26]

ii. Increased release of tissue factor from adipose tissue, resulting in increased thrombin generation[27]

iii. Higher levels of PAI-1 with increasing visceral fat, which counteract the effect of tPA released during haemorrhagic shock[28]

iv. Prevents prolongation of clot initiation, improves fibrin crosslinking due to an increased level of fibrinogen concentration and factor XII and thereby improves clot strength following haemorrhagic shock[29-31]

v. Counteracts the anti-coagulant activity of activated protein C (aPC)[32]

This propensity towards a hypercoagulable state results in increased rates of venous thromboembolism in obese patients with trauma. Up to 60% of obese patients present with venous thromboembolism in the days following injury, and there is a 2.5-fold increased risk of venous and arterial thromboembolism in this group.[33] It is postulated that the higher rates of multiorgan dysfunction, thromboembolic phenomenon and mortality are secondary to the hypercoagulable state following trauma. Age, gender and partly obesity are non-modifiable risk factors. Modifiable factors like addictions and preventable factors like comorbidities also influence the development of TIC.

ALCOHOL CONSUMPTION

The effects of acute alcohol consumption in TIC is a debatable topic. Heavy drinkers have higher tPA antigen and PAI-1 levels than non-drinkers. Also, they have increased levels of factors VII and VIII, which puts them in a hypercoagulable state.[34] However, the effect of this milieu on trauma is not known. The effect of chronic alcoholism on the liver and subsequent derangements is discussed later in this chapter.

The effect of acute alcohol ingestion in trauma is still under investigation. It is important to identify the relation between alcohol and TIC because motor vehicle collisions are often associated with alcohol intoxication. Alcohol ingestion blunts the physiologic response to trauma, resulting in greater resuscitative requirements.[35]

The effect of alcohol on coagulation parameters is described as multifaceted. It alters the platelet function, prolongs bleeding time, inhibits platelet adhesion to fibrinogen, decreases fibrinogen and fibrin functionality, impairs fibrinolysis and slows the rate of fibrin formation and crosslinking.[36] Fibrinogen activity 10 minutes after the start of clotting was better in females who had elevated blood ethanol levels compared to their male counterparts.[36] *In vitro*, it was found to increase the clot formation time.[37] Howard *et al.*, in their rotational thromboelastometry (ROTEM)-based study on the effect of alcohol in trauma, found a bidirectional effect. There was impaired clot formation initially followed by subsequent inhibition of fibrinolysis.[38] Another study by the same author on 264 trauma patients with increased ethanol levels showed impaired clot formation in the thromboelastography (TEG) assay. However, this was not predictive of transfusion or early or late mortality.[39] To summarize, studies on the effect of acute alcohol ingestion in trauma have produced conflicting evidence and its true impact in TIC is yet to be ascertained.

SMOKING

A very interesting hypothesis has been postulated regarding the effect of smoking in cardiovascular disease, termed the "smokers' paradox".[40] This postulates that smokers have improved survivability after an acute myocardial infarction when compared to non-smokers because they have better tolerance to decreased oxygen delivery and hypoxia. Along similar lines, it is proposed that smoking might have a protective effect against TIC. Smoking is known to induce platelet hyperactivity, increase platelet count and modify platelet adhesion and aggregation.[41] This is postulated to have some survival benefit when definitive care or administration of blood components is delayed.[42] Alternatively, there is also evidence suggesting that smokers have an increased possibility of developing acute respiratory distress syndrome (ARDS) following blood transfusion for haemorrhagic shock because cigarette smokers have an exaggerated response to inflammatory stimuli, thereby resulting in increased mortality following major trauma.[43] At present, there is no concrete evidence to suggest a significant effect of smoking on trauma, haemorrhagic shock and TIC.

COMORBIDITIES

Patients with comorbidities have a higher chance of mortality after trauma, even after adjusting for the effects of ageing and severity of injury. Physiologic reserve of a person is influenced by intrinsic factors like age, gender and pre-injury health status. The presence of a sound physiologic reserve influences the outcome of minor and moderate injury. Those who are elderly and have comorbidities have a poor reserve and have a possibility of worse outcome.[44] The mortality in this group might not be immediate after trauma, but later during the hospital stay. However, with severe trauma, the effect of physiologic reserve has a lesser impact as the severity of injury overwhelms the response of a sound physiologic reserve. Studies have shown increased mortality with conditions like chronic obstructive pulmonary disease, congenital coagulopathy, diabetes, cirrhosis and ischaemic heart disease. Recent studies have also added renal failure to this list.[44,45] Diabetes mellitus, hypertension and cardiovascular disease result in progressive disruption and dysfunction of the endothelium, which favours the development of TIC.[44,45]

CIRRHOSIS LIVER

Cirrhotic patients are often coagulopathic, resulting in higher blood loss resulting in haemorrhagic shock and further hepatic ischaemia. Also, cirrhotic patients have decreased hepatic reserve resulting in impaired synthetic, metabolic, immunologic and secretory function. This makes them less competent in responding to stress or trauma. The overall pooled mortality from meta-analyses was 4.52 times higher in the cirrhosis group when compared to non-cirrhotic group.[46] Similarly, the incidence of coagulopathy was four times higher among cirrhotic compared to non-cirrhotic.[47]

HAEMOPHILIA

Case reports of haemophilia patients presenting with trauma suggest a higher requirement for blood products and a need for factor replacement. Poor patient outcomes are uniformly described in these reports.[48]

DRUGS

NSAIDS

Studies have evaluated the effects of various drugs in traumatic haemorrhage and their role in TIC. A retrospective study assessing the role of 15 drugs commonly prescribed, including nonsteroidal anti-inflammatory drugs (NSAIDs), aspirin, other antiplatelet agents, beta-blockers etc., was done. It was found that NSAID use was associated with a reduction in the incidence of TIC and clinically significant coagulopathy. The mechanism is not clear, but the effect is proposed due to the attenuation of the platelet activity and anti-inflammatory property of the drug.[49]

ANTICOAGULANTS

Common sense would suggest that patients on anticoagulant drugs would have greater bleeding manifestations following trauma. But studies have shown that pre-injury use of warfarin does not result in a fatal risk of haemorrhagic complications following trauma in the absence of head trauma.[50] A comparison study between warfarin and novel anticoagulant agents

(NOACs) showed that the latter group had decreased mortality and decreased transfused blood products among blunt trauma patients with no intracranial bleed.[51] However, pre-injury anticoagulants can result in worse outcomes in patients with traumatic brain injury.[52] Also, indirectly, they worsen the outcome by delaying the initiation of definitive surgical interventions.[53]

ANTIPLATELETS

Studies have shown that pre-injury antiplatelet drugs do not significantly increase the mortality in patients without head injury.[54] However, similar to anticoagulants, pre-injury anticoagulants result in poorer outcomes in patients with traumatic brain injury.[55]

STATINS

There is conflicting evidence on the effect of pre-injury use of statins. One study had found that the pre-injury statin use was associated with a 67% reduction in mortality following trauma in patients with no cardiovascular comorbidities.[56] However, this study was among patients with a lower severity of injury. Those with higher severity of injury had 80% higher risk of multi-organ dysfunction and mortality following trauma.[57] The causes of the worst performance of patients on statins are even more interesting. It is postulated that the worst outcome is not due to the use of pre-injury statins but due to the withdrawal of statins during the injury period, resulting in a rebound effect and poor outcome. Statins, along with their lipid-lowering effects, also have anti-inflammatory effects as evidenced by lower levels of C-reactive protein (CRP). It was shown earlier that following discontinuation of statins, there is an increase in levels of IL-6 and CRP as early as 3 days. This pro-inflammatory milieu, induced secondary to the withdrawal of statins, is thought to be the reason for increased mortality in these cases.

BETA BLOCKERS

These groups of drugs are the most prescribed ones for cardiovascular illness. Pre-injury use of beta blockers can hurt the compensatory sympathetic activation to hypotension and that can have worse outcomes. However, studies have failed to prove this. Patients who used beta blockers did not differ significantly concerning mortality or blood transfusion requirements.[58] The relation between beta blockers and TIC is unknown, but they are said to harm proinflammatory cytokines like IL-6 and are thereby proposed to blunt the systemic inflammatory response secondary to trauma. Clinical and physiological risk factors contributing to TIC are summarized in Table 3.1.

Table 3.1   Risk factors contributing to TIC

Risk factor	Mechanism	Clinical implication	Key references
Age (elderly)	Endothelial dysfunction Decreased platelets Altered coagulation proteins	Dysregulated coagulation, poorer outcomes	Curry *et al.*[5]
Gender (female)	Estrogen-mediated hypercoagulability, better clot stability	Better protection from TIC	Coleman *et al.*[13]
Obesity	Pro-inflammatory state, altered fibrinolysis	Higher risk of thromboembolism	McCully *et al.*[32]
Diabetes/hypertension/ cardiovascular diseases	Endothelial dysfunction Platelet activation	Favour the development of TIC	Hollis *et al.*[44]
NSAIDs	Attenuation of platelet activity Anti-inflammatory	Reduced tendency for TIC	Neal *et al.*[49]
Acute alcohol use	Still under investigation	No evidence of any effect	Eismann *et al.*[36]
Chronic alcohol use	Platelet dysfunction, liver dysfunction	Increased risk of coagulopathy	Morrison *et al.*[47]

INJURY CHARACTERISTICS AND SEVERITY

SEVERITY OF INJURY

Injury severity can be assessed using the following:

i. *Anatomical criteria:* Injury Severity Score (ISS), Abbreviated Injury Scale (AIS).

ii. *Physiological criteria:* Classes of haemorrhage, shock index (SI).

iii. *Biochemical criteria:* Lactate and base excess levels.

Relationship of the severity of injuries to development of TIC is summarized in Table 3.2.

SPECIFIC INJURIES

The prevalence of TIC based on body region was studied by Hess *et al.*, who found TIC prevalence to be 7.6% for isolated head injury, 4.8% for thoracic trauma and 5% for abdominal

Table 3.2 Relationship of injury severity with TIC

Evidence	What was studied?	Inference
Hess *et al.*[58]	Investigated the prevalence of abnormal coagulation tests in trauma patients	Prevalence of abnormal PT ranged from 5% to 43% as ISS increased from 5 to > 45 1. The prevalence of thrombocytopenia also ranged from 4% to 18% as ISS increased
Cohen *et al.*[59]	Studied the role of activated protein C in early coagulopathy of trauma	Significant association of coagulopathy with the combined presence of hypo-perfusion (base deficit > 6) and severe Injury (ISS > 15)
Savioli *et al.*[60]	Investigated characteristics and outcomes of trauma coagulopathy and its correlation with the SI and ISS	1. High SI and ISS are strong indicators of trauma coagulopathy. 2. The incidence of trauma coagulopathy is higher when 3 or more body regions are involved

Bunch *et al.*[61]	White paper on shock-induced endotheliopathy (SHINE)	1. SHINE is a contributing factor to coagulopathy
		2. SHINE is caused by hypoperfusion (base deficit > 6 or high SI) by various mechanisms
		  1. Sympathetic nervous system activation and catecholamine release damaging endothelium.
		  2. Inflammatory cytokines and other mediators injuring endothelial cells.
		  3. Reduced oxygen delivery contributing to endothelial injury.

Moore *et al.*[62]	Studied patterns of fibrinolysis in severe trauma	In victims with high ISS, and high base deficit 1. Fibrinolytic shutdown was seen in 64% of patients (17% mortality). 2. Hyperfibrinolysis was seen in 18% of patients (the highest mortality rate of 44%).

Table 3.3 Injury types and their association with TIC

Injury type	TIC mechanism involved	Predictors of TIC
Traumatic brain injury	Damage to blood–brain barrier and release of brain-derived molecules, tissue factor release[58]	Severe traumatic brain injury (TBI) (Glasgow Coma Scale [GCS] < 8) is an independent risk factor for TIC. Early coagulopathy
Thoracic trauma	Related to hypoxia rather than hypoperfusion[58]	Pulmonary contusion identified on admission chest X-ray (CXR) is a powerful predictor of TIC
Abdominal trauma	Haemorrhagic shock leading to hypoperfusion[58]	FASILA score, which includes Focused Assessment with Sonography in Trauma (FAST) status, SI and lactate, predicts TIC with higher scores (> 4)[63]
Orthopedic trauma	Fat embolism, extensive soft tissue damage, endotheliopathy, and bone marrow contamination[58]	Any injury that is Gustilo Anderson type 3, multiple long bone fractures, and mangled extremities
Spinal cord injury	Early phase: Hypoperfusion from neurogenic shock. Late phase: Venous stasis and consumptive coagulopathy[58]	A high level of injury (above T6 level) implies a higher chance of TIC.

trauma.[58] Mechanisms involved in the development of TIC and predictors of TIC associated with injury to specific regions are given in Table 3.3.

MECHANISM OF INJURY AND COAGULATION

i. In severe blunt trauma, massive tissue injury speeds up thrombin generation, leading to more TIC.

ii. Penetrating trauma (e.g., stab wounds) causes less tissue injury than blunt trauma, resulting in lower procoagulant production and coagulation activation.

iii. Early coagulopathy of trauma is seen in 38% of combat casualties; 92% of these involve penetrating injuries, with 65% due to explosions.

iv. Crush or explosion injuries can cause extensive tissue damage.

v. Widespread crush injury with generalized coagulation activation may lead to significant consumption of clotting factors and clinical coagulopathy, but this is likely rare in isolation and has not been specifically reported.[64]

Wohlauer *et al.* found platelet dysfunction upon admission in severe blunt trauma patients with a mean ISS of 19.[65] Coleman *et al.* found that all patients with blunt solid organ injury were hypercoagulable upon ICU admission, but of these, 58% had fibrinolytic shutdown and 50% showed resistance to tPA.[66]

PRE-HOSPITAL AND ED RESUSCITATION

A retrospective analysis of the German Trauma Registry database, which included 17,200 patients with multiple injuries, demonstrated that the incidence of coagulopathy increased with the volume of intravenous fluids administered pre-clinically. Coagulopathy was observed in over 40% of patients who received more than 2,000 ml of IV fluids, over 50% of those who received more than 3,000 ml, and over 70% of those who received more than 4,000 ml.[67] A summary of the prehospital management intervention and its possible effect on the development of TIC is given in Table 3.4.

Table 3.4 Influence of prehospital and ED resuscitation on TIC development

Intervention	Potential TIC effect	Best practices
Inadequate haemorrhage control	Continuous loss of platelets and coagulation factors, consumptive coagulopathy	Early control of haemorrhage using direct pressure, or tourniquet, or a haemostatic dressing
Excessive crystalloids	Haemodilution, leading to hypocoagulability	Limit to 1–1.5 L, prefer balanced solutions, and early blood product administration
Colloid usage	Disruption of clot formation, decreased strength of the clot formed, and haemodilution	Avoid colloids during initial phases of resuscitation
Delayed transfusion and transfusion-induced dilutional coagulopathy	Haemodilution decreases clot formation.	Initiate blood products based on a TEG-based algorithm or in a ratio of 1:1:1 for PRBC:FFP:Platelets
Permissive hypotension	Prevents dislodging clots, minimizes hypothermia and acidosis associated with large volume IV fluid therapy	1. Permissive hypotension only in the absence of TBI 2. Prolonged permissive hypotension may exacerbate coagulopathy, so early definitive management is necessary.

CONCLUSION

With the increasing age of the world population, the possibility of elderly patients with a history of substance abuse, having multiple comorbidities on multiple drugs, presenting with trauma is only going to increase. Severity of the injury, delay in receiving initial resuscitation, and resuscitation methods also influence the development of TIC. Different categories of health-related risk factors—physiological, comorbidities, and injury- and treatment-related risks—interact and overlap to influence a patient's overall risk profile. Along with this, the paucity of evidence on the effect of many of these factors in the development of TIC is worth noting.

TAKE-HOME MESSAGE

There is a complex interplay of various factors that results in the development of TIC following major trauma. This includes patient characteristics like age and body habitus, the underlying health conditions, the physiologic reserve of the patient and the effect of different medications the patient is taking; trauma characteristics like severity of trauma and body regions involved in trauma; and factors related to prehospital and intra-hospital resuscitation.

REFERENCES

1. American College of Surgeons Committee on Trauma. Geriatric trauma. In: ATLS Student course manual. Chicago, Illinois; 2018. p. 216–7.
2. Lesbo M, Hviid CV, Brink O, Juul S, Borris LC, Hvas A-M. Age-dependent thrombin generation predicts 30-day mortality and symptomatic thromboembolism after multiple trauma. Scientific Reports. 2023 Jan 30;13(1). doi: 10.1038/s41598-023-28474-7

3. Savioli G, Ceresa IF, Caneva L, Gerosa S, Ricevuti G. Trauma-induced coagulopathy: Overview of an emerging medical problem from pathophysiology to outcomes. Medicines. 2021 Mar 24;8(4):16. doi:10.3390/medicines8040016

4. Balvers K, Wirtz MR, van Dieren S, Goslings JC, Juffermans NP. Risk factors for trauma-induced coagulopathy- and transfusion-associated multiple organ failure in severely injured trauma patients. Frontiers in Medicine. 2015 Apr 24;2. doi:10.3389/fmed.2015.00024

5. Curry NS, Davenport R, Wong H, Gaarder C, Johansson P, Juffermans NP. Traumatic coagulopathy in the older patient: Analysis of coagulation profiles from the activation of coagulation and inflammation in trauma-2 (ACIT-2) observational, Multicenter Study. Journal of Thrombosis and Haemostasis. 2023 Feb;21(2):215–26. doi:10.1016/j.jtha.2022.11.005

6. Franchini M, Lippi G, Favaloro E. Aging hemostasis: Changes to laboratory markers of hemostasis as we age—A narrative review. Seminars in Thrombosis and Hemostasis. 2014 Aug 6;40(06):621–33. doi:10.1055/s-0034-1384631

7. Johansson PI, Sørensen AM, Perner A, Welling K, Wanscher M, Larsen CF. Elderly trauma patients have high circulating noradrenaline levels but attenuated release of adrenaline, platelets, and leukocytes in response to increasing injury severity. Critical Care Medicine. 2012 Jun;40(6):1844–50. doi:10.1097/ccm.0b013e31823e9d15

8. Ohmori T, Kitamura T, Tanaka K, Saisaka Y, Ishihara J, Onishi H. Admission fibrinogen levels in severe trauma patients: A comparison of elderly and younger patients. Injury. 2015 Sept;46(9):1779–83. doi:10.1016/j.injury.2015.04.007

9. Cardenas JC, Rahbar E, Pommerening MJ, Baer LA, Matijevic N, Cotton BA. Measuring thrombin generation as a tool for predicting hemostatic potential and transfusion requirements following trauma. Journal of Trauma and Acute Care Surgery. 2014 Dec;77(6):839–45. doi:10.1097/ta.0000000000000348

10. Coleman JR, Moore EE, Samuels JM, Cohen MJ, Silliman CC, Ghasabyan A. Whole blood thrombin generation in severely injured patients requiring massive transfusion. Journal of the American College of Surgeons. 2021 May;232(5):709–16. doi:10.1016/j.jamcollsurg.2020.12.058

11. Mari D, Ogliari G, Castaldi D, Vitale G, Bollini EM, Lio D. Hemostasis and ageing. Immunity & Ageing. 2008 Oct 23;5(1). doi:10.1186/1742-4933-5-12

12. Wang J, Lim HY, Nandurkar H, Ho P. Age, sex and racial differences in fibrin formation and fibrinolysis within the healthy population. Blood Coagulation & Fibrinolysis. 2022 Jan 25;33(2):141–4. doi:10.1097/mbc.0000000000001115

13. Coleman JR, Gumina R, Hund T, Cohen M, Neal MD, Townsend K. Sex dimorphisms in coagulation: Implications in trauma-induced coagulopathy and trauma resuscitation. American Journal of Hematology. 2024 Apr;99(S1). doi:10.1002/ajh.27296

14. McCrum ML, Leroux B, Fang T, Bulger E, Arbabi S, Wade CE. Sex-based differences in transfusion need after severe injury: Findings of the PROPPR study. Surgery. 2019 Jun;165(6):1122–7. doi:10.1016/j.surg.2018.12.023

15. Gee AC, Sawai RS, Differding J, Muller P, Underwood S, Schreiber MA. The influence of sex hormones on coagulation and inflammation in the trauma patient. Shock. 2008 Mar;29(3):334–41. doi:10.1097/shk.0b013e3181506ee5

16. Gang W, Limin X, Yang W, Zhanzhi W, Lijun X. The effects of craniocerebral and extracranial trauma on the changes in serum testosterone and estradiol in the early stage and their clinical significance. Journal of Trauma and Acute Care Surgery. 2013 Jan;74(1):254–8. doi:10.1097/ta.0b013e318270db12

17. Favaloro EJ, Soltani S, McDonald J, Grezchnik E, Easton L. Cross-laboratory audit of normal reference ranges and assessment of ABO blood group, gender and age on detected levels of plasma coagulation factors. Blood Coagulation & Fibrinolysis. 2005 Nov;16(8):597–605. doi:10.1097/01.mbc.0000187250.32630.56

18. Silliman CC, Dzieciatkowska M, Moore EE, Kelher MR, Banerjee A, Liang X. Proteomic analyses of human plasma: Venus versus Mars. Transfusion. 2011 Aug 31;52(2):417–24. doi:10.1111/j.1537-2995.2011.03316.x

19. Miyoshi T, Oku H, Asahara S, Okamoto A, Kokame K, Nakai M. Effects of low-dose combined oral contraceptives and protein S k196e mutation on anticoagulation factors: A prospective observational study. International Journal of Hematology. 2019 Mar 19;109(6):641–9. doi:10.1007/s12185-019-02633-x

20. Coleman JR, Moore EE, Kelher MR, Samuels JM, Cohen MJ, Sauaia A. Female platelets have distinct functional activity compared with male platelets: Implications in transfusion practice and treatment of trauma-induced coagulopathy. Journal of Trauma and Acute Care Surgery. 2019 Jun 3;87(5):1052–60. doi:10.1097/ta.0000000000002398

21. Kain K, Carter AM, Bamford JM, Grant PJ, Catto AJ. Gender differences in coagulation and fibrinolysis in white subjects with acute ischemic stroke. Journal of Thrombosis and Haemostasis. 2003 Feb;1(2):390–2. doi:10.1046/j.1538-7836.2003.00040.x

22. Coleman JR, Moore EE, Schmitt L, Hansen K, Dow N, Freeman K. Estradiol provokes hypercoagulability and affects fibrin biology: A mechanistic exploration of sex dimorphisms in coagulation. Journal of Trauma and Acute Care Surgery. 2022 Oct 20;94(2):179–86. doi:10.1097/ta.0000000000003822

23. Obesity and Overweight [Internet]. World Health Organization; 2024 [cited 2024 Aug 20]. Available from: https://www.who.int/news-room/fact-sheets/detail/obesity-and-overweight

24. Blokhin IO, Lentz SR. Mechanisms of thrombosis in obesity. Current Opinion in Hematology. 2013 Sept;20(5):437–44. doi:10.1097/moh.0b013e3283634443

25. Levi M, van der Poll T, Schultz M. Infection and inflammation as risk factors for thrombosis and atherosclerosis. Seminars in Thrombosis and Hemostasis. 2012 Mar 7;38(05):506–14. doi:10.1055/s-0032-1305782

26. Liu T, Chen J, Bai X, Zheng G, Gao W. The effect of obesity on outcomes in trauma patients: A meta-analysis. Injury. 2013 Sept;44(9):1145–52. doi:10.1016/j.injury.2012.10.038

27. Faber DR, De Groot PG, Visseren FL. Role of adipose tissue in haemostasis, coagulation and fibrinolysis. Obesity Reviews. 2009 Aug 26;10(5):554–63. doi:10.1111/j.1467-789x.2009.00593.x

28. Shimomura I, Funahasm T, Takahashi M, Maeda K, Kotani K, Nakamura T. Enhanced expression of pai-1 in visceral fat: Possible contributor to vascular disease in obesity. Nature Medicine. 1996 Jul;2(7):800–3. doi:10.1038/nm0796-800

29. Nakata M, Yada T, Soejima N, Maruyama I. Leptin promotes aggregation of human platelets via the long form of its receptor. Diabetes. 1999 Feb 1;48(2):426–9. doi:10.2337/diabetes.48.2.426

30. Bodary PF. Effect of leptin on arterial thrombosis following vascular injury in mice. JAMA. 2002 Apr 3;287(13):1706. doi:10.1001/jama.287.13.1706

31. Samuels JM, Moore EE, Coleman JR, Sumislawski JJ, Cohen MJ, Silliman CC. Obesity is associated with Postinjury hypercoagulability. Journal of Trauma and Acute Care Surgery. 2019 Jun 24;87(4):876–82. doi:10.1097/ta.0000000000002414

32. McCully BH, Dean RK, McCully SP, Schreiber MA. Diet-induced obesity prevents the development of acute traumatic coagulopathy. Journal of Trauma and Acute Care Surgery. 2014 Dec;77(6):873–8. doi:10.1097/ta.0000000000000461

33. Kornblith LZ, Howard B, Kunitake R, Redick B, Nelson M, Cohen MJ. Obesity and clotting. Journal of Trauma and Acute Care Surgery. 2015 Jan;78(1):30–8. doi:10.1097/ta.0000000000000490

34. Mukamal KJ, Jadhav PP, D'Agostino RB, Massaro JM, Mittleman MA, Lipinska I. Alcohol consumption and hemostatic factors. Circulation. 2001 Sept 18;104(12): 1367–73. doi:10.1161/hc3701.096067

35. Bilello J, McCray V, Davis J, Jackson L, Danos LA. Acute ethanol intoxication and the trauma patient: Hemodynamic pitfalls. World Journal of Surgery. 2011;35:2149–53.

36. Eismann H, Sieg L, Ahmed H, Teske J, Behrendt P, Friedrich L, *et al.* Influence of alcohol consumption on blood coagulation in rotational thromboelastometry (rotem): An in-vivo study. Korean Journal of Anesthesiology. 2020 Aug 1;73(4):334–41. doi:10.4097/kja.20071

37. Engström M, Schött U, Reinstrup P. Ethanol impairs coagulation and fibrinolysis in whole blood: A study performed with rotational thromboelastometry. Blood Coagul Fibrinolysis. 2006;17:661–5.

38. Howard BM, Kornblith LZ, Redick BJ, Conroy AS, Nelson MF, Calfee CS. Exposing the bidirectional effects of alcohol on coagulation in trauma: Impaired clot formation and decreased fibrinolysis in rotational thromboelastometry. The Journal of Trauma and Acute Care Surgery. 2018;84:97–103.

39. Howard BM, Kornblith LZ, Redick BJ, Vilardi RF, Balhotra KS, Crane JM. The effects of alcohol on coagulation in trauma patients. Journal of Trauma and Acute Care Surgery. 2014 Dec;77(6):865–72. doi:10.1097/ta.0000000000000357

40. Andrikopoulos G. In-hospital mortality of habitual cigarette smokers after acute myocardial infarction. The "Smoker's paradox" in a countrywide study. European Heart Journal. 2001 May 1;22(9):776–84. doi:10.1053/euhj.2000.2315

41. Glynn MF, Mustard JF, Buchanan MR, Murphy EA. Cigarette smoking and platelet aggregation. Canadian Medical Association Journal. 1966;95(11):549–53.

42. Bell TM, Bayt DR, Zarzaur BL. "Smoker's Paradox" in patients treated for severe injuries: Lower risk of mortality after trauma observed in current smokers. Nicotine & Tobacco Research. 2015 Feb 2;17(12):1499–504. doi:10.1093/ntr/ntv027

43. Moazed F, Hendrickson C, Conroy A, Kornblith LZ, Benowitz NL, Delucchi K. Cigarette smoking and ARDS after blunt trauma. Chest. 2020 Oct;158(4):1490–8. doi:10.1016/j.chest.2020.05.603

44. Hollis S, Lecky F, Yates DW, Woodford M. The effect of pre-existing medical conditions and age on mortality after injury. The Journal of Trauma: Injury, Infection, and Critical Care. 2006 Nov;61(5):1255–60. doi:10.1097/01.ta.0000243889.07090.da

45. Morris JA. The effect of preexisting conditions on mortality in trauma patients. JAMA: The Journal of the American Medical Association. 1990 Apr 11;263(14):1942–6. doi:10.1001/jama.263.14.1942

46. Serrano E, Liu P, Nwabuo AI, Langness S, Juillard C. The effect of cirrhosis on trauma outcomes: A systematic review and meta-analysis. Journal of Trauma and Acute Care Surgery. 2019 Aug 6;88(4):536–45. doi:10.1097/ta.0000000000002464

47. Morrison CA, Wyatt MM, Carrick MM. The effects of cirrhosis on trauma outcomes: An analysis of the National Trauma Data Bank. Journal of Surgical Research. 2008 May. doi:10.1016/j.jss.2008.04.034

48. Reinke C, Spodeck A, Schildhauer TA, Swol J. Haemophilia A in A major trauma patient. BMJ Case Reports. 2015 Dec 16. doi:10.1136/bcr-2015-211694

49. Neal MD, Brown JB, Moore EE, Cuschieri J, Maier RV, Minei JP. Prehospital use of nonsteroidal anti-inflammatory drugs (NSAIDs) is associated with a reduced incidence of trauma-induced coagulopathy. Annals of Surgery. 2014 Aug;260(2):378–82. doi:10.1097/sla.0000000000000526

50. Mina AA, Bair HA, Howells GA, Bendick PJ. Complications of preinjury warfarin use in the trauma patient. The Journal of Trauma: Injury, Infection, and Critical Care. 2003 May;54(5):842–7. doi:10.1097/01.ta.0000063271.05829.15

51. Feeney JM, Neulander M, DiFiori M, Kis L, Shapiro DS, Jayaraman V. Direct oral anticoagulants compared with warfarin in patients with severe blunt trauma. Injury. 2017 Jan;48(1):47–50. doi:10.1016/j.injury.2016.08.016

52. Bhogadi SK, Alizai Q, Colosimo C. Not all traumatic brain injury patients on preinjury anticoagulation are the same. The American Journal of Surgery. 2023;226(6):785–9.

53. Bhogadi SK, Nelson A, Hosseinpour H, Anand T, Hejazi O, Colosimo C. Effect of PCC on outcomes of severe traumatic brain injury patients on preinjury anticoagulation. The American Journal of Surgery. 2024 Jun;232:138–41. doi:10.1016/j.amjsurg.2024.01.035

54. Ott MM, Eriksson E, Vanderkolk W, Christianson D, Davis A, Scholten D. Antiplatelet and anticoagulation therapies do not increase mortality in the absence of traumatic brain injury. Journal of Trauma: Injury, Infection & Critical Care. 2010 Mar;68(3):560–3. doi:10.1097/ta.0b013e3181ad6600

55. Beynon C, Hertle DN, Unterberg AW, Sakowitz OW. Clinical review: Traumatic brain injury in patients receiving antiplatelet medication. Critical Care. 2012 Jul 26;16(4):228. doi: 10.1186/cc11292

56. Efron DT, Sorock G, Haut ER, Chang D, Schneider E, MacKenzie E. Preinjury statin use is associated with improved in-hospital survival in elderly trauma patients. Journal of Trauma: Injury, Infection & Critical Care. 2008 Jan;64(1):66–74. doi:10.1097/ta.0b013e31815b842a

57. Neal MD, Cushieri J, Rosengart MR, Alarcon LH, Moore EE, Maier RV. Preinjury statin use is associated with a higher risk of multiple organ failure after injury: A propensity score adjusted analysis. Journal of Trauma: Injury, Infection & Critical Care. 2009 Sept;67(3):476–84. doi:10.1097/ta.0b013e3181ad66bb

58. Hess JR, Lindell AL, Stansbury LG, Dutton RP, Scalea TM. The prevalence of abnormal results of conventional coagulation tests on admission to a trauma center. Transfusion. 2009;49(1):34–9.

59. Cohen MJ, Call M, Nelson M, Calfee CS, Esmon CT, Brohi K, *et al.* Role of activated protein c in early coagulopathy and later organ failure, infection and death in trauma patients. Annals of Surgery. 2012;255(2):379–85.

60. Savioli G, Ceresa IF, Macedonio S, Gerosa S, Belliato M, Iotti GA, *et al.* Trauma coagulopathy and its outcomes. Medicina. 2020;56(4):205.

61. Bunch CM, Chang E, Moore EE, Moore HB, Kwaan HC, Miller JB, *et al.* Shock-induced endotheliopathy (SHINE): A mechanistic justification for viscoelastography-guided resuscitation of traumatic and non-traumatic shock. Frontiers in Physiology. 2023;14:1094845.

62. Moore HB, Moore EE, Gonzalez E, Chapman MP, Chin TL, Silliman CC, *et al.* Hyperfibrinolysis, physiologic fibrinolysis, and fibrinolysis shutdown: The spectrum of postinjury fibrinolysis and relevance to antifibrinolytic therapy. Journal of Trauma and Acute Care Surgery. 2014;77(6):811–7.

63. El-Menyar A, Abdelrahman H, Al-Thani H, Mekkodathil A, Singh R, Rizoli S. The FASILA Score: A novel bio-clinical score to predict massive blood transfusion in patients with abdominal trauma. World Journal of Surgery. 2020 Apr;44(4):1126–36. doi:10.1007/s00268-019-05289-0

64. Niles SE, McLaughlin DF, Perkins JG, Wade CE, Li Y, Spinella PC, *et al.* Increased mortality associated with the early coagulopathy of trauma in combat casualties. Journal of Trauma: Injury, Infection & Critical Care. 2008;64(6):1459–65.

65. Wohlauer MV, Moore EE, Thomas S, Sauaia A, Evans E, Harr J, *et al.* Platelet dysfunction: An unrecognized role in the acute coagulopathy of trauma. Journal of the American College of Surgeons. 2012;214(5):739–46.

66. Coleman JR, Kay AB, Moore EE, Moore HB, Gonzalez E, Majercik S, *et al.* It's sooner than you think: Blunt solid organ injury patients are already hypercoagulable upon hospital admission – Results of a bi-institutional, prospective study. The American Journal of Surgery. 2019;218(6):1065–73.

67. Wafaisade A, Lefering R, Tjardes T, Wutzler S, Simanski C; Trauma Registry of DGU, *et al.* Acute coagulopathy in isolated blunt traumatic brain injury. Neurocritical Care. 2010;12(2):211–9.

Chapter 4

TRAUMATIC BRAIN INJURY–ASSOCIATED COAGULOPATHY

Venencia Albert, Arulselvi Subramanian,
and Deepak Agrawal

DOI: 10.1201/9781003711070-4

INTRODUCTION

Traumatic brain injury (TBI) is defined as "an alteration in brain function or other evidence of brain pathology caused by an external force."[1] It is a major cause of death and disability worldwide, affecting all age groups and populations. Often described as "the most complex disease in the most complex organ," TBI is highly heterogeneous in its cause, mechanism, severity, and outcome.[2] The blood–brain barrier (BBB), which maintains homeostasis between blood circulation and the central nervous system, is frequently disrupted after injury. TBI involves both primary and secondary brain injuries. The primary injury occurs at the moment of impact, leading to shearing, compression, or contusion of brain tissue and vascular structures. This initial insult can damage endothelial cells, disrupt vascular integrity, and alter metabolic processes. The pattern of primary injury depends on the intensity and direction of force. Secondary brain injury develops over time due to processes such as inflammation, oxidative stress, metabolic failure, or ischaemia. These secondary insults, both intracranial and systemic, can exacerbate the initial injury. Primary injuries include contusions, lacerations, diffuse axonal injury (DAI), and lesions such as epidural haemorrhages (EDHs), subdural haemorrhages (SDHs), subarachnoid haemorrhages (SAHs), and intracerebral haemorrhages (ICHs). Focal injuries are localized, while diffuse injuries involve widespread damage. Cerebral contusions are cortical bruises caused by brain impact against the skull and countercoup forces. EDH occurs above the dura, usually from middle meningeal artery rupture, accounting for about 1.5% of head injury admissions and predominantly affecting males.[3] SDH develops below the dura and is often identified by haematoma thickness >10 mm or midline shift >20 mm. SAH occurs in the subarachnoid space between the pia and arachnoid membranes. DAI, a hallmark of severe TBI, presents with petechial haemorrhages at the grey and white matter junction, corpus callosum, and brainstem. Beyond cerebral damage, systemic complications such as hypertension, metabolic imbalance, and coagulopathy often accompany TBI (Figure 4.1).

TBI remains a global health challenge, causing significant disability and economic burden. The World Health Organization (WHO) projected that by 2020, TBI would surpass many diseases as a leading cause of death and disability.[4] About 54–60 million people sustain brain injury each year, with reported incidence rates of 180–250 per 100,000 in the United States and Europe, and up to 500 per 100,000 in some regions,[5,6] compared with about 50 per 100,000 in China.[7] It predominantly affects young adults (15–24 years), especially males, and the elderly above 50 years. Low- and middle-income countries bear a higher burden than high-income nations. In India, road accidents cause about 1,374 crashes and 400 deaths daily, with Delhi reporting the highest fatalities.[8,9] Despite the scale of the problem, comprehensive epidemiological data from India remain limited. TBI is the leading cause of early trauma-related deaths, second only to haemorrhagic shock.[10] While haemorrhagic shock contributes to 30–40% of trauma mortality, its outcomes can be improved through early haemostasis and rational transfusion. About one-quarter of TBI patients experience concurrent haemorrhagic shock, which doubles or triples mortality.[10] Traumatic intracranial haemorrhage, including epidural, subdural, subarachnoid, or parenchymal bleeding occurs in about 50% of cases. Moreover, TBI-associated coagulopathy contributes to the progression of haemorrhagic lesions, with an overall prevalence of 32.7%.[11] Even in isolated TBI without significant blood loss, coagulopathy remains a major determinant of outcome[12] seen in polytrauma. Unlike TIC in multisystem injuries, TBI-related coagulopathy can develop without major external bleeding.[13] It arises from the unique vascular and molecular responses of the injured brain. Disruption of the BBB allows tissue factor (TF) and other procoagulant substances to enter systemic circulation, activating coagulation cascades. Simultaneously, endothelial injury, platelet dysfunction, and release of brain phospholipids

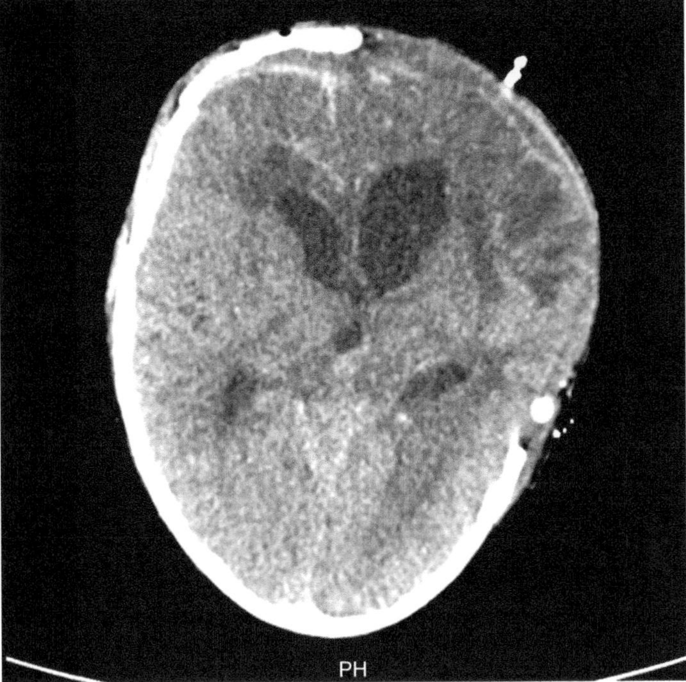

Figure 4.1 Computed tomography (CT) images of an open traumatic brain injury (TBI) patient showing haemorrhage and intracranial haematoma.

promote systemic coagulation abnormalities. The pathophysiology involves a biphasic pattern: an initial hypocoagulable phase followed by a hypercoagulable state. The early phase is marked by prolonged bleeding time and haematoma expansion, contributing to secondary ischemic and haemorrhagic damage.[14] This may progress to disseminated intravascular coagulation (DIC), characterized by widespread microthrombi and paradoxical bleeding.[15] The degree of coagulopathy correlates with the extent of cranial haemorrhage and brain swelling.[16] However, findings across studies are inconsistent. Cohen *et al.*[17] and Genet *et al.*[18] reported that TBI patients showed no significant coagulopathy compared with those having multisystem trauma, unless hypoperfusion was present. Lee *et al.*[19] also observed that coagulopathy was not independently associated with TBI severity, implying systemic factors may play a larger role. Still, many studies demonstrate that isolated TBI can trigger coagulopathy even without hypovolemia or massive transfusion.[20,21] The underlying mechanisms remain incompletely understood. Some evidence suggests that the coagulation abnormalities are integral to TBI pathophysiology rather than secondary systemic effects. The release of brain-derived tissue factor, activation of protein C pathway, and endothelial disruption are central contributors. The resulting imbalance between coagulation and fibrinolysis worsens intracranial bleeding and impairs cerebral perfusion, leading to poor outcomes. TBI-associated coagulopathy is therefore a major risk factor for unfavourable prognosis.[22-24] Early identification of patients at risk is crucial to guide therapy, prevent haematoma expansion, and reduce mortality. Understanding the molecular and systemic links between brain injury and coagulation will help design targeted interventions to improve survival and functional recovery.

THE INCIDENCE OF CLOTTING ABNORMALITIES IN TBI PATIENTS

The incidence of coagulation abnormalities in TBI varies widely, ranging from 15% to 100%.[21] This variation depends on factors such as the severity of injury, timing of testing, sensitivity of assays, and criteria used to define coagulopathy. A meta-analysis of 34 studies[11] in 2008 reported an overall prevalence of 32.7%. Subsequent clinical studies have shown a broad range of rates including Selladurai et al.[25] reported coagulopathy in 38% of patients using the ISTH-DIC criteria, 53% cases with coagulation abnormalities were noted based on six hemostatic parameters by Lozance et al., in 1998. Kuo et al.[26] reported a much higher rate (72.1%) using a modified coagulopathy score; in contrast, Rajajee et al.[27] reported a lower rate (8.4%) using the basic PT, international normalized ratio (INR), and platelet count thresholds. Using the same parameters Chang et al.[28] observed 22% and Zehtabchi et al.[29] found 17.3%. In larger multicentric studies, Wafaisade et al.[30] (2010) reported 22.7% cases with TBI coagulopathy patients (of 3,114), with mortality rate of 17.3%. Similarly, other groups have also associated TBI coagulopathy with high risk of mortality[31-38] regardless of the diagnostic tool. Using rotational thromboelastometry (ROTEM) criteria[33] the prevalence of coagulopathy decreased to 15.8%. More recent data by Chen et al.[39] noted 34.8% coagulopathy with 37% mortality, and Zoghi et al.[40] found 32.6% and 38.1% respectively, both showing mortality rates above 25%. Reported incidence therefore spans from <10% to >70%, underscoring the influence of differing diagnostic definitions and testing time points. Lustenberger et al.[41,42] observed that up to 45% of patients with isolated severe TBI develop coagulopathy, which may appear on admission or emerge several days after injury, correlating closely with injury severity. In our centre we observed[22] coagulopathies in 46% of cases, regardless of severity. A systematic review[43] of coagulopathy isolated TBI revealed wide heterogeneity in definitions but concluded that about 35% of patients present with coagulopathy at hospital arrival. Findings from our group at the All India Institute of Medical Sciences (AIIMS) further reinforce the early and independent occurrence of coagulation dysfunction in isolated TBI, 41% developed early coagulopathy within 3 hours post-injury, unrelated to shock or transfusion[44] with a 2.8-fold higher risk of in-hospital mortality. Acute traumatic endotheliopathy was a key contributor.[45] Additionally, thromboelastography (TEG) proved more sensitive than conventional tests in detecting early trauma-induced coagulopathy (TIC).[46]

PATHOGENESIS OF TBI ASSOCIATED COAGULOPATHY

Early work by Goodnight et al.[47] showed that about 69% of patients with brain tissue injury developed coagulopathy, marked by low fibrinogen, depleted clotting factors, and thrombocytopenia. They proposed that TF released from damaged brain tissue activated the extrinsic pathway, causing consumption coagulopathy.[48] Later studies questioned this as definitive proof remains limited, and inflammatory contributions are not fully understood. Despite high incidence and poor outcomes, data on the mechanisms driving coagulopathy after open or isolated TBI remain incomplete. Isolated severe TBI itself is now recognized as an independent trigger for coagulopathy, seen in about 43% of patients.[43]

KEY MECHANISMS CONTRIBUTING TO TBI-ASSOCIATED COAGULOPATHY

ENDOTHELIAL DYSFUNCTION AND BLOOD–BRAIN BARRIER (BBB) DISRUPTION
Endothelial activation plays a central role in the coagulopathy that follows TBI. Damage to the endothelium triggers coagulation factor activation and thrombin generation, setting

off a cascade that leads to systemic coagulopathy. A strong mechanistic link between endothelial injury and coagulation abnormalities has been established.[49] Elevated plasma syndecan-1, a marker of glycocalyx degradation, has been linked with TBI-associated coagulopathy, increased transfusion requirements, and higher early mortality. In one study, early coagulopathy occurred in 41.6% of patients and independently predicted death (OR = 4.73; 95% CI 1.68–13.3),[44] Morel *et al.*[49] found markedly high concentrations of pro-coagulant microparticles (MPs) in both cerebrospinal fluid (CSF) and peripheral blood shortly after TBI. The abundance of endothelial-derived MPs (EMPs) reflected the severity of vascular damage, and persistently elevated CSF MP levels even 10 days post-injury were associated with poor neurological outcome, suggesting ongoing BBB disruption. This contrasts with observations in polytrauma, where high MP levels have been linked to improved outcomes.[50–52] Our own studies support these findings. We demonstrated that early endothelial injury reflected by elevated soluble thrombomodulin and syndecan-1 levels correlated with poor outcomes in isolated severe TBI.[44] In a later study, we showed that circulating MPs, particularly those derived from endothelium and platelets, were significantly increased during the early phase of isolated severe TBI and were associated with coagulopathy and poor outcome.[53] These findings confirm that early endothelial damage and sustained BBB disruption are major contributors to coagulopathy and adverse prognosis in isolated brain injury.

THE TISSUE FACTOR (TF) HYPOTHESIS

Tissue factor is released into circulation after structural injury to the brain, creating a strong procoagulant state. Normally contained behind the BBB, TF becomes exposed to blood and platelets, binds to factor VIIa, and activates the extrinsic coagulation cascade. This generates thrombin, promotes fibrin formation, and causes microthrombosis and cerebral infarction.[32,39,54] The process also depletes coagulation factors and platelets, leading to platelet exhaustion. However, the role of TF as the main driver of TBI coagulopathy remains uncertain. Some studies found similar TF levels in patients with and without coagulopathy,[38] suggesting other mechanisms are involved. TF has also been identified on platelet and endothelial-derived microparticles, which may amplify coagulation locally and systemically. Hyperfibrinolysis (HF) is an important but underrecognized cause of bleeding after TBI. Although its incidence is relatively low (estimated range 2.5–7%), it is strongly linked with early mortality.[55] Stein *et al.*[56] and Nakae *et al.*[57] reported that HF occurs within hours after severe isolated TBI and contributes to secondary cerebral injury and poor long-term recovery. Unlike in polytrauma, HF in isolated TBI develops independently of systemic hypoperfusion, suggesting that brain injury alone can trigger excessive fibrinolytic activity. Hayakawa *et al.* showed that markers of tissue injury such as lactate dehydrogenase (LDH) and creatine kinase (CK) correlated with HF, while tissue hypoperfusion markers did not, implicating TF and damage-associated molecular patterns (DAMPs) as key drivers.[58] HF leads to degradation of fibrinogen and fibrin clots, impairing clot formation and promoting continued bleeding.[56] Proposed mechanisms include excessive activation of tissue plasminogen activator (tPA), depletion of alpha-2 plasmin inhibitor ($\alpha2AP$), and increased activity of activated protein C (aPC).[13,17] Injury-induced release of tPA and urokinase-type plasminogen activator (uPA) from brain tissue enhances local fibrinolysis, worsening ICH.[58,59] Manoel *et al.*,[37] however, questioned HF as a universal mechanism in isolated TBI, suggesting variability across patient subgroups. Our TEG-based study found HF (lysis at 30 minutes >3%) in 26% of isolated TBI patients, undetected by standard coagulation tests. HF was linked to reduced TF levels, excessive thrombin generation, and impaired anticoagulant response. Mortality in the HF group was 40%, compared with 26% in those with physiological fibrinolysis.[60] Fujiwara *et al.* identified D-dimer >50 µg/mL and fibrinogen <200 mg/dL at admission as predictors of severe HF. Administration of fibrinogen concentrate corrected low fibrinogen levels within hours, but did not significantly improve 30-day survival.[61] Overall, HF in TBI results from local endothelial and neuronal injury rather than systemic shock. It represents a state of uncontrolled fibrin degradation that often escapes routine laboratory detection. TEG enables early identification, while targeted fibrinogen replacement may stabilize clot formation and limit haemorrhage progression. Early detection and individualized treatment are key to managing HF-related coagulopathy in isolated TBI.

PLATELET ACTIVATION AND DYSFUNCTION

Platelet loss and dysfunction in adhesion, activation, and aggregation are major contributors to coagulopathy after TBI.[62-63] In our cohort, 58% of patients had thrombocytopenia at admission, associated with liver dysfunction, higher infection risk, longer intensive care stays, and a fourfold increase in in-hospital mortality. Nearly 46% were non-responders to platelet transfusion, showing higher mortality and altered platelet indices (*unpublished data*). Low platelet count markedly increases bleeding risk in TBI.[62-69] Counts below 175×10^9/L raise the risk of intracranial haemorrhage expansion, and those below 100×10^9/L increase mortality ninefold.[38,65] The IMPACT meta-analysis found thrombocytopenia in 7% of TBI patients on admission.[70] However, several studies found weak correlation between initial platelet count and haemorrhagic progression.[71] Platelet consumption within hours of injury likely reflects early clot formation.[13] Schnüriger *et al.*[68] showed platelet counts $<100 \times 10^9$/L increased mortality ninefold and $<175 \times 10^9$/L predicted haematoma expansion and need for craniotomy, but other studies suggest platelet function, not count, is more relevant.[66] Platelet dysfunction can occur even with normal counts.[72] Sillesen *et al.*[73] demonstrated rapid and persistent platelet dysfunction within 15 minutes of TBI, especially when combined with shock. Endothelial and BBB disruption exposes subendothelial matrix, promoting platelet adhesion and activation. Neurohumoral surges (catecholamines, acetylcholine) further impair platelet function. Overactivated platelets shed microparticles[49,50,53] containing TF, amplifying coagulation and contributing to "platelet exhaustion."[75] where platelets become refractory.[24,74] TF also binds to factor VIIa and integrates into platelet surfaces, enhancing thrombin production and clot propagation.[13,18] Inflammation worsens platelet dysfunction through endothelial injury and complement activation.[76,77] Elevated platelet-to-lymphocyte ratio (PLR) indicates hypercoagulability and inflammation, while low PLR correlates with platelet dysfunction, coagulopathy, and poor neurological outcomes. PLR may thus serve as a simple inflammatory marker in TBI-related coagulopathy.

ACTIVATION OF PROTEIN C PATHWAYS VIA TISSUE HYPOPERFUSION AND SHOCK

Activation of the protein C (PC) pathway plays a key role in coagulopathy following TBI, particularly when systemic hypoperfusion occurs. In a study of 39 isolated TBI patients, Cohen *et al.*[17] found no difference in baseline PC levels between patients and controls [79.4 ± 24.2% vs. 85 ± 36%, p = 0.52]. However, patients with tissue hypoperfusion showed significantly lower inactivated PC levels [56.2 ± 32% vs. 85 ± 35%, p = 0.03], indicating hypoperfusion-driven activation of this pathway. In our study of 120 severe isolated TBI patients, plasma PC and protein S (PS) levels were similar to healthy controls [PC: 85 (43–103) vs. 85.5 (76–109), p = 0.20; PS: 81 (54–102) vs. 91.5 (76–108.5), p = 0.05]. Endothelial protein C receptor (EPCR) levels, however, were markedly lower in patients [47.8 (23.3–76.4) ng/mL] than in controls [85.2 (63.0–103.4) ng/mL, p = 0.0005], suggesting impaired endothelial regulation. When compared by TIC status, PC and PS were significantly reduced in TIC cases [PC: 49.0 (35.5–102.5) vs. 91.0 (55.0–103.0) p = 0.04; PS: 58.5 (34.5–85.5) vs. 89.0 (73.0–115.0) p = 0.002], while EPCR levels showed no difference (p = 0.69).[44] Lustenberger *et al.*[42] also observed that isolated TBI patients with coagulopathy had higher base deficit and lactate levels, further linking hypoperfusion to early protein C activation and TIC.

TISSUE HYPOPERFUSION

Tissue hypoperfusion, along with injury severity, plays an important role in TIC.[78] Jansen *et al.*[79] linked reduced coagulation factor activity with hypoperfusion in severely injured patients, while Wu *et al.*[80] reported lower factor VII activity with greater hypoperfusion. Earlier work suggested that TBI alone does not cause early coagulopathy; hypoperfusion must accompany it to trigger activation of the protein C pathway.[17,18] Lee *et al.*,[19] in a study of 795 trauma patients, found those with a base deficit (BD) ≥6 had lower Glasgow Coma Scale (GCS) scores, lower systolic blood pressure (SBP), higher heart rate, and were more hypocoagulable by both rapid TEG and standard assays. However, coagulopathy patterns did not differ by injury region. Similarly, Cohen *et al.*[17] reported that TBI patients without hypoperfusion (n = 28) did not develop early coagulopathy, whereas those with BD >6 (n = 11) showed prolonged prothrombin and partial thromboplastin times (17.6 ± 3.6 vs. 14.3 ± 2.3, p < 0.005; and 43.1 ± 18.3 vs. 27.4 ± 3.8, p < 0.0001), and elevated aPC levels, supporting the role of hypoperfusion-driven coagulopathy. Talving *et al.*[21] confirmed that coagulopathy often accompanies hypoperfusion in severe TBI. Wafaisade *et al.*[30] identified hypotension (systolic BP <90 mmHg) at the scene or on emergency department arrival as an independent predictor of acute coagulopathy. Dekker *et al.*[20] found TBI-induced coagulopathy associated with systemic hypoperfusion markers, but not all coagulopathic patients had elevated BD or lactate, implying additional mechanisms. In our study, 27.7% of isolated TBI patients showed hypoperfusion; 55% of them developed TIC, but 36.5% without hypoperfusion also did. Though not statistically significant (p = 0.15), this challenges the belief that hypoperfusion is required. TIC occurred early, even without major haemorrhage, hypotension, or fluid resuscitation, suggesting alternative non-hypotensive mechanisms.[44] Similarly, other studies found 60.4% of coagulopathic isolated TBI patients had BD ≤6 mmol/L,[44] and Manoel *et al.*[37] reported higher pH and lower BD in coagulopathic isolated TBI cases, indicating that coagulopathy can arise independent of tissue hypoperfusion.

CELLULAR AND BRAIN-DERIVED MICROPARTICLES (BDMPS)

The pattern of circulating MPs is reported to be altered following brain injury (Figure 4.2), as endothelial, platelet and leukocyte derived microparticles are released due to injury[53] and support microthrombus formation. The injured brain also releases brain derived microparticles released from injured microglia and neurons and mitochondrial microparticles (mtMPs) into the blood stream.[81] These particles are enriched with TF and exposed anionic phospholipids [phosphatidylserine (PS)] and trigger hypercoagulability that shifts to consumptive coagulopathy and hyperfibrinolysis, resulting in exacerbation of brain injury, and secondary insults.[82–84] As the brain tissue is rich in phospholipids (~25% of dry weight),[85] brain-derived microparticles (BDMPs) provide a strong procoagulant platform. The exposure of cardiolipin (CL) on the outer membrane of mtMPs due to TBI, triggers systemic inflammation and procoagulant response. Oxidative stress is also a major driver of secondary injury and inflammation after TBI, mtMPs also generate ROS.[82] Lactoferrin, through its interaction with these microvesicles, has shown promise in mitigating coagulation disturbances and enhancing prognosis in a mouse model of TBI.[86]

THROMBOINFLAMMATION

TBI initiates inflammation coagulation crosstalks a tight interaction between inflammation and coagulation through the BBB, causing secondary insults and delayed recovery. Hyperfibrinolysis and fibrin degradation fragments trigger inflammatory cytokines such as interleukin (IL)-1β, IL-6, and IL-8, causing thrombosis-driven inflammation.[87–90] Activated platelets enhance complement activation, amplifying inflammation, and inflammation in turn also exacerbates thrombosis.[91,92] Following TBI the microglia rapidly migrate to the site of injury in response to damage-associated molecular patterns, while neutrophils and monocytes infiltrate the brain tissue, intensifying local inflammation.[93,94] Persistent or dysregulated immune activity leads to chronic microglial activation and neurodegeneration.[95]

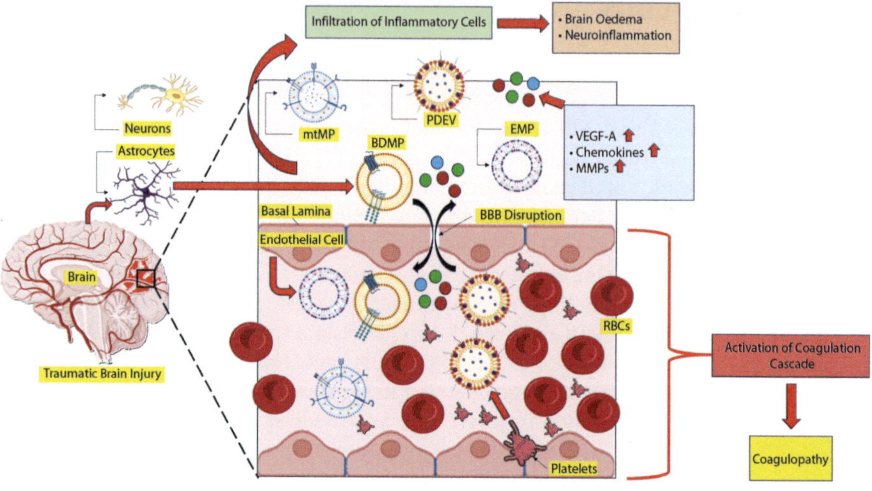

Figure 4.2 Blood–brain barrier disruption and microparticle-mediated pathways after traumatic brain injury.

This figure shows how traumatic brain injury leads to blood–brain barrier disruption and the release of brain-derived, endothelial-derived and mitochondrial microparticles. These particles, along with inflammatory mediators, enter the circulation and trigger endothelial activation, loss of glycocalyx and increased permeability. The process promotes brain oedema, neuroinflammation and downstream platelet activation and coagulation pathway activation. The combined effects contribute to the development of coagulopathy after injury.

Circulating cytokines such as IL-1β, IL-6, IL-10, and tumour necrosis factor alpha (TNF-α) rise within hours of injury,[96–98] reflecting this early systemic response. Activated neutrophils form web like structures known as neutrophil extracellular traps (NETs),[99] which can cross the cerebral endothelium and release procoagulant factors, including BDMPs and DAMPs. Prolonged NET formation, worsens coagulation dysfunction. Platelets can also stimulate NET release via high mobility group box 1 (HMGB1) protein.[100] NETs damage endothelial cells by exposing phosphatidylserine and increasing TF expression,[101] driving a procoagulant phenotype. This cascade contributes to secondary brain injury and neurological decline.[102,103] Targeting NET formation may represent a promising approach for managing TBI-associated coagulopathy (Figure 4.3).

TIME COURSE OF TIC FOLLOWING TBI

Prothrombin time (PT), activated partial thromboplastin time (aPTT) are reported to rise early after injury,[19] PT has been reported in both patients during the first 6–12 hours of injury,[48] aPTT was seen to be elevated in the first 12 hours following injury,[38] and PT/INR was seen to increase in the first 2–6 hours.[21,33,39] A recent systematic review 108 reported normal platelet counts on emergency department arrival, with subsequent drop, and steeper declines were observed to be correlated with more severe TBI,[20] the lowest platelet count (nadir) occurs between 1–5 days,[27–32] followed by recovery in the next 5–9 days.[28,30,31] Contrarily, platelet function was seen to be low on arrival, with continued decline in the first

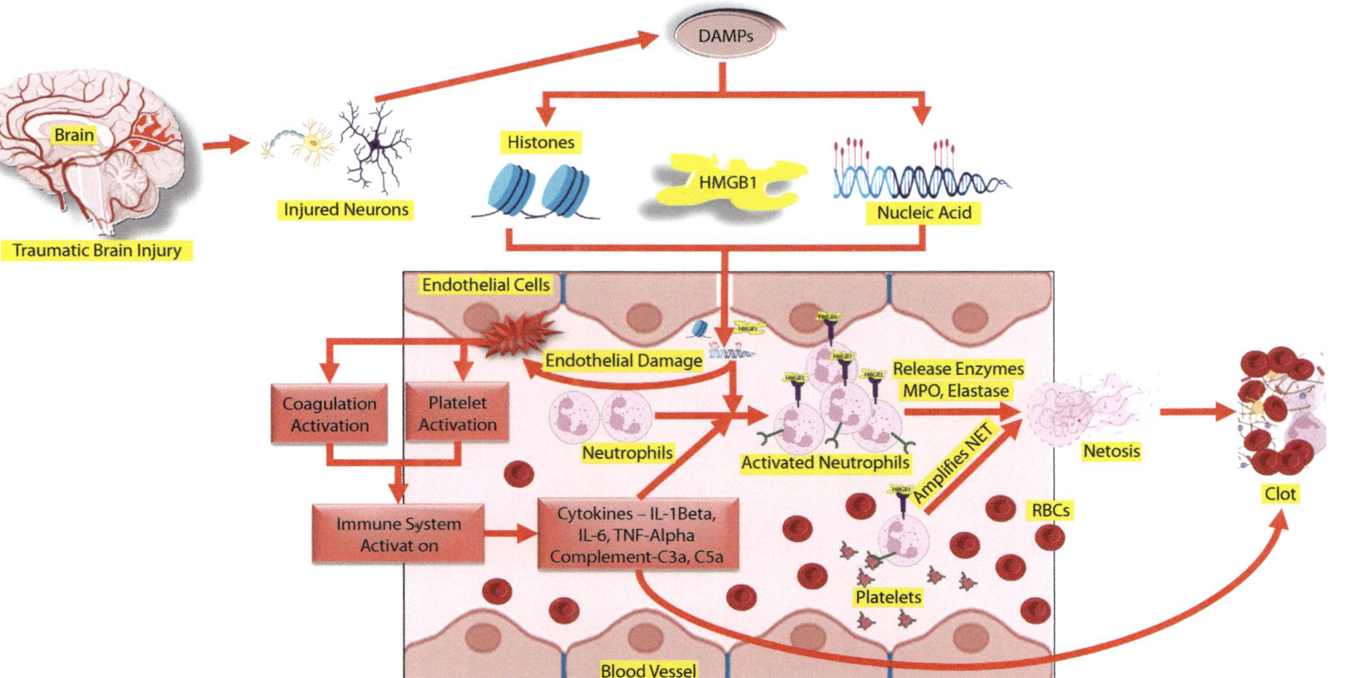

Figure 4.3 Damage associated molecular patterns (DAMPs) and neutrophil-driven pathways linking traumatic brain injury to coagulopathy. Selected elements were sourced from the NIAID NIH BioArt Source (bioart.niaid.nih.gov).

This figure outlines how injured neurons release danger signals, including histones, HMGB1 and nucleic acids. These DAMPs activate endothelial cells, platelets and neutrophils, leading to endothelial injury and immune activation. Neutrophils form extracellular traps and release enzymes that amplify inflammation and promote clot formation. Together, these responses connect traumatic brain injury to dysregulated coagulation and thrombus formation.

Table 4.1 Temporal dynamics of coagulation, platelet, and fibrinolytic markers following TBI[104]

Parameter	Early (0–6 hours)	6–24 hours	Day 1–3	Day 3–7	>7 days
Platelet count	Normal	Starts to fall	Lowest	Recovery	Normal
Platelet function	Low ↓	Lowest	Recovering	Normal/↑	↑ (hyperactive)
PT/APTT	↑	Peak	Normalizing	Normal	—
TAT/F1+2	↑	Decline	Normal	—	—
D-dimer	↑↑	Peak	Decline	Normal (50%)	—

24 hours following injury.[35] The lowest values were observed between 6 and 48 hours,[24,29,36,37] with recovery in the following 2–16 days; some have also reported rebound hyperactive platelets later in the course.[29,36] Thrombin generation (thrombin-antithrombin complex [TAT] and/or F1+2) is reported to be elevated on admission, but returns to normal within 24 hours to 7 days. D-dimer peaks totalling 108 within 3–6 hours with direct correlation to severity of injury;[19,23] however, there is a paucity of follow-up data to report normalization. Pahatouridis *et al.* observed 55% of TBI cases to have normalized d-dimer by day 3109. Similar partners have also been reported in other fibrinolytic markers (PAI-1 and tPA), shown in Table 4.1. The onset of TBI associated coagulopathy ranges from a few hours to 4.5 days post-admission, lasting up to 22 days.[41] About 65% of cases occur within 24 hours, with a second peak at 24–36 hours. In our study, TIC developed in 40% of patients arriving within 1 hour and 47% within 3 hours of injury. Wafaisade *et al.*[30] reported TIC in 22.7% of 3,114 isolated blunt TBI cases upon ED arrival, while Greuters[31] and Franschman[15] observed early abnormalities that persisted up to three days, indicating ongoing coagulation imbalance after injury.

CLINICAL DRIVERS OF ACUTE COAGULOPATHY AFTER TBI

SEVERITY OF INJURY (GCS)

Trauma severity strongly influences the risk of TIC. Earlier studies found larger intracerebral and subarachnoid haemorrhages, and greater midline shifts, associated with TIC.[105] In contrast, our study found no significant difference in computed tomography (CT) scores between coagulopathic and non-coagulopathic isolated severe TBI patients, though midline shift and subdural haematoma were slightly higher in the TIC group (4.0% vs. 1.4% and 46.0% vs. 44.3%).[44] The German Trauma Registry[30] reported that patients with coagulopathy were older and more severely injured, showing higher Abbreviated Injury Scale (AIS) for the head (4.5 vs. 4.2) and lower GCS at the scene (6.8 vs. 9.2, p < 0.001). Coagulopathy correlated with subdural haematoma (43.6% vs. 36.8%), more frequent craniotomies, and increased injury severity (p < 0.001). Similarly, Wu *et al.*[80] and May *et al.*[106] found coagulopathy in patients with lower GCS and higher head AIS scores. In our findings, patients with GCS 3–6 were more common in the TIC group (24–30%) than non-TIC (16–18%), while GCS 7–8 was higher in non-TIC (65.7% vs. 46%, p = 0.07).[44] However, Shaz *et al.*[107] reported no significant correlation between GCS, AIS, and coagulation parameters. Discrepancies across studies may relate to differences in inclusion criteria and injury type. Still, most evidence supports that severe TBI independently increases the risk of early coagulopathy.[39]

AGE

Age-related trends in TIC remain inconsistent. Paediatric studies show mixed results, children with isolated severe TBI had similar or slightly lower TIC frequency compared to adults, likely due to differences in coagulation physiology and assay sensitivity. Chong *et al.*[108] found lower TIC rates in paediatric isolated TBI compared to polytrauma, while James *et al.*[109] found no association between age and coagulopathy in isolated blunt head injuries. Overall, TIC appears to rise with increasing Injury Severity Score (ISS) in children, suggesting that trauma burden rather than age alone drives coagulopathy.

HYPERGLYCAEMIA

Hyperglycaemia is a recognized marker of injury severity and poor outcome after TBI. Elevated admission glucose levels correlate with higher mortality and risk of coagulopathy.[110] Alexiou *et al.* observed that patients with blood glucose $\geq$15.1 g/L were more likely to develop coagulation abnormalities and lower GCS scores. The mechanism is linked to the post-injury stress response catecholamine surge and reduced insulin secretion, which promotes systemic inflammation and endothelial dysfunction. Although glucose control may theoretically mitigate coagulopathy, evidence remains inconclusive.[111,112] Future trials should evaluate whether tight glycaemic management can reduce coagulopathy and improve recovery after open or severe.

TBI
ABNORMALITIES OF SERUM MAGNESIUM LEVELS

Magnesium plays a vital role in haemostasis, influencing platelet aggregation, factor X activation (via factors IXa and VIIa), and regulating anticoagulants such as proteins C and S.[113] Clinical studies show that magnesium sulfate infusion can improve hypocoagulable states and reduce blood loss in surgical settings.[114] However, excess magnesium may inhibit platelet function and prolong bleeding time.[113] Wang *et al.* found both low (<1.7 mg/dL) and high (>2.2 mg/dL) magnesium levels associated with coagulopathy in TBI patients. Low magnesium correlated with larger haemorrhages in aneurysmal subarachnoid haemorrhage and higher haemorrhagic transformation risk in ischaemic stroke,[115] while elevated magnesium related to smaller haematoma volumes.[13] Experimental models also show that magnesium-enriched resuscitation fluids can restore coagulation after haemorrhagic shock.[116] In TBI, magnesium has been studied for neuroprotection through N-methyl-D-aspartate (NMDA) receptor modulation and calcium channel blockade. However, randomized trials and meta-analyses have shown mixed or no survival benefit.[117] The therapeutic impact likely depends on timing, severity, and BBB integrity. The effect of magnesium on coagulopathy after TBI remains unexplored, highlighting the need for targeted studies to determine if correcting hypomagnesemia can stabilize coagulation and improve clinical outcomes.

ASSESSMENT AND MONITORING TOOLS

There is no standard definition for TIC in TBI, leading to wide variation in reported incidence (8.4–2.1%). Our findings showed mortality increased with stricter thresholds for PT, aPTT, or INR. A meta-analysis by Epstein *et al.*[43] of 22 studies found a pooled incidence of 35.2% and mortality ranging from 17% to 86%. In our cohort, mortality in patients with coagulopathy was 37%, compared with 4.7% in those without.[46] These patients also had longer surgeries, prolonged ICU stays (p = 0.003), and lower Glasgow Outcome Scores (3 vs. 5). This supports the need for standardized diagnostic definitions and regular coagulation monitoring in TBI management. Additionally, advanced neurocritical monitoring is essential, especially in moderate to severe TBI.[86] Multimodal monitoring (MMM) integrates several tools to give a real-time view of cerebral physiology. Intracranial pressure (ICP) monitoring remains central, as elevated ICP lowers cerebral perfusion pressure (mean arterial pressure minus ICP), increasing ischaemia and herniation risk.[118]

Guidelines recommend maintaining ICP at 20–25 mmHg and mean arterial pressure (MAP) at 60–70 mmHg.[119] Cerebral microdialysis (CMD) provides biochemical data on cerebral metabolism through hourly sampling.[120] Near-infrared spectroscopy measures oxygenated and deoxygenated haemoglobin levels to assess cerebral oxygenation, though limited to superficial regions such as the frontal cortex. Continuous EEG detects post-traumatic seizures, which occur in about 10–25% of severe TBI patients.[121] Early identification allows timely antiepileptic therapy. In one reported case, MMM-guided care enabled successful management of a comatose TBI patient, demonstrating its clinical value.[122] CT remains the primary imaging modality for rapid detection of intracranial haemorrhage, oedema, or fractures, while magnetic resonance imaging (MRI) offers greater sensitivity for diffuse axonal injury but is slower and less practical for unstable patients. Doppler ultrasound can evaluate cerebral blood flow and vasospasm but depends heavily on operator skill and accessibility of brain regions.[123]

COMPLICATIONS

Coagulopathy after TBI is linked to poor outcomes and several complications, including delayed traumatic intracranial haemorrhage (DTICH), cerebral ischaemia, brain oedema, and acute respiratory distress syndrome. It is an independent predictor of mortality and poor prognosis. Wafaisade *et al.*[30] found a threefold rise in in-hospital deaths, while Talving *et al.*[21] reported up to a tenfold increase. Coagulopathy also correlates with multi-organ failure and progressive haemorrhagic injury. Nearly half of affected patients show worsening intracranial bleeding within 48 hours. Early detection and prompt correction may prevent deterioration and improve outcomes.

CONCLUSION

Coagulopathy following TBI significantly worsens outcomes, increasing risks of delayed haemorrhage, cerebral ischaemia, brain oedema, multi-organ failure, and mortality. Early recognition and correction of coagulation abnormalities are critical to prevent progression, reduce secondary injuries, and improve survival and neurological recovery in affected patients.

TAKE-HOME MESSAGE

TBI causes both immediate structural damage and delayed secondary injury that worsens brain swelling and bleeding. coagulopathy does not always need major bleeding or shock; isolated brain injury alone can cause it. BBB and endothelium disruption is central to early coagulopathy in TBI. Microparticles released from the brain, endothelium and platelets enter the blood after injury and trigger clotting and inflammation. Reported incidence varies widely because studies use different tests and definitions, but about one-third of TBI patients show coagulopathy on arrival. Early recognition is important because coagulopathy strongly predicts haematoma growth, need for surgery and death.

REFERENCES

1. Menon DK, Schwab K, Wright DW, Maas AIR. Position statement: Definition of traumatic brain injury. Arch Phys Med Rehabil. 2010;91(11):1637–40.

2. Maas A. Traumatic brain injury: Changing concepts and approaches. Chin J Traumatol. 2016;19(1):3–6.

3. Tsang KK, Whitfield PC. Traumatic brain injury: Review of current management strategies. Br J Oral Maxillofac Surg. 2012;50(4):298–308.

4. Țolescu RȘ, Zorilă MV, Șerbănescu MS, Kamal KC, Zorilă GL, Dumitru I *et al*. Severe traumatic brain injury (TBI) - A seven-year comparative study in a Department of Forensic Medicine. Rom J Morphol Embryol. 2020;61(1):95–103. doi:10.47162/RJME.61.1.10

5. GBD 2016 traumatic brain injury and spinal cord injury collaborators. GBD 2016 traumatic brain injury and spinal cord injury collaborators, global, regional, and national burden of traumatic brain injury and spinal cord injury, 1990–2016: A systematic analysis for the global burden of disease study 2016. Lancet Neurol. 2019;18(1):56–87.

6. Maas AIR, Menon DK, Manley GT, Abrams M, Åkerlund C, Andelic N, *et al*. Traumatic brain injury: Progress and challenges in prevention, clinical care, and research. Lancet Neurol. 2022;21(11):1004–60. doi:10.1016/S1474-4422(22)00309-X

7. Zou JF, Fang HL, Zheng J, Ma YQ, Wu CW, Su GJ, *et al*. The epidemiology of traumatic brain injuries in the fastest-paced city in China: A retrospective study. Front Neurol. 2023;14:1255117. Published 2023 Nov 9. doi:10.3389/fneur.2023.1255117

8. Mahata D, Narzary PK, Govil D. Spatio-temporal analysis of road traffic accidents in Indian large cities. Clin Epidemiol Glob Health. 2019;7(4):586–91.

9. Kamal VK, Agrawal D, Pandey RM. Epidemiology, clinical characteristics and outcomes of traumatic brain injury: Evidences from integrated level 1 trauma center in India. J Neurosci Rural Pract. 2016;7(4):515–25. doi:10.4103/0976-3147.188637

10. Kauvar DS, Lefering R, Wade CE. Impact of haemorrhage on trauma outcome: An overview of epidemiology, clinical presentations, and therapeutic considerations. J Trauma. 2006;60:S3–11.

11. Harhangi BS, Kompanje EJ, Leebeek FW, Maas AI. Coagulation disorders after traumatic brain injury. Acta Neurochir. 2008;150:165–75.

12. Zhang J, Jiang R, Liu L, Watkins T, Zhang F, Dong J. Traumatic brain injury-associated coagulopathy. J Neurotrauma. 2012;29(17):2597–605.

13. Laroche M, Kutcher ME, Huang MC, Cohen MJ, Manley GT. Coagulopathy after traumatic brain injury. Neurosurgery. 2012;70:1334–45.

14. Mc Mahon A, Weiss L, Bennett K, Curley G, Ainle N, Maguire FP. Extracellular vesicles in disorders of hemostasis following traumatic brain injury. Front Neurol. 2024;15:1373266. doi:10.3389/fneur.2024.1373266. Published 2024 May 9.

15. Franschman G, Greuters S, Jansen WH, Posthuma LM, Peerdeman SM, Wattjes MP, *et al*. Haemostatic and cranial computed tomography characteristics in patients with acute and delayed coagulopathy after isolated traumatic brain injury. Brain Inj. 2012;26:1464–71.

16. Allard CB, Scarpelini S, Rhind SG, Baker AJ, Shek PN, Tien H, *et al*. Abnormal coagulation tests are associated with progression of traumatic intracranial hemorrhage. J Trauma. 2009;67(5):959–67.

17. Cohen MJ, Brohi K, Ganter MT, Manley GT, Mackersie RC, Pittet JF. Early coagulopathy after traumatic brain injury: The role of hypoperfusion and the protein C pathway. J Trauma. 2007;63:1254–62.

18. Genét GF, Johansson PI, Meyer MA, Sølbeck S, Sørensen AM, Larsen CF, *et al.* Trauma-induced coagulopathy: Standard coagulation tests, biomarkers of coagulopathy, and endothelial damage in patients with traumatic brain injury. J Neurotrauma. 2013;30:301–6.

19. Lee TH, Hampton DA, Diggs BS, McCully SP, Kutcher M, Redick BJ, *et al.* Traumatic brain injury is not associated with coagulopathy out of proportion to injury in other body regions. J Trauma Acute Care Surg. 2014;77:67–72.

20. Dekker SE, Duvekot A, de Vries HM, Geeraedts LM Jr, Peerdeman SM, de Waard MC, *et al.* Relationship between tissue perfusion and coagulopathy in traumatic brain injury. J Surg Res. 2016;205(1):147–54.

21. Talving P, Benfield R, Hadjizacharia P, Inaba K, Chan LS, Demetriades D. Coagulopathy in severe traumatic brain injury: A prospective study. J Trauma. 2009 Jan;66(1):55–61. doi: 10.1097/TA.0b013e318190c3c0; discussion 61–2.

22. Chhabra G, Rangarajan K, Subramanian A, Agrawal D, Sharma S, Mukhopadhayay AK. Hypofibrinogenemia in isolated traumatic brain injury in Indian patients. Neurol India. 2010;58(5):756–7. doi: 10.4103/0028-3886.72175

23. Yang F, Peng C, Peng L, Wang J, Li Y, Li W. A machine learning approach for the prediction of traumatic brain injury induced coagulopathy. Front Med (Lausanne). 2021;8:792689. doi: 10.3389/fmed.2021.792689

24. Maegele M. Coagulopathy and progression of intracranial hemorrhage in traumatic brain injury: Mechanisms, impact, and therapeutic considerations. Neurosurgery. 2021;89(6):954–66.

25. Selladurai BM, Vickneswaran M, Duraisamy S, Atan M. Coagulopathy in acute head injury—A study of its role as a prognostic indicator. Br J Neurosurg. 1997;11(5): 398–404.

26. Kuo JR, Chou TJ, Chio CC. Coagulopathy as a parameter to predict the outcome in head injury patients–analysis of 61 cases. J Clin Neurosci. 2004;11(7):710–4.

27. Rajajee V, Brown DM, Tuhrim S. Coagulation abnormalities following primary intracerebral hemorrhage. J Stroke Cerebrovasc Dis. 2004;13(2):47–51.

28. Chang EF, Meeker M, Holland MC. Acute traumatic intraparenchymal hemorrhage: Risk factors for progression in the early post-injury period. Neurosurgery. 2006;58(4):647–56.

29. Zehtabchi S, Soghoian S, Liu Y, Carmody K, Shah L, Whittaker B, Sinert R. The association of coagulopathy and traumatic brain injury in patients with isolated head injury. Resuscitation. 2008;76:52–6.

30. Wafaisade A, Lefering R, Tjardes T, Wutzler S, Simanski C; Trauma Registry of DGU. Acute coagulopathy in isolated blunt traumatic brain injury. Neurocrit Care. 2010;12:211–9.

31. Greuters S, van den Berg A, Franschman G, *et al.* Acute and delayed mild coagulopathy are related to outcome in patients with isolated traumatic brain injury. Critical Care. 2011;15(1):R2.

32. Sun Y, Wang J, Wu X, Xi C, Gai Y, Liu H, *et al.* Validating the incidence of coagulopathy and disseminated intravascular coagulation in patients with traumatic brain injury: Analysis of 242 cases. Br J Neurosurg. 2011;25:363–8.

33. Schöchl H, Solomon C, Traintinger S, Nienaber U, Tacacs-Tolnai A, Windhofer C, Bahrami S, Voelckel W. Thromboelastometric (ROTEM) findings in patients suffering from isolated severe traumatic brain injury. J Neurotrauma. 2011;28(10):2033–41.

34. Shrestha A, Man Joshi R, Devkota PU. Coagulation disorder in moderate to severe traumatic brain injuries. Asian J Med Sci. 2014;6(3):22–5.

35. Joseph B, Aziz H, Zangbar B, Kulvatunyou N, Pandit V, O'Keeffe T, *et al.* Acquired coagulopathy of traumatic brain injury defied by routine laboratory tests: Which laboratory values matter? J Trauma Crit Care Surg. 2014;76:121–5.

36. Abdelmalik PA, Boorman DW, Tracy J, Jallo J, Rincon F. Acute traumatic coagulopathy accompanying isolated traumatic brain injury is associated with worse long-term functional and cognitive outcomes. Neurocrit Care. 2016;24(3):361–70.

37. de Oliveira Manoel AL, Neto AC, Veigas PV, Rizoli S. Traumatic brain injury associated coagulopathy. Neurocrit Care. 2015;22(1):34–44.

38. Di Battista AP, Rizoli SB, Lejnieks B, Min A, Shiu MY, Peng HT, *et al.* Sympathoadrenal activation is associated with acute traumatic coagulopathy and endotheliopathy in isolated brain injury. Shock (Augusta, Ga). 2016;46(3 Suppl):96–103.

39. Chen Y, Tian J, Chi B, Zhang S, Wei L, Wang S. Factors associated with the development of coagulopathy after open traumatic brain injury. J Clin Med. 2021;11(1):185. doi:10.3390/jcm11010185

40. Zoghi S, Ansari A, Azad TD, Niakan A, Kouhpayeh SA, Taheri R, *et al.* Early hypocoagulable state in traumatic brain injury patients: Incidence, predisposing factors, and outcomes in a retrospective cohort study. Neurosurg Rev. 2024;47(1):297. doi:10.1007/s10143-024-02523-9. Published 2024 Jun 26.

41. Lustenberger T, Talving P, Kobayashi L, Inaba K, Lam L, Plurad D, Demetriades D. Time course of coagulopathy in isolated severe traumatic brain injury. Injury. 2010;41:924–8.

42. Lustenberger T, Talving P, Kobayashi L, Barmparas G, Inaba K, Lam L, *et al.* Early coagulopathy after isolated severe traumatic brain injury: Relationship with hypoperfusion challenged. J Trauma. 2010;69(6):1410–4.

43. Epstein DS, Mitra B, O'Reilly G, Rosenfeld JV, Cameron PA. Acute traumatic coagulopathy in the setting of isolated traumatic brain injury: A systematic review and meta-analysis. Injury. 2014;45(5):819–24.

44. Albert V, Arulselvi S, Agrawal D, Pati HP, Pandey RM. Early posttraumatic changes in coagulation and fibrinolysis systems in isolated severe traumatic brain injury patients and its influence on immediate outcome. Hematol Oncol Stem Cell Ther. 2019 Mar;12(1):32–43. doi: 10.1016/j.hemonc.2018.09.005. Epub 2018 Sep 27.

45. Albert V, Subramanian A, Agrawal D, Pati HP, Gupta SD, Mukhopadhyay AK. Acute traumatic endotheliopathy in isolated severe brain injury and its impact on clinical outcome. Med Sci (Basel). 2018 Jan 16;6(1).5. doi: 10.3390/medsci6010005

46. Albert V, Subramanian A, Pati HP, Agrawal D, Bhoi SK. Efficacy of thromboelastography (TEG) in predicting acute trauma-induced coagulopathy (ATIC) in isolated severe traumatic brain injury (iSTBI). Indian J Hematol Blood Transfus. 2019 Apr;35(2):325–31. doi: 10.1007/s12288-018-1003-4

47. Goodnight SH, Kenoyer G, Rapaport SI, Patch MJ, Lee JA, Kurze T. Defibrination after brain-tissue destruction: A serious complication of head injury. N Engl J Med. 1974;290(19):1043–7.

48. Halpern CH, Reilly PM, Turtz AR, Stein SC. Traumatic coagulopathy: The effect of brain injury. J Neurotrauma. 2008;25(8):997–1001.

49. Morel N, Morel O, Petit L, Hugel B, Cochard JF, Freyssinet JM, Sztark F, Dabadie P. Generation of procoagulant microparticles in cerebrospinal fluid and peripheral blood after traumatic brain injury. J Trauma. 2008;64:698–704.

50. Windeløv NA, Johansson PI, Sørensen AM, Perner A, Wanscher M, Larsen CF, *et al.* Low level of procoagulant platelet microparticles is associated with impaired coagulation and transfusion requirements in trauma patients. J Trauma Acute Care Surg. 2014;77(5):692–700.

51. Matijevic N, Wang YW, Wade CE, Holcomb JB, Cotton BA, Schreiber MA, *et al.* PROMMTT study group. Cellular microparticle and thrombogram phenotypes in the prospective observational multicenter major trauma transfusion (PROMMTT) study: Correlation with coagulopathy. Thromb Res. 2014;134(3):652–8.

52. Curry N, Raja A, Beavis J, Stanworth S, Harrison P. Levels of procoagulant microvesicles are elevated after traumatic injury and platelet microvesicles are negatively correlated with mortality. J Extracell Vesicles. 2014;3:25625.

53. Albert V, Subramanian A, Pati HP. Impact of early microparticle release during isolated severe traumatic brain injury: Correlation with coagulopathy and mortality. Neurol India. 2024;72(2):285–91. doi:10.4103/ni.ni_1159_21

54. Hoffman M, Monroe DM. Tissue factor in brain is not saturated with factor VIIa: Implications for factor VIIa: Dosing in intracerebral hemorrhage. Stroke. 2009; 40:2882–4.

55. Schoechl H, Voelkel W, Maegele M, Solomon C. Trauma - Associate hyperfibrinolysis. Hämostaseology 2012;32:22–7.

56. Stein SC, Smith DH. Coagulopathy in traumatic brain injury. Neurocrit Care. 2004;1(4):479–88.

57. Nakae R, Takayama Y, Kuwamoto K, Naoe Y, Sato H, Yokota H. Time course of coagulation and fibrinolytic parameters in patients with traumatic brain injury. J Neurotrauma. 2016;33(7):688–95.

58. Hayakawa M. Pathophysiology of trauma-induced coagulopathy: Disseminated intravascular coagulation with the fibrinolytic phenotype. J Intensive Care. 2017;5:14.

59. Gando S. Hemostasis and thrombosis in trauma patients. Semin Thromb Hemost. 2015;41:26–34.

60. Albert V, Arulselvi S. Study of hyperfibrinolysis in acute traumatic brain injury (TBI) patients using thromboelastography (TEG) and its correlation with coagulation markers. In: Abstracts of the 58th Annual Conference of the Indian Society of Hematology & Blood Transfusion (ISHBT); November 2017; Guwahati, India, 2017, 33(Suppl 1), 1–126. doi:10.1007/s12288-017-0893-x

61. Fujiwara G, Murakami M, Ishii W, Maruyama D, Iizuka R, Murakami N, *et al.* Effectiveness of administration of fibrinogen concentrate as prevention of hypofibrinogenemia in patients with traumatic brain injury with a higher risk for severe hyperfibrinolysis: Single center before-and-after study. Neurocrit Care. 2023;38(3):640–9. doi:10.1007/s12028-022-01626-9

62. Andersson AS, Hossain I, Marklund N. Contusion expansion, low platelet count and bifrontal contusions are associated with worse patient outcome following traumatic brain injury-a retrospective single-center study. Acta Neurochir (Wien). 2024;166(1):377. doi:10.1007/s00701-024-06269-7. Published 2024 Sep 24.

63. Levy M, Arfi Levy E, Marianayagam NJ, Frolov V, Maimon S, Salomon O. Distinctive patterns of sequential platelet counts following blunt traumatic brain injury predict outcomes. Brain Inj. 2024;38(10):818–26. doi:10.1080/02699052.2024.2347571

64. Bradbury JL, Thomas SG, Sorg NR, Mjaess N, Berquist MR, Brenner TJ, *et al.* Viscoelastic testing and coagulopathy of traumatic brain injury. J Clin Med. 2021;10:5039. doi: 10.3390/jcm10215039

65. Briggs A, Gates JD, Kaufman RM, Calahan C, Gormley WB, Havens JM. Platelet dysfunction and platelet transfusion in traumatic brain injury. J Surg Res. 2015 Feb;193(2):802–6. doi: 10.1016/j.jss.2014.08.016

66. Castellino FJ, Chapman MP, Donahue DL, Thomas S, Moore EE, Wohlauer MV, *et al.* Traumatic brain injury causes platelet adenosine diphosphate and arachidonic acid

receptor inhibition independent of hemorrhagic shock in humans and rats. J Trauma Acute Care Surg. 2014;76:1169–76.

67. Wohlauer MV, Moore EE, Thomas S, Sauaia A, Evans E, Harr J, Silliman CC, *et al.* Early platelet dysfunction: An unrecognized role in the acute coagulopathy of trauma. J Am Coll Surg. 2012;214:739–46.

68. Schnüriger B, Inaba K, Abdelsayed GA, Lustenberger T, Eberle BM, Barmparas G, *et al.* The impact of platelets on the progression of traumatic intracranial hemorrhage. J Trauma. 2010;68:881–5.

69. Davis PK, Musunuru H, Walsh M, Cassady R, Yount R, Losiniecki A, *et al.* Platelet dysfunction is an early marker for traumatic brain injury-induced coagulopathy. Neurocrit Care. 2012;18:201–8.

70. Van Beek JG, Mushkudiani NA, Steyerberg EW, Butcher I, McHugh GS, Lu J, Marmarou A, Murray GD, Maas AI. Prognostic value of admission laboratory parameters in traumatic brain injury: Results from the IMPACT study. J Neurotrauma. 2007;24:315–28.

71. Engstrom M, Romner B, Schalen W, Reinstrup P. Thrombocytopenia predicts progressive hemorrhage after head trauma. J Neurotrauma. 2005;22:291–6.

72. Riojas CM, Ekaney ML, Ross SW, Cunningham KW, Furay EJ, Brown CVR, Evans SL. Platelet dysfunction after traumatic brain injury: A review. J Neurotrauma. 2021 Apr 1;38(7):819–29. doi: 10.1089/neu.2020.7301

73. Sillesen M, Rasmussen LS, Jin G, Jepsen CH, Imam A, Hwabejire JO, *et al.* Assessment of coagulopathy, endothelial injury, and inflammation after traumatic brain injury and hemorrhage in a porcine model. J Trauma Acute Care Surg. 2014;76(1):12–9; discussion 19–20.

74. Matthay ZA, Fields AT, Nunez-Garcia B, Park JJ, Jones C, Leligdowicz A, *et al.* Importance of catecholamine signaling in the development of platelet exhaustion after traumatic injury. J Thromb Haemost. 2022 Sep;20(9):2109–18. doi: 10.1111/jth.15763. Epub 2022 May 30.

75. Davizon P, Munday AD, López JA. Tissue factor, lipid rafts, and microparticles. Semin Thromb Hemost. 2010;36:857–64.

76. Gong P, Liu Y, Gong Y, Chen G, Zhang X, Wang S, *et al.* The association of neutrophil to lymphocyte ratio, platelet to lymphocyte ratio, and lymphocyte to monocyte ratio with post-thrombolysis early neurological outcomes in patients with acute ischemic stroke. J Neuroinflamm. 2021;18:51. doi: 10.1186/s12974 021-02090-6

77. Idowu OE, Oyeleke SO, Vitowanu JM. Impact of inflammatory cell ratio, biomarkers, activated partial thromboplastin time and prothrombin time on chronic subdural haematoma severity and outcome. Eur J Trauma Emerg Surg. 2021:1–8. doi: 10.1007/s00068-021-01665-5

78. Brohi K, Cohen MJ, Ganter MT, Matthay MA, Mackersie RC, Pittet JF. Acute traumatic coagulopathy: Initiated by hypoperfusion: Modulated through the protein C pathway? Ann Surg. 2007;245(5):812–8.

79. Jansen JO, Scarpelini S, Pinto R, Tien HC, Callum J, Rizoli SB. Hypoperfusion in severely injured trauma patients is associated with reduced coagulation factor activity. J Trauma. 2011;71(5 Suppl 1):S435–40.

80. Wu X, Du Z, Yu J, Sun Y, Pei B, Lu X, *et al.* Activity of factor VII in patients with isolated blunt traumatic brain injury: Association with coagulopathy and progressive hemorrhagic injury. J Trauma Acute Care Surg. 2014;76(1):114–20.

81. Tian Y, Salsbery B, Wang M, Yuan H, Yang J, Zhao Z, *et al.* Brain-derived microparticles induce systemic coagulation in a murine model of traumatic brain injury. Blood. 2015;125:2151–9. doi: 10.1182/blood-2014-09-598805

82. Zhao Z, Zhou Y, Tian Y, Li M, Dong JF, Zhang J. Cellular microparticles and pathophysiology of traumatic brain injury. Protein Cell. 2017;8(11):801–10. doi:10.1007/s13238-017-0414-6

83. Hou H, Qu Z, Liu R, Jiang B, Wang L, Li A. Traumatic brain injury: Advances in coagulopathy (review). Biomed Rep. 2024;21(5):156. doi:10.3892/br.2024.1844

84. Suzuki J, Umeda M, Sims PJ, Nagata S. Calcium-dependent phospholipid scrambling by TMEM16F. Nature. 2010;468:834–8.

85. Sparvero LJ, Amoscato AA, Kochanek PM, Pitt BR, Kagan VE, Bayir H. Mass-spectrometry based oxidative lipidomics and lipid imaging: Applications in traumatic brain injury. J Neurochem. 2010;115:1322–36.

86. Zhou Y, Cai W, Zhao Z, Hilton T, Wang M, Yeon J, et al. Lactadherin promotes microvesicle clearance to prevent coagulopathy and improves survival of severe TBI mice. Blood. 2018;131:563–72. doi: 10.1182/blood-2017-08-801738

87. Hubbard WB, Dong JF, Cruz MA, Rumbaut RE. Links between thrombosis and inflammation in traumatic brain injury. Thromb Res. 2021 Feb;198:62–71. doi: 10.1016/j.thromres.2020.10.041. Epub 2020 Nov 25.

88. Libby P, Simon DI. Inflammation and thrombosis: The clot thickens. Circulation. 2001;103(13):1718–20.

89. Lee ME, Kweon SM, Ha KS, Nham SU. Fibrin stimulates microfilament reorganization and IL-1beta production in human monocytic THP-1 cells. Mol Cells. 2001 Feb 28;11(1):13–20.

90. Liu X, Piela-Smith TH. Fibrin(ogen)-induced expression of ICAM-1 and chemokines in human synovial fibroblasts. J Immunol. 2000 Nov 1;165(9):5255–61. doi: 10.4049/jimmunol.165.9.5255

91. Yang Z, Simovic MO, Liu B, Burgess MB, Cap AP, DalleLucca JJ, et al. Indices of complement activation and coagulation changes in trauma patients. Trauma Surg Acute Care Open. 2022 Sep 14;7(1):e000927. doi: 10.1136/tsaco-2022-000927

92. Hammad A, Westacott L, Zaben M. The role of the complement system in traumatic brain injury: A review. J Neuroinflammation. 2018 Jan 22;15(1):24. doi: 10.1186/s12974-018-1066-z

93. Davalos D, Grutzendler J, Yang G, Kim JV, Zuo Y, Jung S, et al. ATP mediates rapid microglial response to local brain injury in vivo. Nat Neurosci. 2005;8:752–8.

94. Kumar A, Loane DJ. Neuroinflammation after traumatic brain injury: Opportunities for therapeutic intervention. Brain Behav Immun. 2012;26:1191–201.

95. Loane DJ, Kumar A, Stoica BA, Cabatbat R, Faden AI. Progressive neurodegeneration after experimental brain trauma: Association with chronic microglial activation. J Neuropathol Exp Neurol. 2014;73:14–29.

96. Taşçi A, Okay O, Gezici AR, Ergün R, Ergüngör F. Prognostic value of interleukin-1 beta levels after acute brain injury. Neurol Res. 2003 Dec;25(8):871–4. doi: 10.1179/016164103771953998

97. Venetsanou K, Vlachos K, Moles A, Fragakis G, Fildissis G, Baltopoulos G. Hypolipoproteinemia and hyperinflammatory cytokines in serum of severe and moderate traumatic brain injury (TBI) patients. Eur Cytokine Netw. 2007 Dec;18(4):206–9. doi: 10.1684/ecn.2007.0112. Epub 2007 Nov 12.

98. Santarsieri M, Kumar RG, Kochanek PM, Berga S, Wagner AK. Variable neuroendocrine-immune dysfunction in individuals with unfavourable outcome after severe traumatic brain injury. Brain Behav Immun. 2015;45:15–27.

99. Sollberger G, Tilley DO, Zychlinsky A. Neutrophil extracellular traps: The biology of chromatin externalization. Dev Cell. 2018;44:542–53. doi: 10.1016/j.devcel.2018.01.019

100. Jiao Y, Li W, Wang W, Tong X, Xia R, Fan J, *et al*. Platelet-derived exosomes promote neutrophil extracellular trap formation during septic shock. Crit Care. 2020;24(380). doi: 10.1186/s13054-020-03082-3

101. Frangou E, Chrysanthopoulou A, Mitsios A, Kambas K, Arelaki S, Angelidou I, *et al*. REDD1/autophagy pathway promotes thromboinflammation and fibrosis in human systemic lupus erythematosus (SLE) through NETs decorated with tissue factor (TF) and interleukin-17A (IL-17A) Ann Rheum Dis. 2019;78:238–48. doi: 10.1136/annrheumdis-2018-213181

102. Zhu K, Zhu Y, Hou X, Chen W, Qu X, Zhang Y, *et al*. NETs lead to sympathetic hyperactivity after traumatic brain injury through the LL37-Hippo/MST1 pathway. Front Neurosci. 2021;15(621477) doi: 10.3389/fnins.2021.621477

103. Vaibhav K, Braun M, Alverson K, Khodadadi H, Kutiyanawalla A, Ward A, *et al*. Neutrophil extracellular traps exacerbate neurological deficits after traumatic brain injury. Sci Adv. 2020;6(eaax8847) doi: 10.1126/sciadv.aax8847

104. Fletcher-Sandersjöö A, Thelin EP, Maegele M, Svensson M, Bellander BM. Time course of hemostatic disruptions after traumatic brain injury: A systematic review of the literature. Neurocrit Care. 2021 Apr;34(2):635–56. doi: 10.1007/s12028-020-01037-8

105. MacLeod JB, Lynn M, McKenney MG, Cohn SM, Murtha M. Early coagulopathy predicts mortality in trauma. J Trauma. 2003;55(1):39–44.

106. May AK, Young JS, Butler K, Bassam D, Brady W. Coagulopathy in severe closed head injury: Is empiric therapy warranted? Am Surg. 1997;63(3):233–6.

107. Shaz BH, Winkler AM, James AB, Hillyer CD, MacLeod JB. Pathophysiology of early trauma induced coagulopathy: Emerging evidence for hemodilution and coagulation factor depletion. J Trauma. 2011;70:1401–7.

108. Chong SL, Ong GY, Zheng CQ, Dang H, Ming M, Mahmood M, *et al*. Early coagulopathy in pediatric traumatic brain injury: A pediatric acute and critical care medicine Asian network (PACCMAN) retrospective study. Neurosurgery. 2021;89(2):283–90.

109. James V, Chong SL, Shetty SS, Ong GY. Early coagulopathy in children with isolated blunt head injury is associated with mortality and poor neurological outcomes. J Neurosurg Pediatr. 2020;25:1–7.

110. Yuan Q, Yu J, Wu X, Sun YR, Li ZQ, Du ZY, *et al*. Prognostic value of coagulation tests for in-hospital mortality in patients with traumatic brain injury. Scand J Trauma Resusc Emerg Med. 2018;26:3. doi: 10.1186/s13049-017-0471-0

111. Kurtz P, Rocha EEM. Nutrition therapy, glucose control, and brain metabolism in traumatic brain injury: A multimodal monitoring approach. Front Neurosci. 2020;14:190. doi: 10.3389/fnins.2020.00190

112. Hermanides J, Plummer MP, Finnis M, Deane AM, Coles JP, Menon DK. Glycaemic control targets after traumatic brain injury: A systematic review and meta-analysis. Crit Care. 2018;22:11. doi: 10.1186/s13054-017-1883-y

113. van den Besselaar AM. Magnesium and manganese ions accelerate tissue factor-induced coagulation independently of factor IX. Blood Coagul Fibrinolysis. 2002;13(1):19–23.

114. Aravindan A, Subramanium R, Chhabra A, Datta PK, Rewari V, Sharma SC, *et al*. Magnesium sulfate or diltiazem as adjuvants to total intravenous anesthesia to reduce blood loss in functional endoscopic sinus surgery. J Clin Anesth. 2016 Nov;34:179–85. doi: 10.1016/j.jclinane.2016.03.068

115. Cheng Z, Huang X, Muse FM, Xia L, Zhan Z, Lin X, *et al*. Low serum magnesium levels are associated with hemorrhagic transformation after thrombolysis in acute ischemic stroke. Front Neurol. 2020;11:962. doi: 10.3389/fneur.2020.00962

116. Letson HL, Dobson GP. Correction of acute traumatic coagulopathy with small-volume 7.5% NaCl adenosine, lidocaine, and Mg2+occurs within 5 minutes: A ROTEM analysis. J Trauma Acute Care Surg. 2015;78(4):773–83.

117. Li W, Bai YA, Li YJ, Liu KG, Wang MD, Xu GZ, *et al.* Magnesium sulfate for acute traumatic brain injury. J Craniofac Surg. 2015;26(2):393–8.

118. Depreitere B, Güiza F, Van den Berghe G, Schuhmann MU, Maier G, Piper I, *et al.* Pressure autoregulation monitoring and cerebral perfusion pressure target recommendation in patients with severe traumatic brain injury based on minute-by-minute monitoring data. J Neurosurg. 2014;120:1451–7. doi: 10.3171/2014.3.JNS131500

119. Chesnut RM, Marshall LF, Klauber MR, Blunt BA, Baldwin N, Eisenberg HM, *et al.* The role of secondary brain injury in determining outcome from severe head injury. J Trauma. 1993;34:216–22. doi: 10.1097/00005373-199302000-00006

120. Bernard F, Barsan W, Diaz-Arrastia R, Merck LH, Yeatts S, Shutter LA. Brain oxygen optimization in severe traumatic brain injury (BOOST-3): A multicentre, randomised, blinded-endpoint, comparative effectiveness study of brain tissue oxygen and intracranial pressure monitoring versus intracranial pressure alone. BMJ Open. 2022;12(e060188). doi: 10.1136/bmjopen-2021-060188

121. Okonkwo DO, Shutter LA, Moore C, Temkin NR, Puccio AM, Madden CJ, *et al.* Brain oxygen optimization in severe traumatic brain injury phase-II: A phase II randomized trial. Crit Care Med. 2017;45:1907–14. doi: 10.1097/CCM.0000000000002619

122. Zeiler FA, Thelin EP, Helmy A, Czosnyka M, Hutchinson PJA, Menon DK. A systematic review of cerebral microdialysis and outcomes in TBI: Relationships to patient functional outcome, neurophysiologic measures, and tissue outcome. Acta Neurochir (Wien) 2017;159:2245–73. doi: 10.1007/s00701-017-3338-2

123. Robinson MB, Shin P, Alunday R, Cole C, Torbey MT, Carlson AP. Decision-making for decompressive craniectomy in traumatic brain injury aided by multimodality monitoring: Illustrative case. J Neurosurg Case Lessons. 2021;1(CASE2197). doi: 10.3171/CASE2197

Chapter 5

DIAGNOSTIC ASSESSMENT OF TRAUMA-INDUCED COAGULOPATHY

Venencia Albert and Arulselvi Subramanian

DOI: 10.1201/9781003711070-5

INTRODUCTION

OVERVIEW OF DIAGNOSTIC APPROACHES

The dynamic nature of trauma-induced coagulopathy (TIC), which progresses acutely to various coagulopathic phenotypes, has presented a significant clinical challenge to effectively and rapidly detect it. To date, there are no validated tests for reliably detecting or guiding the treatment of TIC, hindering the implementation of timely and effective goal-directed treatment plans to reduce poor outcomes.

Multiple definitions of TIC have been proposed, and the defining criterion varies considerably, owing to over 20 different proposed parameters of coagulopathy. These parameters include elevated international normalised ratio (INR), prothrombin time (PT), partial thromboplastin time (PTT) or D-dimer, decreased fibrinogen, higher disseminated intravascular coagulation (DIC) score, modified DIC score or modified coagulopathy score, and lower depletion of alpha-2 plasmin inhibitor (α2AP). Conventional coagulation tests such as PT and INR are time-consuming and do not provide a complete picture of the haemostatic process, whereas viscoelastic haemostatic assays (VHAs), such as thromboelastography (TEG) and rotational thromboelastometry (ROTEM), offer a more rapid, holistic view of clot formation, strength, and lysis, enabling more timely and targeted resuscitation. However, several limitations and challenges currently hinder their universal adoption and application across all clinical settings. An ideal coagulation test should be easy to perform and fast and reliable. It should estimate both clotting abnormalities and risk of bleeding, employing real physiology, including flow, endothelial interaction, platelet activity, pH, and temperature.[1]

There are emerging technologies, including novel blood based pathophysiological, metabolomic and genomic biomarkers, and machine learning algorithms, and predictive modelling, that have shown significant potential for the early and accurate prediction of TIC.

CONVENTIONAL COAGULATION TESTS (CCTS)

These include PT, INR, activated PTT (aPTT), fibrinogen concentration, and platelet count. Conventional coagulation tests (CCTs) are widely used across clinical settings to assess coagulation abnormalities. While they offer a quick snapshot of the haemostatic abnormalities after trauma, such as elevated INR, the most commonly used indicator of TIC,[2] they only capture a moment in time. They cannot depict the severity or how rapidly the coagulation phenotypes are shifting in response to injury. They are also limited due to long turnaround times, which range from 30 to 60 minutes.

The PT assay measures the function of the extrinsic coagulation pathway sensitive to clotting factors in the extrinsic and common pathways (factor II, factor VII, and factor X). It measures the time taken for plasma to clot after the addition of tissue factor (thromboplastin) and calcium. The intrinsic coagulation pathway is measured by the aPTT assay, i.e., the time required for plasma to clot after activation of the contact system using an activator and the subsequent addition of phospholipid (partial thromboplastin) and calcium.

The INR and prothrombin time ratio (PTr) are derivatives of PT to standardise the results and ensure comparability across different laboratories and reagents. The observed PT of the patient is divided by the mean normal PT. The INR is considered a surrogate parameter for altered thrombin generation and corresponds to the PTr elevated to the power of the International Sensitivity Index (ISI). The formula is

$$INR = (PT\ Patient/PT\ Normal)\ ISI.$$

Table 5.1 Principles, advantages, and limitations of optical and mechanical clot detection methods

Detection method	Principle	Advantage	Limitation
Optical	Measures the change in light transmission as the clot forms	Noninvasive; standard method	Affected by haemolysis, lipemia, and hyperbilirubinemia
Mechanical	Ball or electrode detects clot impedance	Immune to optical interference	Requires a mechanical probe; less common

Accurate PT/aPTT measurements require strict adherence to standardised collection and handling standard operating procedures (SOPs). Blood must be collected in an anticoagulant vial containing 3.2% buffered sodium citrate, with a citrate-to-blood ratio of 1:9. Maintaining this citrate-to-blood ratio is crucial to prevent *in vitro* clot formation without suppressing coagulation factor activity. Any deviation, including underfilling/overfilling the vial, may cause incorrect estimation. After collection, the vial should be gently inverted 3–4 times, as vigorous shaking may induce haemolysis. The vial should be stored at room temperature; pre-centrifugation refrigeration is contraindicated to avoid loss of both factor VIII and von Willebrand factor (vWF) activity.

The operating principle of endpoint detection for clot formation uses optical density-based chromogenic/immunologic measurements or a mechanical method (detecting a change in viscosity) give in Table 5.1.

Fibrinogen forms fibrin, which is the building block that binds with platelets to form a stable clot. It's the first factor to reach critically low levels, severely impacting clot stability.[3] Fibrin concentration, typically measured using the Clauss method, is a standard laboratory test done in the initial evaluation of TIC. Low fibrin levels upon Emergency Department arrival are independently associated with increased injury, severity, shock, and mortality. Hypofibrinogenemia is commonly defined by a fibrin concentration of <150 mg/dL (1.5 g/dL), and some studies have associated a fibrin level of ≤1.4 g/dL with increased mortality.

Sampling requirements are the same as PT/aPTT, the citrated plasma is diluted (typically 1:1), and the time taken to form a fibrin clot after adding a standard amount of thrombin to the diluted plasma is measured (Clauss method). The clotting time is inversely proportional to the fibrinogen levels. Another technique, the turbidimetric assay, measures the increase in light absorption as fibrin is formed, which is directly proportional to the fibrinogen concentration.

TIC is fundamentally linked to tissue injury and haemorrhagic shock (hypoperfusion). Low haemoglobin and haematocrit serve as critical indicators of massive haemorrhage, shock, and haemodilution. This also correlated with the loss or dilution of key coagulation factors. Haemoglobin at admission has shown a strong statistical link with TIC. Lower values correlate with reduced factor X activity. Patients who develop endogenous auto-heparinization often present with much lower haemoglobin as well, with median levels around 5.8 mmol/L compared with about 8.4 mmol/L in those without this phenotype. Recently, a decline of > 0.5 g/dL in Hb levels within 24 hours of injury, in the absence of hypervolemia or hyperfibrinolysis, was found to indicate auto-heparinization.[4]

While most trauma patients maintain numerically "normal" platelet counts on admission,[5] Platelet count is a critical component in diagnosing and managing TIC, serving both as a traditional laboratory marker of thrombocytopenia and contributing to 70% of the maximum clot strength.[6,7] The standard platelet count only measures the quantity of platelets, not their function. VHAs such as ROTEM provide markers related to platelet function. Thrombocytopenia or low platelet count (normal range 50,000–450,000 cells/uL) is associated with reduced clot strength and increased risk, particularly traumatic brain injury (TBI) (platelet [PLT] <100 × 10 9/L).[6]

Table 5.2 Clinical interpretation of platelet indices in trauma

Parameter	Normal range	TIC-relevant cutoff	What deviation indicates	Clinical interpretation
Platelet count	150–450 ×10⁹/L	<100 ×10⁹/L	Consumption, haemorrhage, dilution	Supports TIC when paired with ↑INR and ↓fibrinogen
MPV	7–11 fL	>11 fL	Larger, younger platelets	Bone marrow response to consumption
PDW	11–16 fL	>16 fL	Platelet size heterogeneity	Regenerative response or immune destruction
P-LCR	27–47%	>50–55%	High proportion of large platelets	Accelerated thrombopoiesis
PCT	0.11–0.28%	<0.08%	Low total platelet mass	Increased bleeding risk
IPF	1–6%	>10% or <2%	>10% = consumptive TIC <2% = inadequate marrow response	Marker for coagulopathy

In addition to the platelet count, platelet indices can also help identify TIC and differentiate whether the thrombocytopenia is due to consumption or impaired platelet production. Mean platelet volume (MPV), platelet distribution width (PDW), and platelet-large cell ratio (P-LCR) increase when the marrow releases larger immature platelets in response to bleeding, while plateletcrit (PCT) offers a measure of total platelet mass and falls as reserve is depleted.[8] The immature platelet fraction (IPF) is the most informative marker that reflects real-time thrombopoiesis. Elevated IPF above 10% along with low platelet count, elevated INR, and fibrinogen strongly supports consumptive TIC with an active marrow response. Typical reference ranges include MPV (7–11 fL), PDW (11–16 fL), P-LCR (27–47%), PCT (0.11–0.28%), and IPF (1–6%). In trauma, elevated MPV, PDW, P-LCR, and IPF indicate accelerated platelet turnover and consumption, whereas low MPV, low P-LCR, and low IPF point to bone marrow suppression or failure (Table 5.2).[9,10]

Blood gas analysis measures [arterial pH and base deficit (BD) or base excess (BE)] serve as critical indicators of tissue hypoperfusion and metabolic acidosis, which are recognised as primary drivers and exacerbating factors of TIC. A BE ≤–6 indicates significant tissue hypoperfusion and strongly predicts early coagulopathy in TBI (OR 3.11).[8,11] Admission BD is an influential continuous variable for estimating TIC risk in Bayesian network models following trauma.[12] An experimental study revealed a decline in factor VIIa activity by almost 90% at pH 7.0 compared with physiological pH 7.4. Hypoperfusion and acidosis also contribute to platelet dysfunction. Trauma patients with high lactate or large base deficits show altered platelet responsiveness, although the exact mechanisms are still under study.[13]

There is still no universal definition of TIC, and the thresholds differ across studies and clinical settings.[14] Many groups define TIC by INR >1.2 or >1.53. While the lower threshold captures a broader group of patients, with some degree of coagulation abnormality, INR >1.5 is a severe threshold, reported to identify a clinically distinct subset of patients at significant risk of worse outcomes.[15] Fibrinogen and platelet counts provide subtle numerical values that alone do not reflect functional activities. Initial haemoglobin low has also been suggested to be an indicator for severe bleeding and coagulopathy.[16]

In 2003, Brohi *et al.*[17] characterised TIC as PT >18s, aPTT >60s or INR >1.5 and MacLeod *et al.* identified TIC as a PT >14s and aPTT >34s.[18] Broader definitions in the literature include a 50% prolongation of aPTT or PT, an INR ≥ 1.5, PT ratio (patient PT/mean laboratory PT)

> 1.5, or fibrinogen < 1 g/.[19,20] A PT ratio > 1.2 has also been shown to predict mortality and transfusion requirements more effectively, and has been suggested as a better marker for defining TIC.[21] Some groups have also applied the International Society on Thrombosis and Haemostasis (ISTH) criteria for DIC to define early coagulopathy.[22,23]

CCTs only assess plasma-based factors and static hypocoagulability; the comprehensive picture may be missed. PT and aPTT were designed for diagnosing factor deficiencies and monitoring anticoagulation, not for TIC, which may occur despite major factor loss, as seen in isolated TBI cases. Prolonged values do not always match bleeding risk. Since these assays are performed at normal pH and 37°C, they do not reflect the effects of hypothermia or acidosis seen in trauma.[17,21,24,25]

VISCOELASTIC TESTING METHODS

VHA provide a dynamic and comprehensive evaluation of the entire coagulation process using whole blood, monitoring the clot initiation, kinetics, firmness over time, and fibrinolysis. It is now recognised as a key tool for the early diagnosis and treatment of TIC.[26]

THE ORIGIN OF VISCOELASTIC TESTING

The foundational concepts for whole blood evaluation of haemostasis using viscoelastic properties were first reported 70 years ago by Dr. Hellmut Hartert in Germany. He developed a mechanism to quantify the dynamics of blood clot formation, using a stainless-steel cup, ~8 × 12 mm, with a surface designed to prevent the blood clot from detaching during rotation, and a concentric pin suspended within by a thin steel wire (0.2 mm in diameter) that functioned as a torsional spring. A layer of paraffin oil covered the blood sample to prevent evaporation. As a clot formed, the fluid became elastic, storing energy that exerted force on the pin, causing small rotations that were transmitted to a film through a mirror coupled to the pin, which was illuminated by a slit lamp (Figure 5.1).[27,28]

Following his initial work, the adoption of TEG grew slowly. Over the next 40 years (1980s), the use of TEG became more widespread, especially in procedures like complex cardiac surgery[29] and liver transplantation.[30] Since then, TEG utilisation has been widely adopted in the fields of trauma and transplant surgery.[31]

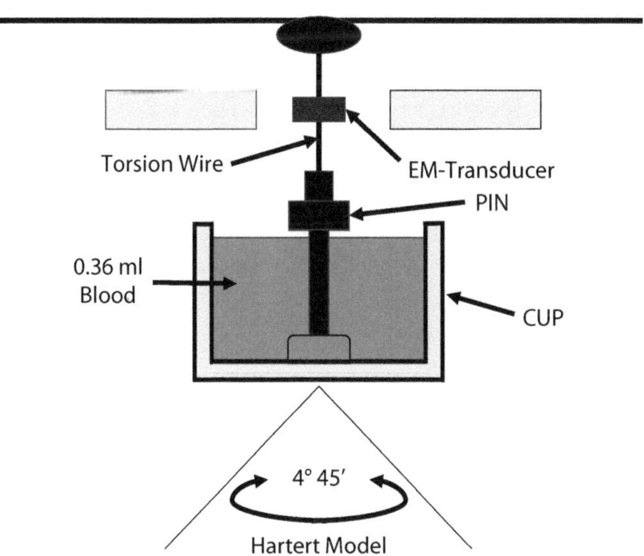

Figure 5.1   Hartert cup and pin model for a viscoelastic assay for haemostasis.

TESTING PRINCIPLE

VHA methodologies utilise the Hartert principle. The fundamental principle is to observe the transition of the blood sample from a viscous to an elastic state. Before clotting, whole blood is purely viscous, and cup rotation results in permanent deformation of the blood, so the pin does not move. As a clot forms, this technology measures the shear elastic modulus (rigidity) of a blood clot by monitoring the changes in torque transmitted to a pin suspended in an oscillating cup.[31]

CORE COMPONENTS AND SETUP

i. *A cup (heated and oscillating):* holds the blood sample and is typically heated to 37°C

ii. *The pin (suspended from a torsion wire):* suspended within the cup, immersed in the blood sample

The sample: a sample of whole blood is placed in the cup, and activated to maximise thrombin generation and platelet activation in the *in vitro* environment.

These techniques monitor the entire clotting process, from initial fibrin formation to eventual clot dissolution, distinguishing them from conventional laboratory tests that only measure the beginning stages of coagulation.[31]

MECHANISM (VISCOUS-TO-ELASTIC TRANSITION)

To measure the shear elastic modulus (rigidity) of the clot. The cup is made to rotate in alternating directions. This rotation occurs in alternating directions. In Hartert's device, the cup rotated by 1/24 radian in each direction, taking 3.5 seconds for one direction, followed by a 1-second stop, for an entire cycle duration of 9 seconds. This oscillating motion simulates the venous flow.[31,32] In the pre-clotting (viscous) phase, the fluid simply flows around the pin, and there is no transfer of force, as the sample cannot pull on the pin, the pin stays still, and the device records no torque or rotation. In the elastic (clotting) phase, as fibrin formation begins, the clot develops structure. The fibrin strands linking the cup and pin allow part of the cup's motion to be transmitted to the pin. The stronger and more organised the clot becomes, the more force it applies to the pin. This causes the pin to rotate in response to the cup's oscillation.

The analyser measures this rotation over time. The size of the pin's deflection reflects the stiffness of the forming clot because the amplitude of movement is proportional to the clot's shear modulus. The greater movement indicates a stronger clot, while reduced movement suggests weak or unstable clot formation. The movement of the cup and pin after clotting is represented as a graphical chart.

FIRST-GENERATION DEVICES

The first 30 years of clinically adopted VHAs were largely defined by two closely related viscoelastic technologies developed as parallel systems, i.e., Thromboelastography (TEG®) and Thromboelastometry (ROTEM®). The two legacy VHAs share the fundamental principle of assessing viscoelasticity (via the cup-and-pin mechanism), but differ primarily in their mechanical actuation (i.e., how the movement is initiated), their detection method, and their nomenclature.[31]

THROMBOELASTOGRAPHY (TEG)

TEG devices deviate from Hartert's model in two major ways: (i) the method to detect and quantify the pin's motion and (ii) overall automation of the testing process (Table 5.3).[31,33] The TEG® 5000 system (thromboelastography; Haemonetics Corporation, Braintree, MA, USA), originally developed by Haemoscope, was the first viscoelastic haemostatic analyser to enter clinical use. The cup oscillates in alternating directions through a 4°45′ rotation, with a cycle duration of 10 seconds. The rotation of the pin is measured via a torsion wire and an electromagnetic transducer, deviating from Hartert's original light-based system. The electric output is directly related to the strength of fibrin-platelet bonds. The resulting movement is plotted as a dynamic tracing[31,33,34] (Figure 5.2A).

Table 5.3   Key parameters of viscoelastic haemostatic assays (VHAs)

TEG parameter	ROTEM parameter	Definition	Haemostatic function
R (Reaction time)	Clotting time (CT)	Period of time from initiation of the test to the initial fibrin formation	Clot initiation (plasma factors)
K (Kinetic time)	Clot formation time (CFT)	Time from the beginning of clot formation until the amplitude reaches 20 mm	Clot propagation/ kinetics (fibrinogen)
α-angle	Alpha angle (α)	Represents the acceleration (kinetics) of fibrin build-up and cross-linking	
MA (Maximum Amplitude)	Maximum clot firmness (MCF)	Maximum amplitude strength of the clot	Clot strength (platelets/fibrinogen)
LY30 (Lysis at 30 min)	Lysis index at 60 minutes (LI60 or LI30)	Measures the rate of amplitude reduction 30 minutes after MA (stability) of the clot	Fibrinolysis (plasmin)

Various additional parameters can be derived from TEG parameters to present a comprehensive picture of the clot behaviour. The clotting index[35] provides an overall assessment of coagulation by combining R, K, α angle, and MA into a single continuous measure.

The coagulation index (CI) for whole blood may be calculated as follows:

$$CI = -0.2454R + 0.0184K + 0.1655MA - 0.0241a - 5.0220$$

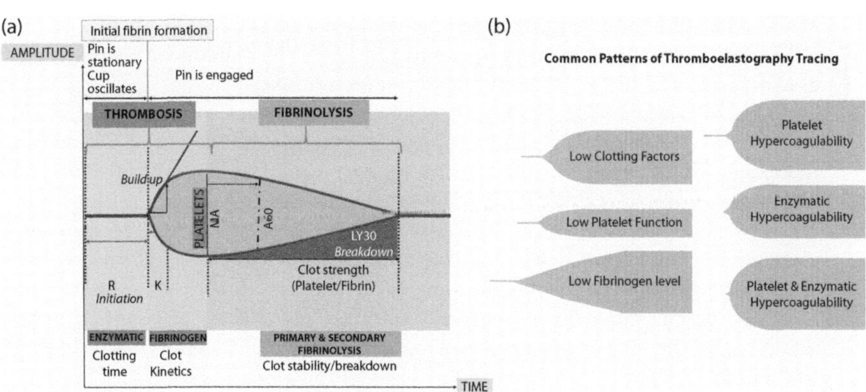

Figure 5.2   (A) Normal dynamic thromboelastography trace demonstrating clot initiation, propagation, strength, and lysis. (B) TEG patterns associated with haemorrhagic and thrombotic states.

A figure showing common thromboelastography (TEG) patterns used to identify coagulation abnormalities. A normal tracing is shown for comparison with the signatures of low clotting factors, impaired platelet function, reduced fibrinogen levels, primary fibrinolysis, and generalised hypocoagulability. Thrombotic patterns display features of platelet hypercoagulability, enzymatic hypercoagulability, combined platelet and enzymatic hypercoagulability, and secondary fibrinolysis. Each tracing highlights characteristic changes in clot initiation, formation, strength, and breakdown that help guide clinical interpretation and management.

Normal values of the coagulation index lie within −3.0 and +3.0, which is 3 standard deviations from the mean of zero. Hypercoagulable (CI > 3.0) or hypocoagulable (CI < −3.0) states can be identified for guiding transfusion.

Other parameters include the shear modulus (G), whicconverts amplitude (A) into a physical measure of firmness to depict clot strength[36] measured in Kdynes/cm^2.

$$\text{Calculated as} = [(5000 \times A)/(100 - A)]/1000.$$

E (Elasticity Constant) is the normalised value of G;

$$\text{expressed as:} [(100 \times A)/(100 - A)]/1000.$$

The thrombodynamic potential index (TPI) is calculated as the E value at MA divided by K and reflects the balance between clot formation and strengthening. Measures of fibrinolysis include the clot lysis indices at 30 and 60 minutes (CL30, CL60), derived from the ratio of the amplitude at those time points to the MA. The estimated percent lysis (EPL) is calculated continuously beginning shortly after the MA is reached and transitions to the standard LY30 value at 30 minutes.[36]

Several variant TEG assays have emerged for targeted assessment of the coagulation process.

- Rapid TEG (rTEG): A modified assay that uses dual activation (tissue factor plus kaolin) to expedite results faster than standard TEG or ROTEM assays, supporting hypotensive resuscitation during trauma, triggering therapeutic action before the completion of the full test run in emergencies. rTEG is crucial for guiding haemostatic resuscitation, delivering real-time results that predict transfusion requirements, <1 hour of admission. Admission rTEG can potentially replace conventional coagulation tests in emergency care.[37,38] rTEG can also rapidly detect hyperfibrinolysis (HF), identifying a rare but highly lethal pattern known as the "black diamond", characterised by a rapid rise to maximum amplitude (TMA ≤14 minutes) and rapid total clot lysis [Time to Total Lysis (TTL) <30 minutes from MA]. The on admission rTEG "black diamond" pattern can be used to identify patients who are at higher risk for mortality.[39]
- The TEG®6s (Haemonetics, Boston, MA, USA) is a fully automated, cartridge-based VHA. It uses resonance-frequency viscoelasticity (Sonic Estimation of Elasticity via Resonance [SEER] sonorheometry), which exposes whole blood to controlled vibration frequencies and measures shifts in resonance as clot stiffness evolves, without physical contact with the sample.[40-43] Its four-channel microfluidic cartridge allows parallel assessment of clot initiation, fibrinogen and platelet contribution, and fibrinolysis using small blood volumes, improving reproducibility and workflow in acute care settings. Although, despite automation, exposure to sustained motion can still significantly alter results, indicating that environmental stability remains important for reliable interpretation in this system.[43]
- Other useful variants include Heparinase TEG (hTEG), which uses kaolin as the activator along with lyophilised heparinase to neutralise unfractionated heparin, and helps identify the presence of heparin. Functional Fibrinogen TEG (FF-TEG) uses tissue factor and the platelet blocker abciximab, a GPIIb/IIIa inhibitor, to assess the fibrin contribution to clot strength.[44]

ROTATIONAL THROMBOELASTOMETRY (ROTEM)

The ROTEM technology followed the TEG system and became one of the first-generation devices that helped bring viscoelastic testing into routine clinical practice. ROTEM® kept the same basic concept but changed the way the system is driven. In the ROTEM® Delta analyser (Werfen, Munich, Germany; rotational thromboelastometry), the cup is held stationary and heated, and a controlled rotational force is applied to the pin. As the clot forms, it restricts

Table 5.4 Description and interpretation of various rotational thromboelastometry variants

ROTEM assay name	Activation agent(s)	Coagulation pathway/ mechanism assessed	Primary diagnostic purpose
INTEM	Ellagic acid	Intrinsic coagulation system	Assesses intrinsic coagulation factors (XII, XI, IX, VIII) and is similar to aPTT; sensitive to heparin
EXTEM	Recombinant tissue factor (plus calcium ions and polybrene)	Extrinsic coagulation system	Assesses extrinsic coagulation factor VII, similar to PT
HEPTEM	Ellagic acid + heparinase	Intrinsic coagulation system with heparin neutralisation	It compares clotting time (CT) results from the intrinsically activated HEPTEM channel (where heparin is neutralised) against the INTEM channel (which is heparin-sensitive), to identify endogenous heparinization/ auto-heparinization.
APTEM	Extrinsically activated test + antifibrinolytic (aprotinin or tranexamic acid)	Fibrinolysis potential	It indicates hyperfibrinolysis if the clot amplitude increases significantly in APTEM. Used for evaluating fibrinolytic activity.

the movement of the pin, and the degree of restriction is inversely related to clot strength. The rotation of the pin is measured utilising a collimated light beam from a light-emitting diode reflected off a mirror coupled to the pin. This motion is then tracked by a photosensor or a charge-coupled device (CCD) image sensor system (Table 5.4).[44–47] A normal dynamic rotational thromboelastometry trace is shown in Figure 5.3.

Other ROTEM assay variations include ARATEM, which activates platelets with arachidonic acid to assess the pathway targeted by cyclooxygenase inhibitors, including acetylsalicylic acid. In the ADPTEM assay, platelets are stimulated with ADP to evaluate the ADP receptor

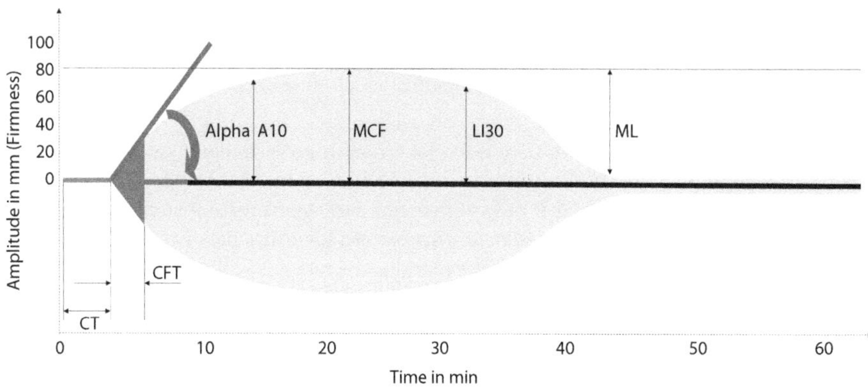

Figure 5.3 Normal dynamic rotational thromboelastometry trace. CT: clotting time; cft: clot formation time; Alpha: angle; MCF: maximum clot firmness; LI30: lysis index 30 min after CT; A10: amplitude 10 min after CT; ML: maximum lysis.

Table 5.5 Viscoelastic haemostatic assay parameters for assessing fibrinogen and platelet contributions to clot strength

VHA parameter/calculation	Description and interpretation
FIBTEM (ROTEM)/Functional fibrinogen (FF) MA	These assays specifically isolate the fibrinogen contribution to clot strength by adding platelet inhibitors. Reagents used are tissue factor + Platelet inhibitor (Cytochalasin D)
Platelet contribution (PC)/PLTEM	Platelet contribution to clot strength is calculated by subtracting the fibrin-only result from the global clot strength. PLTEM (ROTEM): EXTEM – FIBTEM. A decreased PC or PLTEM value suggests low platelet count (thrombocytopenia) or low platelet function.

pathway. The TRAPTEM assay uses a thrombin receptor–activating peptide to examine the PAR-1 pathway.[48]

ASSESSMENT OF PLATELET FUNCTION USING VHAS

VHAs offer a functional, whole-blood evaluation of platelet contribution to clot formation. Maximum amplitude (MA) and MCF, from TEG and ROTEM, respectively, represent the final clot strength. These parameters are primarily driven by platelet–fibrin interactions, as platelets contribute up to 80% of the measured clot strength. Low MA or MCF suggests impairment in platelet quantity, platelet function, and fibrinogen levels. Table 5.5 lists the VHA-based assays used for the evaluation of platelet function and to detect dysfunction.

PLTEM correlates strongly with platelet count. PLTEM is a practical surrogate in acute care settings. Although PLTEM values (A5 and MCF) show meaningful agreement with whole blood aggregometry, its performance may vary across studies.

PLATELET MAPPING ASSAYS

TEG platelet mapping evaluates platelet aggregation in response to specific agonists:[48]

- *ADP pathway:* Assesses responsiveness through the $P2Y_{12}$ receptor.
- *Arachidonic Acid (AA) pathway:* Assesses the thromboxane A_2 pathway, inhibited by aspirin.

In trauma patients, both ADP- and AA-mediated platelet responses are reported to be markedly impaired compared to healthy controls. ADP pathway inhibition has been strongly linked to increased sensitivity to tissue plasminogen activator (tPA), contributing to systemic hyperfibrinolysis. Qualitative platelet dysfunction via ADP-pathway inhibition is a prominent mechanism of TBI-associated coagulopathy, which may occur even in the absence of shock.[49]

The MA-R ratio that links clot initiation to clot strength gives an early snapshot of global coagulation soon after injury. Post hoc analysis of admission TEG by Harrington *et al.*[50] showed an association of low MA-R ratio with major derangements in thrombin generation, clot formation, and inflammatory balance. This pattern identifies patients at high risk who require closer monitoring and targeted intervention. The ratio also aligns with a distinct TIC phenotype marked by impaired thrombin generation and weak clot architecture.

VISCOELASTIC TESTING AND CONVENTIONAL COAGULATION IN TRAUMA

VHA assesses hypocoagulable, hypercoagulable, and hyperfibrinolytic stages, and identifies functional abnormalities that are not visible on plasma-based laboratory tests. In isolated severe TBI patients in India,[51] 45% of TIC patients showed a hypercoagulable profile on TEG, and 37% showed a hypocoagulable profile. CCTs identified coagulopathy in only 16.7% of the patients. In contrast, TEG classified 30% of the no-TIC group (by CCTs) as hypercoagulable

Table 5.6 Key viscoelastic parameter cutoffs for assessing coagulation abnormalities

Condition	Key cutoffs
Hypocoagulability[52,53]	TEG R > 27 s; ROTEM EXTEM CT > 71.5 s; EXTEM CT > 100 s
	TEG MA < 51 mm; < 44 mm (multi-parameter definition); EXTEM A5 < 38.5 mm
	TEG α < 55°; α < 67° in children; K > 3 min
	FIBTEM A5 < 8.5 mm (≈ fibrinogen <150 mg/dL); FIBTEM MCF < 10 mm; FF-TEG MA < 14.9 mm; < 20 mm threshold for fibrinogen replacement
Hypercoagulability[54,55]	TEG R < 9 s
	TEG MA > 69 mm; > 64 mm (alternate definition)
	α > 74°
Hyperfibrinolysis[56–58]	Ly30 ≥ 3%; >10% (suggests need for repeat TXA); EXTEM LI60 < 85%; ML30 > 10%
Fibrinolysis shutdown[59]	Ly30 ≤ 0.8%; ML < 3.5%

and 36% as hypocoagulable, highlighting its greater sensitivity. Correlations between individual CCTs and TEG parameters in this study were weak and insignificant. TEG-based cutoff for κ-time ≥ 3.7 (AUC 0.68; 95% CI 0.54–0.82, specificity 70%, sensitivity 63%) and α angle ≤ 48.0 (AUC 0.66; 95% CI 0.51–0.81, specificity 67%, sensitivity 67%) was established. The diagnostic accuracy of this cutoff for identifying TIC was 55.6% with sensitivity (81.8%) and specificity (14.3%).[51]

The main interpretive cutoffs used in clinical assessment are summarised in Table 5.6. Figure 5.4 shows the flowchart of VHA-defined coagulation abnormalities in trauma.

THROMBIN GENERATION

Thrombin generation was first measured in 1953, by MacFarlane and Biggs using whole blood and by Pitney and Dacie using plasma. The model was time-consuming and required continuous subsampling. A chromogenic method was later developed, but the selected substrate got exhausted quickly, blocking physiological feedback loops of thrombin, leading to incomplete measurement. Another substrate (MeO-mal-AibArg-pNA), was an improvement, but it required optical readings in defibrinated plasma to assess the reaction. This was later replaced by a fluoroscopic agent (Z Gly Gly-Arg), bound to 7-amino-4-methylcoumarin, that enabled automatic fluorescence monitoring. Comparing this with a calibrator of known thrombin activity made a calibrated automated thrombinography (CAT) assay possible.[1] Several commercial fluorogenic and chromogenic systems are now available.

Thrombin generation tests (TGTs) use tissue factor as a trigger to simulate cell wall damage. In platelet-poor plasma, added phospholipids amplify clotting, while in platelet-rich plasma, the platelets provide the surface, allowing the test to reflect platelet and plasma interactions. Key readouts include lag time, time to peak, peak thrombin, and endogenous thrombin potential. Figure 5.5 depicts schematic representation of the output.

Thrombin generation assays present dynamic information that is not captured by PT/INR alone, and adjunct to CCTs, TGT can help massive transfusion protocols after injury. Faster thrombin kinetics and higher INR have been independently linked to higher transfusion rates in patients with the unique phenotype of quick clot initiation and reduced overall thrombin output (consumptive coagulopathy) following severe injury.[60]

Compared to VHAs, TGT captures the full thrombin burst beyond initial fibrin formation, adding value in managing bleeding and predicting surgical bleeding. However, it is limited due to the slow turnaround time, lack of standardisation, preanalytical variability, and absence of clear reference ranges.

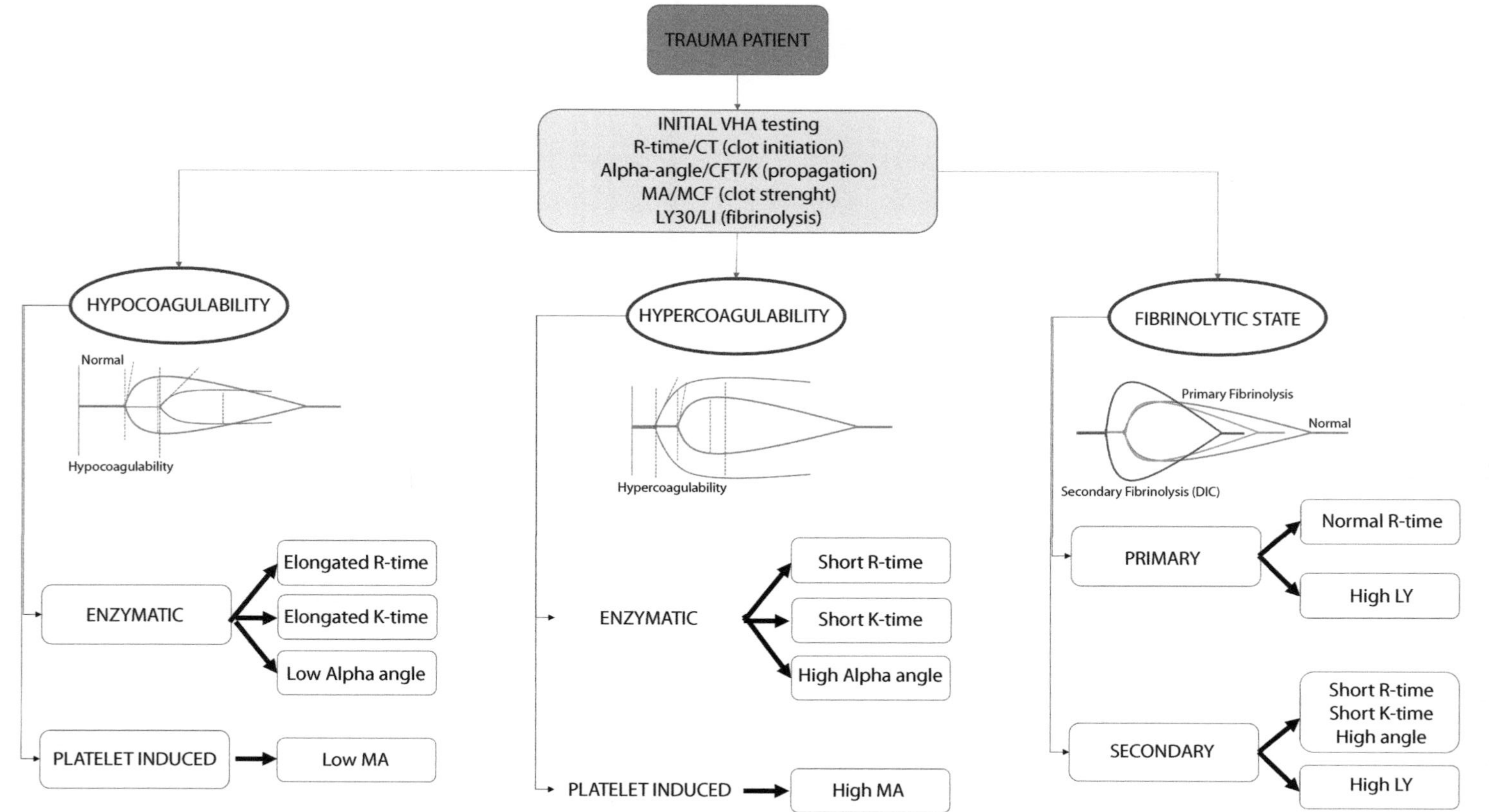

Figure 5.4   Flowchart of VHA-defined coagulation abnormalities in trauma.

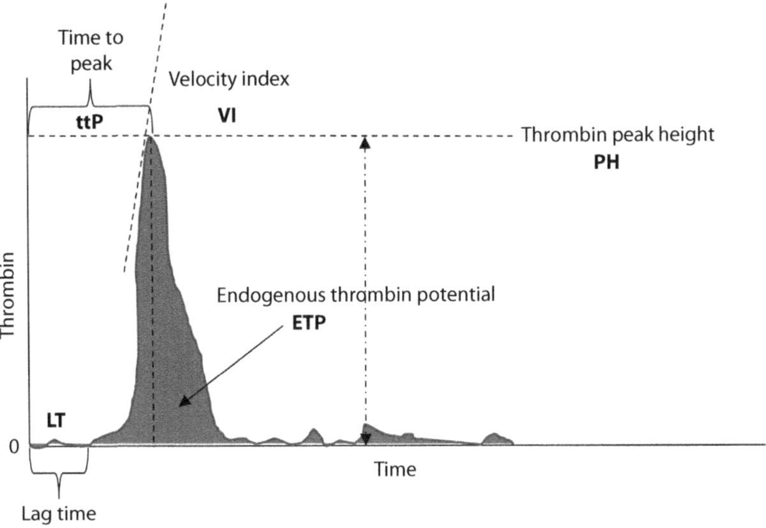

Figure 5.5   Schematic representation of thrombin generation test (TGT) output parameters.

PERIPHERAL BIOMARKERS FOR ASSESSING TRAUMA-INDUCED COAGULOPATHY

Peripheral biomarkers represent measurable indicators of coagulation dysregulation following trauma, and reflect specific pathophysiological mechanisms underlying TIC. These markers span multiple pathways, including thrombin generation, procoagulant activation, anticoagulant depletion, endothelial dysfunction, and fibrinolysis.

Thrombin-antithrombin complex (TAT), formed between active thrombin and its natural inhibitor antithrombin, reflects active thrombin generation. In TBI patients, elevated TAT concentrations were observed compared to controls: 41.3 (17.4–100.2) vs. 12.7 (6.8–20.1) pg/mL (p < 0.0001). Importantly, coagulopathic TBI patients demonstrated further elevated TAT levels, indicating enhanced thrombin generation in association with overt coagulopathy.[61] Marked elevation of soluble fibrin monomers (sFM) levels [38.4 (23.1 123.8) vs. 0.45 (0–5.7) ng/mL] in controls (p < 0.0001) marker of thrombin activity, was also reported. In trauma patients, thrombin generation measured by CAT or other specialised assays has shown independent prognostic value. Thrombin generation profiles, including parameters such as peak thrombin concentration and time-to-peak, have been identified as independent predictors of venous thromboembolism (VTE) after trauma, with time-to-peak demonstrating a hazard ratio of 1.67 (1.29–2.15, p < 0.00001) for symptomatic VTE development.

While tissue factor (TF) activity drives coagulation, alterations involve its carriage on microparticles (tissue factor-bearing microparticles [TFMP]) and the behaviour of its natural inhibitor, tissue factor pathway inhibitor (TFPI). The Prospective Observational Multicenter Major Trauma Transfusion (PROMMTT)[62] study, associated lower levels of TF-bearing MPs (CD41+, CD142+) with substantial bleeding early [206 (43, 270) MP/µL in TIC vs. 60 (33, 195) MP/µL in control; p 0.01] after acute trauma. Additionally, TF bearing platelet microparticles (CD41+CD142+) were independently associated with substantial bleeding [OR 0.892 (95% CI 0.973–0.990, p < 0.0001) and early mortality. Our study showed a significant decline in plasma TF levels in trauma patients compared to controls when sampled before fluid and blood product transfusion: 1.7 (1.02–3.6) vs. 3.9 (3.0–4.7) pg/mL (p = 0.0002). Furthermore, plasma TF was lower in coagulopathic patients compared to non-coagulopathic patients, though this difference approached but did not reach significance: 1.6 (0.8–3.4) vs. 1.9 (1.1–4.3) pg/mL (p = 0.09).

Diagnostic cutoffs for protein C (PC) and protein S (PS) in TIC are not well defined, but the PC pathway shows consistent early changes after injury. Activated protein C (APC) levels between 1.53 and 2.57 ng/mL63 can identify patients at risk for developing coagulopathy (area under the curve [AUC] of 0.83–0.88).[63] APC is noted to increase with injury severity, rising from 0.5 ng/mL (ISS <16) to 1.5 ng/mL (ISS 16–26) and 4.1 ng/mL (ISS >26). Higher APC levels, especially above 1.53 ng/mL, were linked to shock, elevated lactate, longer ICU stay, and greater ventilator dependence.[64] For the zymogen forms, clear diagnostic thresholds have not been defined, but early trauma studies show a steady decline in protein C activity with higher injury severity (median 90.8% for ISS <16 vs. 80% for ISS >26). Patients with acute endogenous heparinization also had lower PC levels (85% vs. 109%).[64] protein S levels fall significantly in TIC, and in isolated severe TBI, a ROC-derived cutoff of PS ≤74% predicted TIC with 72.7% sensitivity and 63.8% specificity.[61] Concurrently, Cohen *et al.* reported no overall change in the PC pathway (79.4±24.2 vs. 85±36, p = 0.52), but hypoperfused patients had significantly reduced unactivated PC (56.2±32 vs. 85±35, p = 0.03).[65] Low levels of PC and PS have been associated with increased risk of VTE, and borderline levels between 61 and 75 IU/dL (OR 1.54–3.18 for PC; PS OR 1.84, 1.31–2.59).[66] These patterns highlight early depletion of natural anticoagulants as a consistent feature of TIC, even though formal diagnostic cutoffs for PC and PS zymogens are still not established.

Endotheliopathy of trauma is reflected by sharp elevation in syndecan-1, soluble thrombomodulin, tPA, vWF, and circulating cell-free DNA levels. Early shedding can appear within minutes. Endogenous heparinization identified on TEG has been linked to a four-fold rise in syndecan-1 [116 (78–140) vs. 31 (18–49) ng/mL, p = 0.02] and higher sTM [4.1 (3.7–4.4) vs. 1.7 (1.0–3.3) ng/mL, p = 0.028].[67] Syndecan-1 thresholds used across studies vary: ≥40 ng/mL predicts 24-hour mortality with reasonable accuracy;[68] ≥30.5 ng/mL identifies TBI-associated coagulopathy,[69] and 92.5 ng/mL predicts disseminated intravascular coagulation (DIC) progression [AUC of 0.862, 100% sensitivity, and 67.8% specificity].[70] Patients with TIC [26 (14–79) vs. 23 (12–50) ng/mL, p = 0.01] and DIC [218.8 (134.5–798.2) vs. 67.2 (39.6–114.5) ng/mL, p < 0.001] showed elevated syndecan-1 levels compared to those who did not.

Endothelial activation following trauma leads to a surge of vWF, while ADAMTS13 activity falls transiently. This imbalance, along with consumptive coagulopathy, has been linked to TIC pathology, especially in TBI.[71] As specific thresholds for vWF alone are not established, the ADAMTS13 activity to vWF antigen ratio is a practical indicator of imbalance. This ratio is markedly reduced in paediatric trauma patients at admission compared with controls.[72]

PROTEOMETABOLOMIC MAKERS OF TIC

Recent untargeted metabolomics studies have identified lysophosphatidylethanolamines as potential biomarkers for distinguishing TIC. The diagnostic performance of both LysoPE (20:4/0:0)(AUC = 0.933, 95% CI: 0.849–0.995) and LysoPE (0:0/18:2) (AUC = 0.916, 95% CI: 0.818–0.914) surpassed both conventional coagulation tests and admission assessment scores. Lysophosphatidylethanolamines (LysoPEs) are bioactive lipids generated when cell membranes are broken down (hydrolysed) by phospholipase A2 (PLA2) during inflammation. In TIC, massive tissue injury and immune activation trigger a "lipid storm" that disrupts platelet and endothelial membranes, altering their ability to support coagulation complexes. The LysoPEs offer a rapid, highly specific "yes/no" test for TIC that is far more accurate than current clotting times (PT/PTT) in the first hour of injury.[73]

THE "SUCCINATE-LIPID-SHEDDASE" AXIS

While succinate was previously known as a marker of ischaemia (lack of oxygen), it has recently emerged as a critical driver (ischaemia signal) of downstream pathology of ischaemia at the cellular level.[74] Succinate accumulation in endothelial cells directly causes endotheliopathy, leading to coagulopathy in trauma patients. In trauma, hypoxia triggers calcium-dependent

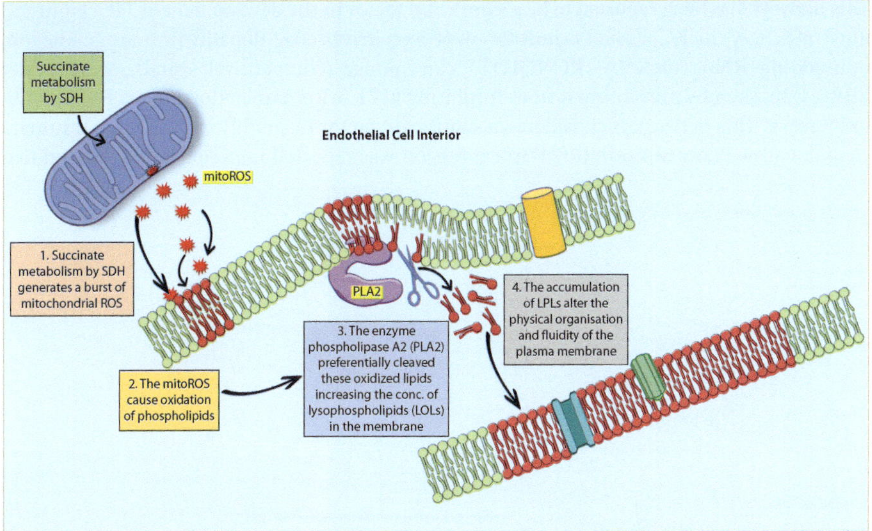

Figure 5.6 Succinate lipid sheddase pathway driving endothelial injury in trauma-induced coagulopathy.

This figure illustrates the hypoxia-induced succinate build-up in endothelial cells. Reperfusion triggers succinate dehydrogenase to produce a burst of mitochondrial ROS, which oxidises membrane lipids. Phospholipase A2 converts these into lysophospholipids, disrupting the membrane and promoting glycocalyx shedding through MMP24 and MMP25. The loss of glycocalyx leads to the release of heparin-like molecules, factor consumption, and elevated syndecan-1, contributing to trauma-induced coagulopathy.

pathways in endothelial cells, leading to a build-up of intracellular succinate. When blood flow is restored, succinate is rapidly metabolised by succinate dehydrogenase, producing a surge of mitochondrial reactive oxygen species. These oxidants attack membrane lipids and generate oxidised lipid products. Phospholipase A2 targets these damaged lipids and converts them into lysophospholipids, which disrupt the organisation of the endothelial cell membrane. This disruption promotes shedding of the glycocalyx by MMP24 and MMP25. The loss of glycocalyx contributes to the consumption of clotting factors and the release of heparin-like molecules, resulting in auto-heparinization. This process plays a central role in TIC and is accompanied by elevated levels of syndecan-1 in the circulation. Targeting succinate metabolism with subdural haematoma (SDH) inhibitors, to preserve vascular integrity, represents a transformative therapeutic strategy for preventing TIC[74] (Figure 5.6).

RNA REGULATORS: THE "ceRNA NETWORK" HYPOTHESIS

MicroRNA (miRNA) plays a crucial, multifaceted role in the regulation of coagulation[75] and inflammatory pathways following trauma. Previous studies have identified several specific miRNAs that contribute to the pathogenesis of trauma outcomes. MicroRNAs in trauma are associated with the suppressed expression of clotting factors and proteins. miR-24 has been linked with a hypocoagulation state by inhibiting the synthesis of factor X. Expression of miR-24 was found to be 3.17-fold elevated in trauma compared to controls. This level was significantly higher in patients with TIC as compared to those without TIC. *In vitro* studies have shown that miR-24 transduction significantly reduces the factor X levels.[76]

Hsa-miR-24-3p targets vWF and inhibits its expression by binding directly to the 3′untranslated region (3′UTR) of vWF and impacts platelet aggregation and haemostasis through the competitive endogenous RNA (ceRNA) network, the KCNQ1OT1-hsa-miR-24-3p-VWF axis.

This network has been reported to be a significant factor in the development of TIC. Figure 5.7 illustrates how the KCNQ1OT1–miR-24–vWF axis drives coagulopathy in trauma. The long non-coding RNA (lncRNA) KCNQ1OT1 can sponge (competitively bind), or sequester, miR-24-3p, thereby preventing it from inhibiting vWF mRNA and allowing vWF expression to increase. This network is considered a significant factor in conditions like acute traumatic coagulopathy. Elevated hsa-miR-24-3p expression was reported in peripheral blood and liver

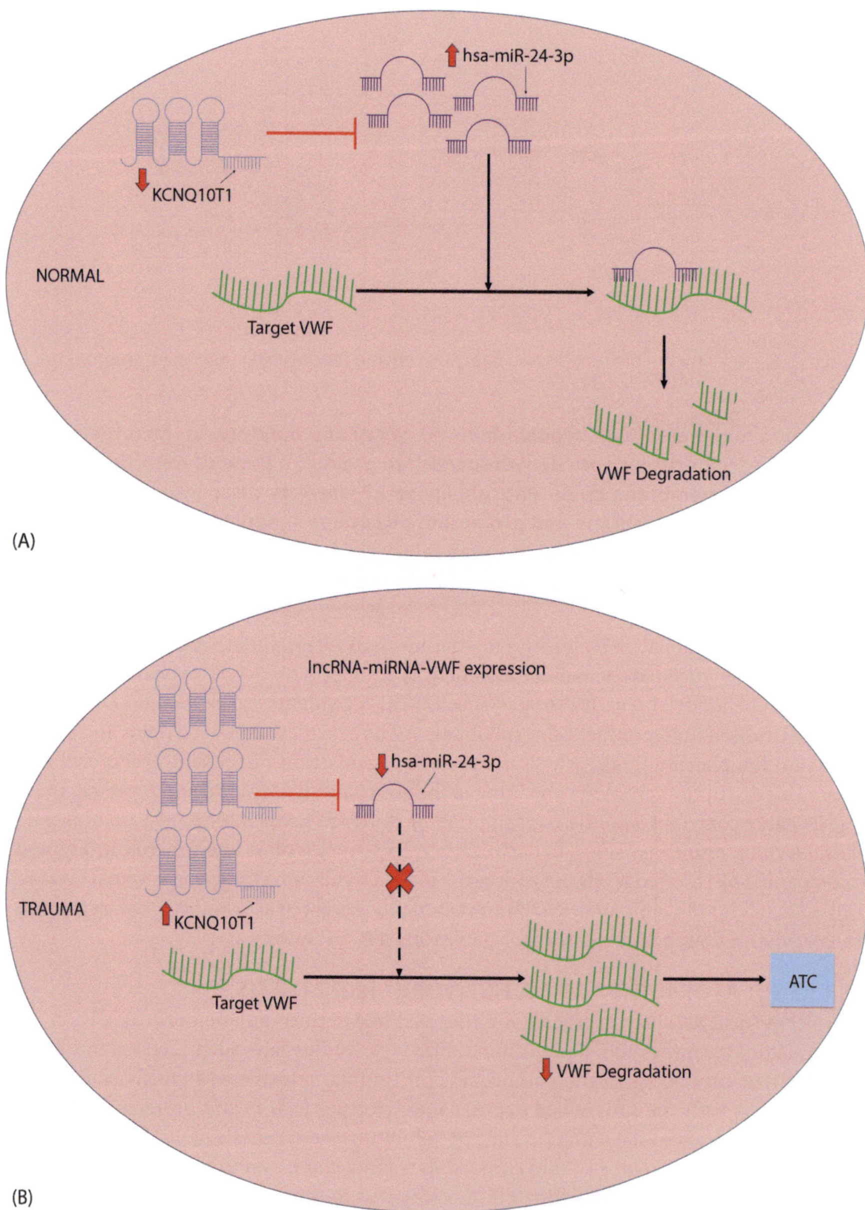

Figure 5.7 Illustration of how KCNQ1OT1-miR-24-vWF axes drive coagulopathy in Trauma. (A) Normal vWF levels support platelet adhesion and haemostasis; (B) trauma leads to suppressed vWF synthesis, causing lower vWF levels and impaired haemostasis.

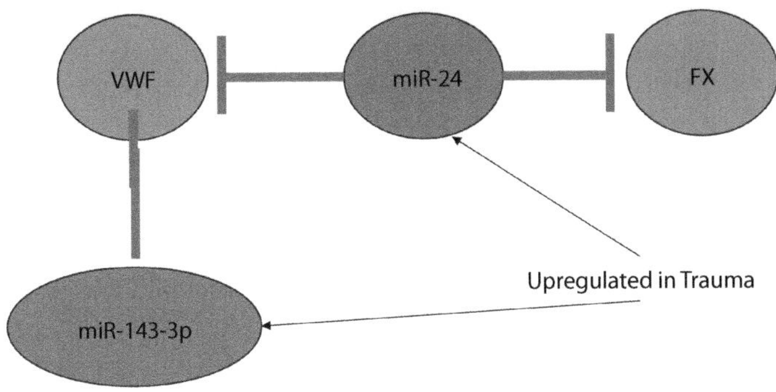

Figure 5.8 MicroRNA-mediated haemostatic dysregulation in trauma.

tissue, while vWF and KCNQ1OT1 expression were observed to be decreased in patients and rat models.[73,76]

Another pathway involves miR-143-3p, which also negatively regulates vWF, contributing to coagulation dysfunction in TIC.[77] MicroRNA-mediated haemostatic dysregulation in trauma is shown in Figure 5.8. vWF is a key glycoprotein essential for haemostasis as it helps platelets adhere to the injured vessel wall and averts factor VIII degradation. TIC is linked with low vWF levels and reduced clot formation. Recent work examining the circRNA-miRNA-mRNA ceRNA network identified vWF as a key gene in TIC pathogenesis, particularly through the circ_0001274 axis. The study demonstrated that miR-143-3p directly targets and suppresses vWF, whereas circ_0001274 can competitively bind to miR-143-3p. By acting as a molecular sponge, circ_0001274 reduces the inhibitory effect of miR-143-3p and increases vWF expression, which may help improve coagulation in TIC. These findings suggest that the circ_0001274/miR-143-3p/VWF pathway could serve as a promising therapeutic target in TIC.

Restoring the "sponge" RNAs (e.g., KCNQ1OT1 mimics) or using "antagomirs" (to block miR-24-3p) could theoretically restore factor X and vWF levels without transfusion.

The markers listed in Table 5.7 represent a shift from traditional clotting tests (like PT/APTT) toward understanding metabolic exhaustion and gene regulation failure as the molecular

Table 5.7 Novel omics and molecular markers associated with TIC

Marker	Type	Mechanistic link	Diagnostic/prognostic performance
LysoPE (20:4/0:0)[73,74]	Metabolite (LysoPE)	Membrane lipid perturbation: links to platelet/endothelial signalling	AUC 0.933 (95% CI 0.849–0.995) for TIC vs. non-TIC
LysoPE (0:0/18:2)[73-74]	Metabolite (LysoPE)	Lipid remodelling; decreased in some TIC cohorts	AUC 0.916 (95% CI 0.818–0.914)
Succinate[73]	Metabolites	Correlates with platelet dysfunction (inverse with ADP-MA)	Significant negative correlations with ADP-MA
miR-24-3p[76]	miRNA	Suppresses FX synthesis; targets vWF via ceRNA network	↑ in TIC (≈3.17-fold); negative correlation with factor X (rho ≈ −0.40)
miR-143-3p[77]	miRNA	Direct inhibitor of vWF	↑ in TIC; inhibition restores vWF
circ_0001274/ KCNQ1OT1[73,77]	circRNA/ lncRNA (ceRNA)	Sponge miRNAs (miR-143-3p, miR-24-3p), thereby protecting vWF	Downregulation in TIC → loss of vWF regulation

drivers of TIC. These markers reveal a groundbreaking concept in TIC; the body does not just "consume" coagulation factors; it actively stops producing them. This is driven by a failure in the ceRNAregulatory network. In a healthy individual, high levels of "Sponges" (lncRNA/circRNA/circ_0001274) keep the "Silencers" (like miR-24-3p) in check, ensuring normal production of the coagulation factors. In trauma, the "sponges" are downregulated, leaving the "silencers" unchecked, causing a drop in coagulation factor production. This could explain why some patients remain coagulopathic even after massive transfusion. Future therapies may involve lncRNA mimics (artificial sponges) to soak up these miRNAs and restart the patient's own coagulation factor production.[73-78]

FUTURE DIRECTIONS IN TIC DIAGNOSTICS

New technologies are now pushing diagnostics toward faster, smaller, and more precise platforms that may redefine how TIC is detected. Diagnostics in TIC is moving beyond slow static laboratory assays to platforms that can make real vascular conditions give molecular profiling output that exposes the pathology behind coagulopathy.

NEXT-GENERATION VHAS: QUANTRA SEER SONORHEOMETRY

The Quantra System is a cartridge-based point-of-care (POC) device that uses sonorheometry, a technology based on Sonic Estimation of Elasticity via Resonance (SEER). High-frequency ultrasound measures clot stiffness without any physical contact. The velocity of these waves correlates directly with clot shear modulus (stiffness) measured in hectopascals (hPa). The system uses QStat cartridges, which can differentiate the specific contribution of fibrinogen and platelets to the clot strength, as well as measure clot stability to lysis. It measures clot stability to lysis (CSL), clot stiffness (CS), and breaks down clot stiffness into fibrinogen contribution to stiffness (FCS) and platelet contribution to clot stiffness (PCS).[79,80]

MICROFLUIDIC AND "ORGAN-ON-A-CHIP" PLATFORMS

The microfluidic technology incorporates physiological shear stress, endothelial interaction and extremely low sample volumes to overcome the limitations of the current viscoelastic assays.[81,82]

TORTUOSITY-POWERED MICROFLUIDICS:[83]

Recent innovations have introduced devices that can make the tortuous geometry of arterioles. By incorporating stenosed and tortuous channels, these devices generate pathological Shia gradients that can activate platelets and coagulation naturally without the use of exogenous reagents. These tortuosity-based microchannels can induce occlusion in <10 minutes using minimal blood volumes, offering a rapid assessment of thrombotic potential under flow conditions.

ADAPTIVE-BUBBLE HAEMOSTASIS CHIPS:[84]

These devices use microbubbles confined within channels as passive sensors. As coagulation progresses, the forming plot exerts pressure that alters the bubble geometry. Automatic tracking of the bubble deformation yields viscoelastic parameters that are comparable to our time, k time and MA values of TEG, with high diagnostic accuracy.

INJURY-ON-A-CHIP (PINCH):[85]

This system introduces a living endothelial layer within a microchannel. The pneumatic compression creates a controlled "injury", which exposes the procoagulant surfaces and initiates clot formation. This platform captures the critical steps in trauma-induced haemostasis that the static assays cannot reproduce, including endothelial activation and phosphatidylserine exposure.

PRECISION DIAGNOSTICS USING MULTIOMICS

Multiomic approaches are being used to identify molecular endotypes of TIC that have not been captured by the functional assays. Next-generation sequence studies have shown consistent upregulation of Interferon-Stimulated Genes (ISGs) such as OAS2, IFIT1, and RSAD2 in patients with TIC, linking the innate immune activation to coagulation, suggesting that TIC is partly an "immuno-coagulopathy". Integrative analyses using the Weighted Gene Co-expression Network Analysis (WGCNA) and machine learning models have highlighted the potential of biomarkers such as TFPI and MMP9 for diagnostic and prognostic purposes.

CONCLUSION

Diagnostic assessment of TIC is at a critical transition point. Traditional laboratory assays remain important for baseline evaluation, but are insufficient to define the full haemostatic disturbance seen in trauma. Viscoelastic assays have improved real-time assessment but still do not fully account for endothelial injury, platelet dysfunction under flow, immune-coagulation interactions, or metabolic drivers of coagulopathy. Emerging technologies, including microfluidic platforms, endothelial injury-on-a-chip models, and multiomic biomarker profiling, offer a more physiologically relevant and mechanistic view of TIC. When combined with data-driven predictive models, these tools have the potential to identify distinct TIC phenotypes, guide targeted resuscitation, and monitor therapeutic response. Future diagnostic frameworks should move away from single-parameter thresholds toward integrated, multiparametric approaches that reflect the dynamic biology of trauma. Such evolution is essential to improve early recognition, personalise treatment strategies, and reduce preventable mortality associated with TIC.

TAKE-HOME MESSAGE

TIC is a dynamic and heterogeneous condition that cannot be reliably identified using any single diagnostic test. Conventional coagulation tests remain widely available and useful for initial assessment, but they provide delayed results and offer only a limited view of the haemostatic process. Viscoelastic assays have improved functional evaluation of clot formation and breakdown, yet they still fall short in capturing key physiological elements and face operational constraints in routine use. Emerging diagnostic approaches, including microfluidic platforms, endothelial injury models, and multiomic biomarker profiling, better reflect real-world haemostasis and underlying mechanisms. Integrating functional assays with molecular biomarkers and predictive analytics represents the most promising route toward early, precise, and mechanism-based diagnosis of TIC.

Figure Credits: All figures are original and created by the authors. Selected elements were sourced from the NIAID NIH BioArt Source (bioart.niaid.nih.gov/bioart/###). Figures were created by the authors in Microsoft PowerPoint.

REFERENCES

1. Lancé MD. A general review of major global coagulation assays: Thrombelastography, thrombin generation test and clot waveform analysis. *Thromb J.* 2015;13(1). doi: 10.1186/1477-9560-13-1

2. Campbell JE, Aden JK, Cap AP. Acute traumatic coagulopathy: Whole blood thrombelastography measures the tip of the iceberg. *J Trauma Acute Care Surg.* 2015;78(5): 955–961. doi: 10.1097/TA.0000000000000586.

3. Godier A, Mansour A, Garrigue D, Susen S. Fibrinogen: the higher the better?. *Blood Transfus.* 2025;23(1):79–82. doi:10.2450/BloodTransfus.978

4. Ameri M, Schnaars HA, Sibley JR, Honor DJ. Determination of plasma fibrinogen concentrations in beagle dogs, cynomolgus monkeys, New Zealand white rabbits, and Sprague-Dawley rats by using Clauss and prothrombin-time-derived assays. *J Am Assoc Lab Anim Sci.* 2011;50(6):864–867.

5. ăetu AE, Mirea L, Cobilinschi C, Grințescu IC, Grințescu IM. Beyond trauma-induced coagulopathy: Detection of auto-heparinization as a marker of endotheliopathy using rotational thromboelastometry. *J Clin Med.* 2024;13(14):4219. doi:10.3390/jcm

6. Brown LM, Call MS, Margaret Knudson M, Cohen MJ; Trauma Outcomes Group; Holcomb JB, *et al.* A normal platelet count may not be enough: the impact of admission platelet count on mortality and transfusion in severely injured trauma patients. *J Trauma.* 2011;71(2 Suppl 3):S337–S342. doi:10.1097/TA.0b013e318227f67c

7. Kornblith LZ, Kutcher ME, Redick BJ, Calfee CS, Vilardi RF, Cohen MJ. Fibrinogen and platelet contributions to clot formation: implications for trauma resuscitation and thromboprophylaxis. *J Trauma Acute Care Surg.* 2014;76(2):255–263. doi:10.1097/TA.0000000000000108

8. Böhm JK, Güting H, Thorn S, Schäfer N, Rambach V, Schöchl H, *et al.* Global characterisation of coagulopathy in isolated traumatic brain injury (iTBI): A CENTER-TBI analysis. *Neurocrit Care.* 2021;35(1):184–196. doi:10.1007/s12028-020-01151-7

9. Ali I, Graham C, Dempsey-Hibbert NC. Immature platelet fraction as a useful marker in the etiological determination of thrombocytopenia. *Exp Hematol.* 2019;78:56–61. doi:10.1016/j.exphem.2019.09.001

10. Khan MI, Ullah I. Diagnostic importance of mean platelet volume, platelet distribution width and platelet large cell ratio as screening tool in immune thrombocytopenia. *Porto Biomed J.* 2020;5(6):e094. doi:10.1097/j.pbj.0000000000000094

11. Maegele M. Coagulopathy after traumatic brain injury: incidence, pathogenesis, and treatment options. *Transfusion.* 2013;53 Suppl 1:28S–37S. doi:10.1111/trf.12033

12. Sullivan TM, Milestone ZP, Tempel PE, Gao S, Burd RS. Development and validation of a Bayesian belief network predicting the probability of blood transfusion after pediatric injury. *J Trauma Acute Care Surg.* 2023;94(2):304–311. doi:10.1097/TA.0000000000003709

13. Simmons JW, Powell MF. Acute traumatic coagulopathy: pathophysiology and resuscitation. *Br J Anaesth.* 2016;117(suppl 3):iii31–iii43. doi:10.1093/bja/aew328

14. Černý V, Maegele M, Agostini V, Fries D, Leal-Noval SR, Nardai G, *et al.* Variations and obstacles in the use of coagulation factor concentrates for major trauma bleeding across Europe: outcomes from a European expert meeting. *Eur J Trauma Emerg Surg.* 2022;48(2):763–774. doi:10.1007/s00068-020-01563-2

15. Hofmann N, Schöchl H, Oberladstätter D, Zipperle J, Schmitt F, von der Forst M, Martin C, Gratz J. Viscoelastic coagulation testing in bleeding trauma patients: a retrospective

analysis and development of a treatment algorithm. *Br J Anaesth.* 2025;136: 117–125. doi: 10.1016/j.bja.2025.09.040.

16. Knottenbelt JD. Low initial hemoglobin levels in trauma patients: an important indicator of ongoing hemorrhage. *J Trauma.* 1991;31(10):1396–1399. doi:10.1097/00005373-199110000-00015

17. Brohi K, Singh J, Heron M, Coats T. Acute traumatic coagulopathy. *J Trauma.* 2003; 54:1127–1130.

18. MacLeod J, Lynn M, McKenney M, Cohn S, Murtha M. Early coagulopathy predicts mortality in trauma. *J Trauma.* 2003;55(1):39–44.

19. Engels PT, Rezende-Neto JB, Al Mahroos M, Scarpelini S, Rizoli SB, Tien HC. The natural history of trauma-related coagulopathy: implications for treatment. *J Trauma.* 2011;71(5 Suppl 1):S448–S455. doi: 10.1097/TA.0b013e318232e6ac.

20. Maegele M, Paffrath T, Bouillon B. Acute traumatic coagulopathy in severe injury—incidence, risk stratification, and treatment options. Dtsch Arztebl Int 2011;108: 827–835.

21. Frith D, Goslings JC, Gaarder C, Maegele M, Cohen MJ, Allard S, *et al.* Definition and drivers of acute traumatic coagulopathy: clinical and experimental investigations. *J Thromb Haemost.* 2010;8(9):1919–1925. doi:10.1111/j.1538-7836.2010.03945.x

22. Selladurai BM, Vickneswaran M, Duraisamy S, Atan M. Coagulopathy in acute head injury—a study of its role as a prognostic indicator. *Br J Neurosurg.* 1997;11(5):398–404.

23. Sun Y, Wang J, Wu X, Xi C, Gai Y, Liu H, *et al.* Validating the incidence of coagulopathy and disseminated intravascular coagulation in patients with traumatic brain injury: analysis of 242 cases. *Br J Neurosurg.* 2011;25:363–368.

24. Segal JB, Dzik W. Paucity of studies to support that abnormal coagulation test results predict bleeding in the setting of invasive procedures: and evidence-based review. *Transfusion.* 2005;45:1413–1425.

25. Ganter MT, Pittet JF. New insights into acute coagulopathy in trauma patients. *Best Pract Res Clin Anaesthesiol.* 2010;24:15–25.

26. Perkins ZB, Yet B, Marsden M, Glasgow S, Marsh W, Davenport R, *et al.* Early Identification of trauma-induced coagulopathy: Development and validation of a multivariable risk prediction model. *Ann Surg.* 2021;274(6):e1119–e1128. doi:10.1097/SLA.0000000000003771

27. Hartert H. Coagulation analysis with thromboelastography, a new method. *Klin. Wochenschr.* 1948;26:577–658. doi: 10.1007/BF01697545.

28. Hartert H, Schaeder JA. The physical and biological constants of thrombelastography. *Biorheology.* 1962;1:31–39. doi: 10.3233/BIR-1962-1105.

29. Shore-Lesserson L, Manspeizer HE, DePerio M, Francis S, Vela-Cantos F, Ergin MA. Thromboelastography-guided transfusion algorithm reduces transfusions in complex cardiac surgery. *Anesth Analg.* 1999 Feb;88(2):312–319.

30. Kang YG, Martin DJ, Marquez J, Lewis JH, Bontempo FA, Shaw BW, Starzl TE, Winter PM. Intraoperative changes in blood coagulation and thrombelastographic monitoring in liver transplantation. *Anesth Analg.* 1985 Sep;64(9):888–896.

31. Hartmann J, Murphy M, Dias JD. Viscoelastic hemostatic assays: moving from the laboratory to the site of care-a review of established and emerging technologies. *Diagnostics (Basel).* 2020;10(2):118. doi:10.3390/diagnostics10020118

32. Roberts TR, Garcia I, Slychko I, Dalton HJ, Batchinsky AI. A deployable viscoelastic coagulation monitor enables point-of-care assessment of coagulopathy in swine with polytrauma. *Mil Med.* 2025;190(5–6):e994–e1003.

33. Nogami K. The utility of thromboelastography in inherited and acquired bleeding disorders. *Br J Haematol.* 2016;174(4):503–514. doi:10.1111/bjh.14148

34. Volod O, Runge A. The TEG 5000 system: System Description and Protocol for Measurements. *Methods Mol Biol.* 2023;2663:725–733. doi:10.1007/978-1-0716-3175-1_48

35. Shaydakov ME, Sigmon DF, Blebea J. Thromboelastography. In: *StatPearls [Internet].* Treasure Island (FL): StatPearls Publishing; 2025 Jan. Available from: https://www.ncbi.nlm.nih.gov/books/NBK537061/

36. Hochleitner G, Sutor K, Levett C, Leyser H, Schlimp CJ, Solomon C. Revisiting Hartert's 1962 calculation of the physical constants of thrombelastography. *Clin Appl Thromb Hemost.* 2017;23(3):201–210. doi:10.1177/1076029615606531

37. Cotton BA, Faz G, Hatch QM, Radwan ZA, Podbielski J, Wade C, *et al.* Rapid thrombelastography delivers real-time results that predict transfusion within 1 hour of admission. *J Trauma.* 2011;71(2):407–417. doi:10.1097/TA.0b013e31821e1bf0

38. Coleman JR, Moore EE, Chapman MP, Banerjee A, Silliman CC, Ghasabyan A, *et al.* Rapid TEG efficiently guides hemostatic resuscitation in trauma patients. *Surgery.* 2018;164(3):489–493. doi:10.1016/j.surg.2018.04.029

39. Chapman MP, Moore EE, Moore HB, Gonzalez E, Morton AP, Chandler J, *et al.* The "Death Diamond": Rapid thrombelastography identifies lethal hyperfibrinolysis. *J Trauma Acute Care Surg.* 2015;79(6):925–929. doi:10.1097/TA.0000000000000871

40. Neal MD, Moore EE, Walsh M, Thomas S, Callcut RA, Kornblith LZ, *et al.* A comparison between the TEG 6s and TEG 5000 analyzers to assess coagulation in trauma patients. *J Trauma Acute Care Surg.* 2020;88(2):279–285. doi:10.1097/TA.0000000000002545

41. Artang R, Anderson M, Nielsen JD. Fully automated thromboelastograph TEG 6s to measure anticoagulant effects of direct oral anticoagulants in healthy male volunteers. *Res Pract Thromb Haemost.* 2019;3(3):391–396. doi:10.1002/rth2.12206

42. Sarani B, Callum J, Neal MD, Meizoso JP, Spinella PC, Leeper C, *et al.* Goal-directed transfusion algorithm for trauma patients with severe hemorrhage using TEG 6S: Results of a Delphi consensus survey and expert panel recommendations. *J Trauma Acute Care Surg.* 2025;98(6):984–991. doi:10.1097/TA.0000000000004606

43. Gill M. The TEG®6s on shaky ground? A novel assessment of the TEG®6s performance under a challenging condition. *J Extra Corpor Technol.* 2017;49(1):26–29.

44. Selby R. "TEG talk": expanding clinical roles for thromboelastography and rotational thromboelastometry. *Hematology Am Soc Hematol Educ Program.* 2020;2020(1):67–75. doi:10.1182/hematology.2020000090

45. Drotarova M, Zolkova J, Belakova KM, Brunclikova M, Skornova I, Stasko J, *et al.* Basic principles of rotational thromboelastometry (ROTEM®) and the role of ROTEM-guided fibrinogen replacement therapy in the management of coagulopathies. *Diagnostics (Basel).* 2023;13(20):3219.

46. Longacre MM, Ibla JC. TEG and ROTEM: Technology and clinical applications, 2026 update. *Am J Hematol.* 2025;100(12):2357–2370. doi:10.1002/ajh.70074

47. Cannata G, Mariotti Zani E, Argentiero A, Caminiti C, Perrone S, Esposito S. TEG® and ROTEM® traces: Clinical applications of viscoelastic coagulation monitoring in neonatal intensive care unit. *Diagnostics (Basel).* 2021;11(9):1642. doi:10.3390/diagnostics11091642

48. Kataria S, Juneja D, Singh O. Redefining haemostasis: Role of rotational thromboelastometry in critical care settings. *World J Crit Care Med.* 2025;14(2):102521.

49. Wohlauer MV, Moore EE, Thomas S, Sauaia A, Evans E, Harr J, *et al.* Early platelet dysfunction: an unrecognized role in the acute coagulopathy of trauma. *J Am Coll Surg.* 2012;214(5):739–746. doi:10.1016/j.jamcollsurg.2012.01.050

50. Harrington J, Zarzaur BL, Fox EE, Wade CE, Holcomb JB, Savage SA. Variations in clot phenotype following injury: The MA-R ratio and fragile clots. *J Trauma Acute Care Surg.* 2022;92(3):504–510. doi:10.1097/TA.0000000000003442

51. Albert V, Subramanian A, Pati HP, Agrawal D, Bhoi SK. Efficacy of thromboelastography (TEG) in predicting acute trauma-induced coagulopathy (ATIC) in isolated severe traumatic brain injury (iSTBI). *Indian J Hematol Blood Transfus.* 2019;35(2):325–331. doi:10.1007/s12288-018-1003-4

52. Spasiano A, Barbarino C, Marangone A, Orso D, Trillò G, Giacomello R, *et al.* Early thromboelastography in acute traumatic coagulopathy: an observational study focusing on pre-hospital trauma care. *Eur J Trauma Emerg Surg.* 2022;48(1):431–439. doi:10.1007/s00068-020-01493-z

53. Matkovic E, Lindholm PF. Role of viscoelastic and conventional coagulation tests for management of blood product replacement in the bleeding patient. *Semin Thromb Hemost.* 2022;48(7):785–795. doi:10.1055/s-0042-1756192

54. Kelly JM, Rizoli S, Veigas P, Hollands S, Min A. Using rotational thromboelastometry clot firmness at 5 minutes (ROTEM® EXTEM A5) to predict massive transfusion and in-hospital mortality in trauma: a retrospective analysis of 1146 patients. *Anaesthesia.* 2018;73(9):1103–1109. doi:10.1111/anae.14297

55. Morrow GB, Carlier MSA, Dasgupta S, Craigen FB, Mutch NJ, Curry N. Fibrinogen replacement therapy for traumatic coagulopathy: Does the fibrinogen source matter?. *Int J Mol Sci.* 2021;22(4):2185. doi:10.3390/ijms22042185

56. Stettler GR, Moore EE, Moore HB, Nunns GR, Silliman CC, *et al.* Redefining postinjury fibrinolysis phenotypes using two viscoelastic assays. *J Trauma Acute Care Surg.* 2019;86(4):679–685. doi:10.1097/TA.0000000000002165

57. Chapman MP, Moore EE, Ramos CR, Ghasabyan A, Harr JN, Chin TL, *et al.* Fibrinolysis greater than 3% is the critical value for initiation of antifibrinolytic therapy. *J Trauma Acute Care Surg.* 2013;75(6):961–967. doi:10.1097/TA.0b013e3182aa9c9f

58. Vasovic LV, Littlejohn J, Alqunaibit D, Dillard A, Qiu Y, Rand S, *et al.* Rotational thromboelastometry in patients with acute respiratory distress syndrome owing to coronavirus disease 2019: Is there a viscoelastic fingerprint and a role for predicting thrombosis?. *Surgery.* 2022;171(4):1092–1099. doi:10.1016/j.surg.2021.08.051

59. Creel-Bulos C, Sniecinski R. Fibrinolysis Shutdown and Thrombosis in a COVID-19 ICU. Shock. 2021 Jun 1;55(6):845–846. doi: 10.1097/SHK.0000000000001666.

60. MacArthur TA, Spears GM, Kozar RA, Dong JF, Auton M, Jenkins DH, *et al.* Thrombin generation kinetics are predictive of rapid transfusion in trauma patients meeting critical administration threshold. *Shock.* 2021;55(3):321–325. doi:10.1097/SHK.0000000000001633

61. Albert V, Arulselvi S, Agrawal D, Pati HP, Pandey RM. Early posttraumatic changes in coagulation and fibrinolysis systems in isolated severe traumatic brain injury patients and its influence on immediate outcome. *Hematol Oncol Stem Cell Ther.* 2019;12(1):32–43. doi:10.1016/j.hemonc.2018.09.005

62. Matijevic N, Wang YW, Wade CE, Holcomb JB, Cotton BA, Schreiber MA, *et al.* Cellular microparticle and thrombogram phenotypes in the prospective observational multicenter major trauma transfusion (PROMMTT) study: correlation with coagulopathy. *Thromb Res.* 2014;134(3):652–658. doi:10.1016/j.thromres.2014.07.023

63. Caspers M, Schäfer N, Bouillon B, Schaeben V, Ciorba MC, Maegele M, *et al.* Protein C in adult patients with sepsis: from pathophysiology to monitoring and supplementation. *J Anesth Analg Crit Care.* 2025;5(1):21. doi:10.1186/s44158-025-00243-0

64. Caspers M, Schäfer N, Bouillon B, Schaeben V, Ciorba MC, Maegele M, *et al.* Plasmatic coagulation profile after major traumatic injury: a prospective observational study. *Eur J Trauma Emerg Surg.* 2022;48(6):4595–4606. doi:10.1007/s00068-022-01971-6

65. Cohen MJ, Call M, Nelson M, Calfee CS, Esmon CT, Brohi K, Pittet JF. Critical role of activated protein C in early coagulopathy and later organ failure, infection and death in trauma patients. *Ann Surg.* 2012;255(2):379.

66. Bucciarelli P, Passamonti SM, Biguzzi E, Gianniello F, Franchi F, Mannucci PM, *et al.* Low borderline plasma levels of antithrombin, protein C and protein S are risk factors for venous thromboembolism. *J Thromb Haemost.* 2012;10(9):1783–1791. doi:10.1111/j.1538-7836.2012.04858.x

67. Johansen ME, Johansson PI, Ostrowski SR, Bestle MH, Hein L, Jensen AL, *et al.* Profound endothelial damage predicts impending organ failure and death in sepsis. *Semin Thromb Hemost.* 2015;41(1):16–25.

68. Gonzalez Rodriguez E, Ostrowski SR, Cardenas JC, Baer LA, Tomasek JS. Syndecan-1: A Quantitative Marker for the Endotheliopathy of Trauma. *J Am Coll Surg.* 2017; 225:419–427.

69. Albert V, Subramanian A, Agrawal D, Pati HP, Gupta SD, Mukhopadhyay AK. Acute traumatic endotheliopathy in isolated severe brain injury and its impact on clinical outcome. *Med Sci (Basel).* 2018;6(1):5. doi:10.3390/medsci6010005

70. Wada H, Yamamoto A, Tomida M, Ichikawa Y, Ezaki M, Masuda J, *et al.* Proposal of quick diagnostic criteria for disseminated intravascular coagulation. *J Clin Med.* 2022;11(4):1028. doi:10.3390/jcm11041028

71. Zeineddin A, Dong JF, Wu F, Terse P, Kozar RA. Role of Von Willebrand factor after injury: It may do more than we think. *Shock.* 2021;55(6):717–722. doi:10.1097/ SHK.0000000000001690

72. Russell RT, McDaniel JK, Cao W, Shroyer M, Wagener BM, Zheng XL, *et al.* Low plasma ADAMTS13 activity is associated with coagulopathy, endothelial cell damage and mortality after severe paediatric trauma. *Thromb Haemost.* 2018;118(4):676–687. doi:10.1055/s-0038-1636528

73. Xu X, Ouyang Q, Shao M, Yi Q, Liu S, Huang Y, *et al.* Screening of biomarkers for early diagnosis of trauma-induced coagulopathy based on untargeted metabolomics. *Front Endocrinol (Lausanne).* 2025;16:1632694. doi:10.3389/fendo.2025.1632694

74. Abdullah S, Ghio M, Cotton-Betteridge A, Vinjamuri A, Drury R, Packer J, *et al.* Succinate metabolism and membrane reorganization drives the endotheliopathy and coagulopathy of traumatic hemorrhage. *Sci Adv.* 2023;9(24):eadf6600. doi:10.1126/sciadv.adf6600

75. Jankowska KI, Sauna ZE, Atreya CD. Role of microRNAs in Hemophilia and Thrombosis in Humans. *Int J Mol Sci.* 2020;21(10):3598. doi:10.3390/ijms21103598

76. Chen LJ, Yang L, Cheng X, Xue YK, Chen LB. Overexpression of miR-24 Is involved in the formation of hypocoagulation state after severe trauma by inhibiting the synthesis of coagulation factor X. *Dis Markers.* 2017;2017:3649693. doi:10.1155/2017/3649693

77. Luo Y, Liu S, Li Q, Zhang Y, Fu Y, Yang N, *et al.* circ_0001274 competitively binds miR-143-3p to upregulate VWF expression to improve acute traumatic coagulopathy. *Oxid Med Cell Longev.* 2023;2023:9650323. doi:10.1155/2023/9650323

78. Zanza C, Romenskaya T, Racca F, Rocca E, Piccolella F, Piccioni A, *et al.* Severe trauma-induced coagulopathy: Molecular mechanisms underlying critical illness. *Int J Mol Sci.* 2023;24(8):7118. doi:10.3390/ijms24087118

79. Corey FS, Walker WF. Sonic estimation of elasticity via resonance: A new method of assessing hemostasis. *Ann Biomed Eng.* 2016;44(5):1405–1424. doi:10.1007/s10439-015-1460-y

80. Rossetto A, Wohlgemut JM, Brohi K, Davenport R. Sonorheometry versus rotational thromboelastometry in trauma: a comparison of diagnostic and prognostic performance. *J Thromb Haemost.* 2023;21(8):2114–2125. doi:10.1016/j.jtha.2023.04.031

81. Paloschi V, Sabater-Lleal M, Middelkamp H, Vivas A, Johansson S, van der Meer A, *et al.* Organ-on-a-chip technology: a novel approach to investigate cardiovascular diseases. *Cardiovasc Res.* 2021;117(14):2742–2754. doi:10.1093/cvr/cvab088

82. Sakurai Y, Hardy ET, Lam WA. Hemostasis-on-a-chip/incorporating the endothelium in microfluidic models of bleeding. *Platelets.* 2023;34(1):2185453. doi:10.1080/09537104.2023.2185453

83. Luna DJ, R Pandian NK, Mathur T, *et al.* Tortuosity-powered microfluidic device for assessment of thrombosis and antithrombotic therapy in whole blood. *Sci Rep.* 2020;10(1):5742. doi:10.1038/s41598-020-62768-4

84. Chen L, Yu L, Chen M, Liu Y, Xu H, Wang F, *et al.* A microfluidic hemostatic diagnostics platform: Harnessing coagulation-induced adaptive-bubble behavioral perception. *Cell Rep Med.* 2023;4(11):101252. doi:10.1016/j.xcrm.2023.101252

85. Deal H, Byrnes EM, Pandit S, Sheridan A, Brown AC, Daniele M. Injury-on-a-chip for modelling microvascular trauma-induced coagulation. *Lab Chip.* 2025;25(3):440–453. doi:10.1039/d4lc00471j

Chapter 6

SCORING SYSTEMS TO ASSESS PROBABILITY OF MASSIVE TRANSFUSION IN TRAUMA

Joses Dany James, Vignesh Kumar, and Sruthi Kandaswamy

DOI: 10.1201/9781003711070-6

INTRODUCTION

Uncontrollable haemorrhage remains the primary preventable cause of death after critical injury.[1,2] In the era of damage control resuscitation (DCR), balanced resuscitation using blood and blood products, minimal crystalloid usage, early haemorrhage control, prevention and correction of coagulopathy, and restoration of tissue perfusion and oxygen delivery ensure the best probability of survival. A recent Delphi analysis of blood transfusion requirements estimated that 44.2% (CI 36.3–52.2) of polytrauma patients are expected to require blood transfusions, amounting to ~122,000 units (CI 95.7–165.3 × 1000).[3] Considering this dichotomy, transfusions should be used both prudently and liberally. This chapter emphasises the relevance of multiple scoring systems in trauma management.

PHYSIOLOGICAL AND CLINICAL INDICATORS OF MASSIVE TRANSFUSION

A recent systematic review[4] revealed that more than 20 scores have been validated for use in trauma to determine the need for transfusions. Two clinical signs are consistently present in nearly all of these: heart rate (HR) and systolic blood pressure (SBP). Another typical clinical indicator is the evidence of ongoing bleeding. This could be a positive Focused Assessment with Sonography in Trauma (FAST), indicating intraperitoneal bleeding, an unstable pelvic fracture indicating retroperitoneal bleeding, and femur fractures, especially bilateral ones. From simple clinical signs, scoring systems for massive transfusion (MT) have evolved to using advanced tools, such as point-of-care (POC) labs and viscoelastic assays. While modern methods improve accuracy by incorporating markers such as pH, lactate, and coagulopathy tests, they are more complex and less widely accessible globally.

SCORES UTILISING ONLY CLINICAL INDICATORS

SHOCK INDEX (SI)

Ever since its introduction by Allgower and Burri,[5] the shock index (SI) has been utilised in multiple ways. The SI, calculated as the ratio of HR to SBP, quantifies hypoperfusion. An SI >0.9 predicts mortality, Massive Haemorrhagic Protocol (MHP) activation, and haemostatic intervention. The Shock Index Paediatric Age-Adjusted (SIPA) similarly predicts transfusion needs in severely injured children.[6] The SI is simple to use but may overestimate MHP needs in cases like obstructive or cardiogenic shock. It is less reliable in the elderly, hypertensive patients, or those on beta or calcium channel blockers. A review suggests SI alone isn't the best predictor for MHP.[7]

FIELD TRIAGE SCORE

The Field Triage Score (FTS) simplifies the Revised Trauma Score (RTS) by using SBP (≤100 mmHg) and motor GCS (<6). Designed for military use, it estimates blood pressure (BP) via radial pulse and links low m-GCS to hypoperfusion. FTS and RTS are both strong MHP predictors, with FTS being simpler to apply.[8] Developed as a military score to be used in the field, an SBP of 100 mmHg was chosen as the cut-off, as this was widely understood to be the BP at which the radial pulse disappears, and the score does not directly need the SBP to be measured. Any low score of m-GCS < 6 was considered indicative of decreased mentation secondary to hypoperfusion. In comparing RTS and a modified version of the FTS (where total GCS was used), both were good predictors of the need for MHP activation among combat casualties, with the FTS having its obvious advantage of being easier to use.[9]

Table 6.1   The trauma-induced coagulopathy clinical score (TICCS)

Criteria	Points
General Severity	2
Admitted to the resuscitation room with trauma team activation	0
Non-critical (regular ED room)	
Blood Pressure	5
SBP * fell below 90 mmHg at least once	0
SBP * always above 90 mmHg	
Extent of Significant Injuries	1
Head and neck	1
Upper extremity (left)	1
Upper extremity (right)	1
Lower extremity (left)	1
Lower extremity (right)	2
Torso	2
Abdomen	2
Pelvis	
Total possible score	0–18

TRAUMA-INDUCED COAGULOPATHY CLINICAL SCORE (TICCS)

Trauma-Induced Coagulopathy Clinical Score (TICCS) is a relatively new score developed for use in the pre-hospital setting to identify patients who may develop TIC and require DCR. It consists of three parameters:

i. The severity of injuries necessitating a triage to the resuscitation room

ii. SBP < 90 mmHg

iii. The anatomical extent of injuries

All evaluated by the paramedic on the scene or the clinician in the ER (Table 6.1). The total score can range from 0 to 18, and a TICCS score of ≥10 has been shown to predict TIC and the need for MT in a prospective single-centre study involving 82 patients.[10] Retrospective validation of TICCS was performed using data from 33,385 patients in the German Trauma Registry (TR-DGU). It showed an area under the curve (AUC) of 0.7 (95% CI: 0.69–0.70), with a cut-off value of ≥12 yielding the best trade-off between true positives and false positives.[11] The m-TICCS score, with an AUC of 0.77, demonstrated accuracy comparable to that of the Trauma Associated Severe Haemorrhage (TASH) score (0.78). Despite being easy to use, it is subjective and validated mainly for blunt injuries, limiting broader application.

CODE RED ACTIVATION

Developed by the emergency medicine and pre-hospital care team at Royal London Hospital,[12] the Code Red activation (CRA) uses three triggers: (1) active haemorrhage, (2) SBP <90 mmHg, and (3) no response to fluid bolus to alert hospitals to potential transfusion needs. A total of 91% of CRA patients required transfusions. Retrospective and prospective validations showed improved outcomes, though CRA predicts general transfusion needs, not massive transfusions specifically.[13,14]

MODIFIED EARLY WARNING SCORE (MEWS)

Modified Early Warning Score (MEWS) was initially modified from the Early Warning Score to identify the need for ICU admission among medically ill patients.[15] Since then, it has also been shown to predict mortality among polytrauma patients.[16] In addition to the common clinical variables, since MEWS uses the AVPU (alert, verbal response, pain response, and unresponsive) scale, which has generated interest in its ability to predict outcomes among patients with traumatic brain injury (TBI) and polytrauma, with most of the data coming out of Asia (Table 6.2).[17,18]

Table 6.2 The modified early warning score (MEWS)

Variable	Value	Score
SBP	≤70 mmHg	+3
	71–80 mmHg	+2
	81–100 mmHg	+1
	101–199 mmHg	0
	≥200 mmHg	+2
Heart rate	<40 bpm	+2
	41–50 bpm	+1
	51–100 bpm	0
	101–110 bpm	+1
	11–129 bpm	+2
	≥130 bpm	+3
Respiratory rate	<9 bpm	+2
	9–14 bpm	0
	15–20 bpm	+1
	21–29 bpm	+2
	≥30 bpm	+3
Temperature (°C)	<35°C/95°F	+2
	35–38.4°C/95–101.1°F	0
	≥38.5°C/101.3°F	+2
AVPU scale	Alert	0
	Reacts to voice	+1
	Reacts to pain	+2
	Unresponsive	+3

A retrospective study of patients with TBI and polytrauma revealed that MEWS was able to predict the need for MT among this subset reasonably well (OR, 1.42; 95% CI, 1.25–1.61), area under the receiver operating characteristic curve (AUROC) 0.80 (95% CI, 0.78–0.83). Usually, scores developed with one indication do not do well for another, and using MEWS in the trauma setting will require further prospective validation. However, at present, it remains one of the few scoring systems studied for application among patients with TBI.

SCORES UTILISING CLINICAL INDICATORS AND POINT-OF-CARE (POC) TESTS

ASSESSMENT OF BLOOD CONSUMPTION (ABC) SCORE AND THE REVISED ASSESSMENT OF BLOOD TRANSFUSION (RABT) SCORE

Initially developed at Vanderbilt Hospital, the assessment of blood consumption (ABC) score, published in 2009, has stood the test of time primarily due to its simplicity and ease of use. It consists of only two clinical variables (HR and SBP), one mechanism of injury (one point for penetrating mechanism), and one POC test (FAST) (see Table 6.3). Initially

Table 6.3 The assessment of blood consumption (ABC) score

Variable	Value	Score
SBP	≤90 mmHg	+1
Heart rate	≥120/min	+1
Mechanism of injury	Penetrating	+1
FAST	Positive	+1
Total possible score		4

developed from a retrospective cohort,[19] the score has been prospectively validated in multiple centres.[20] However, many of these studies had a sizeable proportion of patients with penetrating trauma, and the scores were applied retrospectively. ABC score has not shown the same sensitivity and specificity when tested in other institutionsm and has been shown to overestimate the need for MT. It has also been shown to have limitations, especially in a predominantly blunt trauma population.[2,21]

Recently, a modification of the ABC score, called the revised assessment of blood transfusion (RABT) score, was formulated. It replaces HR and SBP with the shock index (+1 for SI > 1) and adds pelvic fractures to the score (+1).[23] Retrospective validation of RABT from two Canadian Level 1 Trauma centres showed predictive value equal to SI and ABC scores, with an AUROC of 0.67 (0.61–0.73).[24]

TRAUMA-ASSOCIATED SEVERE HAEMORRHAGE (TASH) SCORE

The authors believe that, at present, Trauma-Associated Severe Haemorrhage (TASH) is the best available score to predict MT. This is because it is a weighted score validated in large trauma databases, and it includes most of the common indicators of haemorrhage and hypoperfusion.[25] The score includes seven independent variables, including anatomical injuries, sex, POC radiology, and POC laboratory investigations (see Table 6.4). The overall score ranges from 0 to 28, with each cumulative point increasing the risk of MT, and each numerical score assigning a specific percentage of need for MT. The score was generated and validated using data from over 6,000 patients in the TR-DGU. The score has been revalidated in multiple countries and has consistently demonstrated high predictive value.[26-28] The obvious disadvantage of TASH is that it has multiple parameters.

The calculation of the score is thus cumbersome and depends on the speed at which POC investigations can be done. It is thus a valuable tool in high-quality Level 1 trauma centres, but may be of limited value in resource-limited settings.

Table 6.4   Trauma-associated severe haemorrhage (TASH) score

Variable	Value	Score
Sex	Male	+1
Haemoglobin	<7 g/dL	+8
	<9 g/dL	+6
	<10 g/dL	+4
	<11 g/dL	+3
	<12 g/dL	+2
	≥12 g/dL	0
Base deficit	<10 mmol/L	+4
	<6 mmol/L	+3
	<2 mmol/L	+1
	≥2 mmol/L	0
SBP	<100 mmHg	+4
	<120 mmHg	+1
	≥120 mmHg	0
Heart rate	>120 bpm	+2
	≤120 bpm	0
FAST	Positive for intra-abdominal fluid	+3
Pelvis	Clinically unstable pelvic fracture	+6
Femur	Open or Dislocated Femur fracture	+3
Total possible score		28

Table 6.5 McLaughlin score

Variable	Value	Score
Heart rate	>105/min	1
SBP	<110 mmHg	1
pH	<7.25	1
Haematocrit	<32%	1
Total possible score		4

MCLAUGHLIN SCORE

The McLaughlin score[29] (Table 6.5) was developed from retrospective data of 302 patients treated at a single combat hospital with data obtained through the Joint Theatre Trauma Registry (JTTR) maintained at the United States Army Institute of Surgical Research.

The score identified four independent risk factors for MT:

i. HR >105 bpm,

ii. SBP <110 mmHg,

iii. pH <7.25, and

iv. Haematocrit <32.0%.

The components are non-weighted and are simply identified as 'yes' or 'no' (see Figure 6.1).

The incidence of MT increases from 20% if the patient has one of these variables present upon admission to 80% if all four are present. The algorithm yielded an AUC of 0.83.

TRAUMA BLEEDING SEVERITY SCORE (TBSS)

The Traumatic Bleeding Severity Score (TBSS) (Table 6.6) was developed with retrospective data from a single centre in Japan. The score was created using data from 119 severely injured trauma patients, with predictive variables assigned a simple score based on the odds ratio from a multivariate logistic regression analysis.

The TBSS was calculated as the sum of the component scores, ranging from 0 to 57. It included the following components:

i. Age

ii. SBP after infusion of 1 L of crystalloids

Iii. Number of region points on the FAST scan

iv. Pelvic fracture

v. Serum lactate

The predictive value of the TBSS was then validated using data from 113 severely injured trauma patients. The AUROC, sensitivity, and specificity for a TBSS >15 points were 0.98, 97.4%, and 96.2%, respectively.[30] A modified version of the score, where SBP was calculated at admission before crystalloid administration, was compared with other existing scores and found to have an excellent predictive value, comparable to TASH (AUROC: 0.92).[31] The score has been helpful in the Japanese population, which has a higher proportion of aged patients among its trauma patients.

$$\log [p/(1 - p)] = 42.1 + [0.7 \times (\text{points for ISS})] - [5.6 \times (\text{min pH during 1st hour})] - [0.04 \times (\text{min SBP during 1st hour})]$$

Figure 6.1 Algorithm suggesting how to select a scoring system for clinical usage.

Table 6.6 The trauma bleeding severity score (TBSS)

Variable	Value	Score
Age	≥60 years	6
SBP	≥110 mmHg	0
	100 ≤ to <110 mmHg	4
	90 ≤ to <100 mmHg	8
	<90 mmHg	12
FAST	Positive	3
Pelvic fracture	AO classification	3
	Type A	6
	Type B	9
	Type C	
Lactate	0 ≤ 2.5 mmol/L	0
	2.5 ≤ 5 mmol/L	4
	5 ≤ 7.5 mmol/L	8
	>7.5 mmol/L	12

VISCOELASTIC ASSAYS

Thromboelastography (TEG) and rotational thromboelastometry (ROTEM) have been studied to guide the need for MT in trauma. A retrospective single-centre study on 53 patients revealed that an abnormal maximum clot firmness (MCF) value predicted the need for MT (AUROC 0.83, 95% CI 0.71–0.94).[32] A prospective study on rapid TEG (rTEG) in 583 major trauma activations revealed that an activated clotting time (ACT) of >128 predicted the need for MT (≥10 U) in the first 6 hours (OR 5.15, 95% CI, 1.36–19.49). In addition, an ACT <105 also predicted patients who did not receive any transfusions within the first 24 hours (OR 2.80, CI 1.02–7.07). Another prospective cohort study out of the UK revealed that clot amplitude at 5 minutes could identify patients requiring MT (detection rate of 71%).[33] Viscoelastic assays appear to have a definite role in predicting the need for MT. Its incorporation with other clinical indicators needs further research.

SCORES UTILISING CLINICAL INDICATORS, ROUTINE LABORATORY TESTS, AND INJURY SCORES

CINCINNATI INDIVIDUAL TRANSFUSION TRIGGERS (CITT)

Looking at the vast number of scoring systems available, Callcut *et al.*[34] hypothesised that it is more important to understand the predictive value of individual variables rather than collate them into a score. Analysing data from ~170 patients requiring immediate surgery after trauma, the study aimed to identify the predictive capabilities of five transfusion triggers, such as:

i.   SBP <90 mmHg,

ii. Hb <11 g/dL,

iii. Temperature <35.5°C,

iv. INR >1.5, and

v.   Base deficit (BD) > 6.

The study demonstrated that an international normalised ratio (INR) value >1.5 indicates the need for an MT of more than 10 units of blood within 6 hours in a patient requiring surgical intervention. INR (OR 11.3, 95% CI 2.7–47) and SBP (OR 8.5, 95% CI 3.4–21) were highly predictive, while temperature was least predictive [OR 3.4 (95% CI 1.5–7.7)].

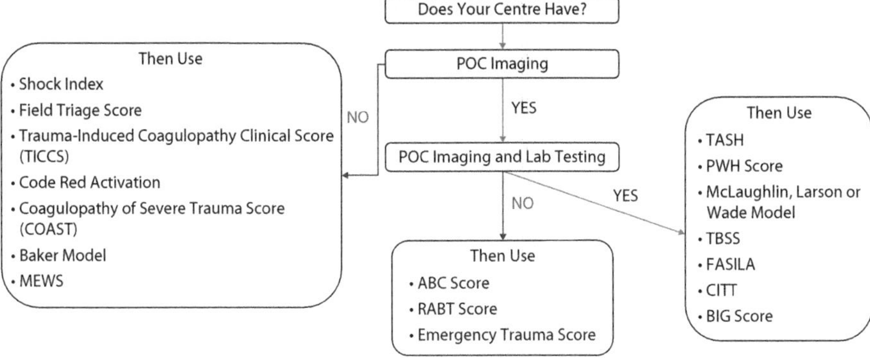

Figure 6.2 Formula for the Moore model.

The study emphasised the need to look at individual transfusion triggers rather than composite scores.

MOORE MODEL

Using retrospective data from 383 patients entered in a prospective multicentre database, the Moore model developed a final predictive model including the following variables: Injury Severity Score (ISS) $\leq$ 25 gives 0 points; ISS > 25 gives 1 point; minimum pH during the first hour of arrival, and minimum systolic blood pressure during the first hour after arrival in mmHg. The values of these variables were entered into a formula to give the probability of MT (see Figure 6.2).

SCHREIBER MODEL

Another military score developed with data from 558 combat victims from Iraq, the Schreiber model[35] identified the following variables:

i. Haemoglobin $\leq$ 11 g/dl,

ii. INR > 1.5, and

iii. Penetrating mechanism of injury.

Haemoglobin $\leq$ 11 g/dl (OR 7.7) was the single best predictor for MT. Using the three variables as a predictive model, the model had a good AUROC of 0.80. The need for the INR value made the model difficult to use quickly upon patient arrival.

VANDROMME SCORE

Vandromme and team attempted to create a predictive model using available triggers from other scoring systems, including the following:

i. Blood lactate $\geq$ 5 mMol/L,

ii. HR > 105 beats/min,

iii. INR > 1.5,

iv. haemoglobin $\leq$ 11g/dL, and

v. SBP <110 mmHg

in a prospective manner.[36] While they could not construct a final predictive model, the best-fit model included three or more positive clinical measures (Sensitivity: 53%, Specificity: 98%, positive predictive value [PPV]: 33%, negative predictive value [NPV]: 99%). There was increased PPV when all clinical measurements were positive (Sensitivity: 9%, Specificity: 100%, PPV: 86%, NPV: 98%).

THE BIG SCORE (BASE DEFICIT, INR, AND GCS SCORE)

The admission base deficit, INR, and GCS, or BIG, score has been shown to predict mortality among paediatric and adult trauma patients.[37] The BIG score was calculated using the following formula: [base deficit + (2.5 × INR) + (15 − GCS)]. A retrospective single-centre study attempted to study the use of the BIG score to predict mortality and MT in 5605 patients. The study showed that the AUROC of the BIG score for MT was 0.84 (95% CI, 0.83–0.85).[38] The need for an admission INR value hampers the use of the score to guide transfusion. However, adding to the previously discussed scores, this remains among the few to consider GCS and associated head injury.

SCORING SYSTEMS AND COAGULOPATHY

Trauma-induced coagulopathy (TIC) is a complex, early onset condition that impairs the body's ability to form stable blood clots after injury. TIC significantly increases the risk of uncontrolled bleeding and is associated with higher mortality in trauma patients.[39] Early identification of coagulopathy is crucial, as timely correction with haemorrhage control and the use of blood products, tranexamic acid, and viscoelastic testing can reduce bleeding and improve outcomes. In this context, the early identification of TIC is likely to become a crucial component of future trauma scoring systems, identifying the need for massive transfusion. At this point, however, the widespread utilisation of scoring systems with POC viscoelastic assay results is limited by availability and cost in low- and middle-income countries (LMICs).

CHALLENGES AND FUTURE PERSPECTIVES

MT management faces challenges due to the lack of a standardised definition and limited usability of scoring systems in LMICs (Tables 6.7 and 6.8). The traditional definition of MT,

Table 6.7 Comparative table of commonly used scoring systems with accuracy, strengths, and limitations

Score	Parameters	Predictive value	Strengths	Limitations
Shock index (SI)	HR/SBP, SI > 0.9	Predicts mortality, MHP activation, haemostatic intervention; SIPA for paediatric transfusion prediction.	Simple and widely used.	Overestimates in obstructive/ cardiogenic shock, less reliable for elderly, hypertensive patients, and those on beta/ calcium blockers.
Field triage score (FTS)	SBP ≤100 mmHg, motor GCS <6	Predicts MHP activation; simpler than RTS.	Easy to apply in military and pre-hospital settings.	Needs refinement for civilian settings; uses proxy SBP (e.g., radial pulse).
TICCS	Severity of injuries, SBP <90 mmHg, and anatomical extent of injuries	Predicts TIC and MT (AUC 0.7, best cutoff ≥12).	Subjectively assessed; validated for blunt injuries.	Limited data for broader applications; subjective nature reduces reproducibility.

(Continued)

Table 6.7   (*Continued*)

Score	Parameters	Predictive value	Strengths	Limitations
Code red activation (CRA)	Active haemorrhage, SBP <90 mmHg, no response to fluid bolus	91% of CRA patients require transfusion; this improves outcomes.	Simple, pragmatic tool; validated retrospectively and prospectively.	Predicts general transfusion needs, not specific to MT.
Coagulopathy of severe trauma (COAST)	Entrapment, temperature, SBP, abdominal/ pelvic injuries, chest decompression	Highly specific (94.2%) but low sensitivity (21.6%) for TIC prediction; MT incidence 15.3% in COAST-positive patients.	High specificity; focuses on TIC.	Low sensitivity; not well-suited for MHP activation.
Baker model	SBP <90 mmHg, GCS <9, HR >120 bpm, high-risk injury mechanism	Transfusion rates: 100% (4 factors), 68% (3 factors), 42% (2 factors), 12% (1 factor), 2% (none).	Effective in trauma centers with detailed pre-hospital injury histories.	Requires accurate injury histories, limiting use in underdeveloped pre-hospital systems.
MEWS	HR, SBP, RR, temperature, AVPU scale	Predicts ICU admission, mortality, and MT for TBI/ polytrauma (AUC 0.80).	Simple; AVPU scale accommodates TBI patients.	Needs further validation for trauma use.
ABC score	HR, SBP, penetrating mechanism, FAST	Predicts MT but overestimates in blunt trauma populations.	Easy to use; validated in multiple centres.	Limitations in blunt trauma populations; retrospective application biases.
TASH	Anatomical injuries, sex, radiology, and laboratory parameters	AUROC: 0.78–0.83; highly predictive of MT in multiple validations.	Comprehensive; validated across various settings.	Complex; depends on rapid POC testing; limited in resource-constrained settings.
Emergency transfusion score (ETS)	Age, primary arrival, mechanism, SBP, FAST, pelvic stability	High NPV (0.998) for transfusion needs in ER settings.	Cost-effective for transfusion prediction in the ER.	Not designed for MT contexts.
Prince of Wales Hospital (PWH) score	Similar to TASH with added GCS	Cut-off ≥6: PPV 82.9%, NPV 96.6%.	Includes GCS, helpful for mentation.	Inferior to TASH; lacks detailed validation for head injuries.
Wade model	SBP, HR, pH, hematocrit	$\pi > 0.5$ predicts MT (PPV 75%, NPV 72%).	Uses a straightforward formula.	Modest specificity; may not generalise well across different populations.

(*Continued*)

Table 6.7 (*Continued*)

Score	Parameters	Predictive value	Strengths	Limitations
McLaughlin score	HR >105 bpm, SBP <110 mmHg, pH <7.25, hematocrit <32%	Incidence of MT: 20% (1 factor), 80% (4 factors).	Simple, strong prediction for MT.	Derived from a single combat hospital dataset; needs broader validation.
Larson score	HR >110 bpm, SBP <110 mmHg, hemoglobin ≤11 g/dl, BD ≤6 mmol/l	Predicts MT with sensitivity 69%, specificity 65%, and incidence of 54% in COAST-positive patients.	Military-focused; decent predictive value.	Limited specificity; moderate sensitivity.
TBSS	Age, SBP after 1L crystalloid, FAST, pelvic fracture, serum lactate	AUC: 0.98; highly predictive for MT (AUROC 0.92 in modified version).	Excellent prediction in the Japanese trauma population.	Population-specific; needs global validation.
FASILA score	FAST, SI, lactate	AUROC: 0.87; developed for abdominal trauma.	Unique to abdominal trauma; simple and specific.	Needs further validation outside the initial study population.
Viscoelastic assays	TEG, ROTEM	Predicts MT with good sensitivity and specificity (AUC 0.83 for clot firmness).	Real-time coagulation analysis aids in MT decisions.	Resource-intensive; integration into clinical workflows requires further study

10 or more units of packed red blood cells (PRBCs) in 24 hours, excludes critically bleeding patients who die early or stabilise without reaching the threshold.

Revised definitions, such as requiring 3–5 PRBCs within 1–6 hours or 4 or more units of blood components within 2 hours, aim to address survivorship bias and align with DCR. Existing scoring systems often rely on complex radiological and POC tests, which are unavailable in many LMIC hospitals.

This reliance delays MHP activation, increasing mortality risk. Systems must instead focus on accessible clinical and POC indicators (see Figure 6.1). Trauma patterns vary widely. High-income countries manage high-velocity injuries in advanced centres, while LMICs face severe blunt trauma and delayed presentations. Smaller hospitals often lack the resources for rapid coagulation tests, which complicates MT activation in these settings. Future systems should incorporate tools such as TEG or ROTEM to enhance predictions. Head injuries, a major cause of trauma, remain understudied in MT contexts. Artificial intelligence shows promise in creating adaptive, locally relevant predictive models for MHP activation. MT scoring success depends on tailoring to local resources, patient patterns, and injury mechanisms. Customisation ensures better outcomes than adopting universal systems, advancing global trauma care.

Table 6.8 Comparative table of some hybrid scoring systems

Model/study	Focus/key	Variables	AUROC	Notes
Callcut (CITT)	Individual transfusion triggers rather than composite scores.	SBP <90 mmHg, Hb <11 g/dL, Temp <35.5°C, INR >1.5, Base Deficit (BD) >6.	INR >1.5 (OR 11.3, CI 2.7–47) and SBP (OR 8.5, CI 3.4–21) were most predictive. Temp was least (OR 3.4).	Highlights the predictive value of individual triggers over composite scoring.
Moore model	Retrospective analysis for developing a predictive MT model.	Injury Severity Score (ISS), minimum pH, and minimum SBP during the first hour.	Generated a probability model for MT using ISS and early arrival vitals.	Uses a formula for MT probability but lacks real-time rapid assessment tools.
Schreiber model	Military model focusing on combat trauma data.	Hb ≤11 g/dL (OR 7.7), INR >1.5, penetrating injury mechanism.	Haemoglobin ≤11 g/dL was the best predictor for MT. Model AUROC = 0.80.	Dependence on INR limits quick usability upon patient arrival.
Vandromme score	Combined variables from existing systems for predictive modelling.	Lactate ≥5 mMol/L, HR >105 bpm, INR >1.5, Hb ≤11 g/dL, SBP <110 mmHg.	Sensitivity: 53%, Specificity: 98%, PPV: 33%, NPV: 99%. Increased PPV when all measurements are positive.	Could not finalise a predictive model; findings had mixed sensitivity and specificity.
BIG score	Predicting mortality and MT in pediatric and adult trauma patients using a composite score.	Base deficit, INR, GCS: [Base Deficit + (2.5 × INR) + (15 - GCS)].	AUROC for MT: 0.84 (95% CI 0.83– 0.85). Incorporates GCS and head injury.	Dependence on INR reduces immediate applicability

CONCLUSION

Multiple scoring systems are currently available to predict the need for MT among trauma patients. However, their use must be personalised from centre to centre. The majority of them use common clinical indicators, and it's always better for trauma centres to develop their scores based on these for their usage.

TAKE-HOME MESSAGE

Selecting the right scoring system to predict the need for MT in trauma depends heavily on the clinical setting, available resources, and the types of injuries encountered. Simple tools like the SI and FTS are easy to apply and work well in pre-hospital or resource-limited environments, but their predictive accuracy is modest, and they perform poorly in older adults, patients on cardiovascular medications, and those with non-haemorrhagic shock. Scores that incorporate anatomical injury patterns or subjective assessments, such as the TICCS, offer some value but suffer from variability and limited generalisability. Activation tools like Code Red are good for identifying patients who need blood early, yet they do not reliably distinguish who will require MT.

REFERENCES

1. Injuries and violence [Internet]. 2024. [cited 2024 Oct 14]. Available from: https://www.who.int/news-room/fact-sheets/detail/injuries-and-violence

2. Eastridge BJ, Holcomb JB, Shackelford S. Outcomes of traumatic hemorrhagic shock and the epidemiology of preventable death from injury. Transfusion. 2019;59(S2):1423–8.

3. Mammen JJ, Asirvatham ES, Lakshmanan J, Sarman CJ, Mani T, Charles B, et al. A national level estimation of population need for blood in India. Transfusion. 2021;61(6):1809–21.

4. El-Menyar A, Mekkodathil A, Abdelrahman H, Latifi R, Galwankar S, Al-Thani H, et al. Review of existing scoring systems for massive blood transfusion in trauma patients: Where do we stand? Shock. 2019 Sept;52(3):288.

5. Allgöwer M, Burri C. "Schockindex" ["Shock index"]. Dtsch Med Wochenschr. 1967;92(43):1947–50. doi:10.1055/s-0028-1106070

6. Acker SN, Ross JT, Partrick DA, Tong S, Bensard DD. Pediatric specific shock index accurately identifies severely injured children. J Pediatr Surg. 2015 Feb;50(2):331–4.

7. Carsetti A, Antolini R, Casarotta E, Damiani E, Gasparri F, Marini B, et al. Shock index as predictor of massive transfusion and mortality in patients with trauma: A systematic review and meta-analysis. Crit Care. 2023 Mar 5;27(1):85.

8. Eastridge BJ, Butler F, Wade CE, Holcomb JB, Salinas J, Champion HR, et al. Field triage score (FTS) in battlefield casualties: Validation of a novel triage technique in a combat environment. Am J Surg. 2010 Dec 1;200(6):724–7.

9. Cancio LC, Wade CE, West SA, Holcomb JB. Prediction of mortality and of the need for massive transfusion in casualties arriving at combat support hospitals in Iraq. J Trauma Acute Care Surg. 2008 Feb;64(2):S51.

10. Tonglet ML, Minon JM, Seidel L, Poplavsky JL, Vergnion M. Prehospital identification of trauma patients with early acute coagulopathy and massive bleeding: Results of a prospective non-interventional clinical trial evaluating the trauma induced coagulopathy clinical score (TICCS). Crit Care. 2014 Nov 26;18(6):648.

11. Tonglet M, Lefering R, Minon JM, Ghuysen A, D'Orio V, Hildebrand F, et al. Prehospital identification of trauma patients requiring transfusion: Results of a retrospective study evaluating the use of the trauma induced coagulopathy clinical score (TICCS) in 33,385 patients from the TraumaRegister DGU®. Acta Chir Belg. 2017 Nov 2;117(6):385–90.

12. Weaver AE, Hunter-Dunn C, Lyon RM, Lockey D, Krogh CL. The effectiveness of a 'Code Red' transfusion request policy initiated by pre-hospital physicians. Injury. 2016;47(1):3–6.

13. Cole E, Weaver A, Gall L, West A, Nevin D, Tallach R, et al. A decade of damage control resuscitation: New transfusion practice, new survivors, new directions. Ann Surg. 2021;273(6):1215.

14. Reed MJ, Glover A, Byrne L, Donald M, McMahon N, Hughes N, et al. Experience of implementing a national pre-hospital code red bleeding protocol in Scotland. Injury. 2017 Jan 1;48(1):41–6.

15. Subbe CP, Kruger M, Rutherford P, Gemmel L. Validation of a modified Early warning score in medical admissions. QJM Mon J Assoc Physicians. 2001 Oct;94(10):521–6.

16. Jiang X, Jiang P, Mao Y. Performance of modified early warning score (MEWS) and circulation, respiration, abdomen, motor, and speech (CRAMS) score in trauma severity and in-hospital mortality prediction in multiple trauma patients: A comparison study. PeerJ. 2019;7:e7227.

17. Kim DK, Lee DH, Lee BK, Cho YS, Ryu SJ, Jung YH, *et al.* Performance of modified early warning score (MEWS) for predicting in-hospital mortality in traumatic brain injury patients. J Clin Med. 2021 Apr 28;10(9):1915.

18. Yu Z, Xu F, Chen D. Predictive value of modified early warning score (MEWS) and revised trauma score (RTS) for the short-term prognosis of emergency trauma patients: A retrospective study. BMJ Open. 2021 Mar 15;11(3):e041882.

19. Nunez TC, Voskresensky IV, Dossett LA, Shinall R, Dutton WD, Cotton BA. Early prediction of massive transfusion in trauma: Simple as ABC (assessment of blood consumption)? J Trauma Acute Care Surg. 2009 Feb;66(2):346.

20. Cotton BA, Dossett LA, Haut ER, Shafi S, Nunez TC, Au BK, *et al.* Multicenter Validation of a simplified score to predict massive transfusion in trauma. J Trauma Acute Care Surg. 2010 July;69(1):S33.

21. Costa A, Carron PN, Zingg T, Roberts I, Ageron FX; for the Swiss Trauma Registry. Early identification of bleeding in trauma patients: External validation of traumatic bleeding scores in the Swiss Trauma Registry. Crit Care. 2022 Sept 28;26(1):296.

22. Motameni AT, Hodge RA, McKinley WI, Georgel JM, Strollo BP, Benns MV, *et al.* The use of ABC score in activation of massive transfusion: The yin and the yang. J Trauma Acute Care Surg. 2018 Aug;85(2):298.

23. Joseph B, Khan M, Truitt M, Jehan F, Kulvatunyou N, Azim A, *et al.* Massive transfusion: The revised assessment of bleeding and transfusion (RABT) score. World J Surg. 2018;42(11):1.

24. D'Souza K, Norman M, Greene A, Finney CJF, Yan MTS, Trudeau JD, *et al.* Prediction of massive transfusion with the revised assessment of bleeding and transfusion (RABT) score at Canadian level I trauma centers. Injury. 2023 Jan 1;54(1):19–24.

25. Yücel N, Lefering R, Maegele M, Vorweg M, Tjardes T, Ruchholtz S, *et al.* Trauma associated severe hemorrhage (TASH)-score: Probability of mass transfusion as surrogate for life threatening hemorrhage after multiple trauma. J Trauma Acute Care Surg. 2006 June;60(6):1228.

26. Mitra B, Rainer TH, Cameron PA. Predicting massive blood transfusion using clinical scores post-trauma. Vox Sang. 2012;102(4):324–30.

27. Maegele M, Lefering R, Wafaisade A, Theodorou P, Wutzler S, Fischer P, *et al.* Revalidation and update of the TASH-score: A scoring system to predict the probability for massive transfusion as a surrogate for life-threatening haemorrhage after severe injury. Vox Sang. 2011;100(2):231–8.

28. Shih AW, Al Khan S, Wang AYH, Dawe P, Young PY, Greene A, *et al.* Systematic reviews of scores and predictors to trigger activation of massive transfusion protocols. J Trauma Acute Care Surg. 2019 Sept;87(3):717.

29. McLaughlin DF, Niles SE, Salinas J, Perkins JG, Cox ED, Wade CE, *et al.* A predictive model for massive transfusion in combat casualty patients. J Trauma Acute Care Surg. 2008 Feb;64(2):S57.

30. Ogura T, Nakamura Y, Nakano M, Izawa Y, Nakamura M, Fujizuka K, *et al.* Predicting the need for massive transfusion in trauma patients: The traumatic bleeding severity score. J Trauma Acute Care Surg. 2014 May;76(5):1243.

31. Ogura T, Lefor AK, Masuda M, Kushimoto S. Modified traumatic bleeding severity score: Early determination of the need for massive transfusion. Am J Emerg Med. 2016 June 1;34(6):1097–101.

32. Leemann H, Lustenberger T, Talving P, Kobayashi L, Bukur M, Brenni M, *et al.* The role of rotation thromboelastometry in early prediction of massive transfusion. J Trauma Acute Care Surg. 2010 Dec;69(6):1403.

33. Davenport R, Manson J, De'Ath H, Platton S, Coates A, Allard S, *et al.* Functional definition and characterization of acute traumatic coagulopathy. Crit Care Med. 2011;39(12):2652.

34. Callcut RA, Johannigman JA, Kadon KS, Hanseman DJ, Robinson BRH. All massive transfusion criteria are not created equal: Defining the predictive value of individual transfusion triggers to better determine who benefits from blood. J Trauma Acute Care Surg. 2011 Apr;70(4):794.

35. Schreiber MA, Perkins J, Kiraly L, Underwood S, Wade C, Holcomb JB. Early predictors of massive transfusion in combat casualties. J Am Coll Surg. 2007 Oct;205(4):541.

36. Vandromme MJ, Griffin RL, Mcgwin G, Weinberg JA, Rue LW, Kerby JD. Prospective identification of patients at risk for massive transfusion: An imprecise endeavor. Am Surg. 2011 Feb 1;77(2):155–61.

37. Brockamp T, Maegele M, Gaarder C, Goslings JC, Cohen MJ, Lefering R, *et al.* Comparison of the predictive performance of the BIG, TRISS, and PS09 score in an adult trauma population derived from multiple international trauma registries. Crit Care. 2013 Nov 16;17(4):R134.

38. Park S, Wang IJ, Yeom SR, Park SW, Cho SJ, Yang WT, *et al.* Usefulness of the BIG score in predicting massive transfusion and in-hospital death in adult trauma patients. Emerg Med Int. 2023 Oct17:5162050.

39. Mitra B, Cameron PA, Mori A, Maini A, Fitzgerald M, Paul E, *et al.* Early prediction of acute traumatic coagulopathy. Resuscitation. 2011 Sept 1;82(9):1208–13.

TRAUMA-INDUCED COAGULOPATHY

DOI: 10.1201/9781003711070-7

Chapter 7.1: Management Strategies

Sharmishtha Pathak and Babita Gupta

INTRODUCTION

Trauma-induced mortality is a major global health burden, and uncontrolled haemorrhage is one of the most preventable causes of death in these patients.[1] Patients with major haemorrhage present with coagulopathy at the time of presentation to the emergency.

There are several causes for worsening coagulopathy in trauma patients presenting with massive haemorrhage:

i. Consumption of coagulation factors and platelets for clot formation to prevent blood loss

ii. Dilution due to resuscitation with normal saline, crystalloids, and red blood cell transfusion

iii. Hormonal changes, like an increase in vasopressin and adrenaline, and an increased generation of cytokines

iv. Hypoxia, acidosis, and hypothermia predispose to haemostatic defects by impairing the functional ability of platelets, coagulation proteases fall in thrombin generation, and accelerating fibrinolysis.

There has been a significant change in the transfusion support in coagulopathic patients over the last decade, and the recent guidelines and literature suggest early use of high ratios of plasma and platelet components along with red blood cells and limiting colloids and crystalloids, which is known as haemostatic resuscitation.[2] Severely injured patients are more prone to coagulopathy. About 25% of severely injured trauma patients present with haemorrhagic shock and require transfusions and are at risk of coagulopathy, which increases their mortality.[3] Early identification of those patients in coagulopathy will prevent the vicious cycle of hypothermia, acidosis, and bleeding.

Various organisations and expert panels have developed guidelines and consensus statements to standardise the management of trauma-induced coagulopathy (TIC). These documents are essential references for trauma care providers and offer evidence-based recommendations for managing coagulopathy in trauma patients.

MANAGEMENT OF TIC

Damage control haemostatic interventions are essential to cease TIC progression. They include permissive hypotension to minimise fluid infusion and dilution of coagulation factors, early administration of tranexamic acid (TXA) to limit the production of plasmin and reduce fibrinolysis, and early activation of massive haemorrhage protocols (MHPs) employing a balanced transfusion strategy of red blood cells, plasma, and platelets in a predetermined ratio.[4-6] Based on pathophysiology, replacing fibrinogen and calcium as essential components of the coagulation cascade is also necessary. Correcting hypothermia and acidosis helps in facilitating enzymatic coagulation reactions. After the bleeding has ceased, prevention of thrombotic events due to hypercoagulability from late TIC is indicated. Thromboprophylaxis within 24 hours from haemostasis is recommended, provided there is no contraindication.[7,8]

PRE-HOSPITAL CARE

Preventing the progression of haemorrhage to haemorrhagic shock is the primary goal for the initial management of TIC. This is achieved by arresting the bleeding and restoring circulating blood volume. Effective strategies that can be employed in the pre-hospital setting include the use of tourniquets and direct compression of bleeding wounds to slow haemorrhage. Pre-hospital health care providers must also initiate resuscitation of the critically ill patient with traumatic injury to increase intravascular volume to preserve organ perfusion.[9,10] The fluids administered in the pre-hospital setting can significantly help the patient, but can also be potentially harmful. Resuscitation using large volumes of crystalloids may increase the blood pressure but at the cost of exacerbating coagulopathy and clot dislodgement if raised too rapidly. High-volume crystalloid resuscitation has the added risk of hyperfibrinolysis upon presentation to the hospital and is associated with morbidity.[11] Thus, due to the potential problem of coagulopathy, a permissive hypotensive strategy is advocated in actively bleeding patients until definitive bleeding control can be achieved. However, the optimal level of hypotension remains to be established, particularly in patients with associated traumatic brain injury (TBI).[12] Additional therapies in the pre-hospital setting, including transfusion of blood products and TXA are being studied.

HOSPITAL CARE

Globally, there is no accepted single protocol for the treatment of severe traumatic haemorrhage, which is probably due to the difference in availability of resources and the difference in types of injuries received at various centres. However, when resources are available, most guidelines recommend transfusion of high ratios of plasma to red blood cells (RBCs), restricted use of crystalloids, permissive hypotension until active bleeding is controlled (except in the setting of TBI), and goal-directed haemostatic resuscitation with blood components and antifibrinolytics once laboratory test results are available. While European guidelines recommend restricted, balanced crystalloids with inotropic agents to restore volume, and fibrinogen and prothrombin complex concentrate (PCC) to provide clotting factors (provided fibrinogen levels are normal and PCC is given based on viscoelastic haemostatic assay (VHA) showing evidence of delayed coagulation initiation).[9] Figure 7.1.1 describes the management of a bleeding trauma victim in the Emergency Department (ED), and the following section will discuss each aspect in detail.

MASSIVE HAEMORRHAGE PROTOCOLS (MHPS)

The patients who arrive at the hospital in overt haemorrhagic shock must receive empirical blood product resuscitation to restore circulating blood volume and thereby attenuate the development of worsening coagulopathy. It represents a balanced resuscitative strategy for rapid delivery of large volumes of blood products in a pre-defined ratio for the treatment of haemorrhagic shock. There is no single correct strategy, and as such individual institutions differ widely in the trigger threshold for initiation of the massive transfusion protocols as well as the predefined ratios of blood products. The ratio of plasma to RBCs for transfusion remains controversial. The only randomised controlled trial (RCT) evaluating 1:1 and 1:2 ratios demonstrated no benefit in survival with the 1:1 ratio, but suggested a shorter time to haemostasis in this group. It is important to understand that these improved outcomes are limited to patients with severe traumatic injury undergoing a massive transfusion, and there is evidence that patients with less severe traumatic injury who receive a massive transfusion may be harmed by these protocols.

The PROMMTT study demonstrated improved 24-hour survival with transfusions of higher ratios of plasma and platelets at an early stage in resuscitation. The 2015 multicentre PROPPR trial found no difference in the 24-hour or 30-day mortality between a 1:1:1 ratio vs. a 1:1:2 ratio of plasma to platelets to RBCs transfused. However, the group that received a 1:1:1 ratio was more likely to achieve haemostasis and less likely to die from exsanguination. Coagulation factor concentrates are being increasingly used as an alternative to fresh frozen

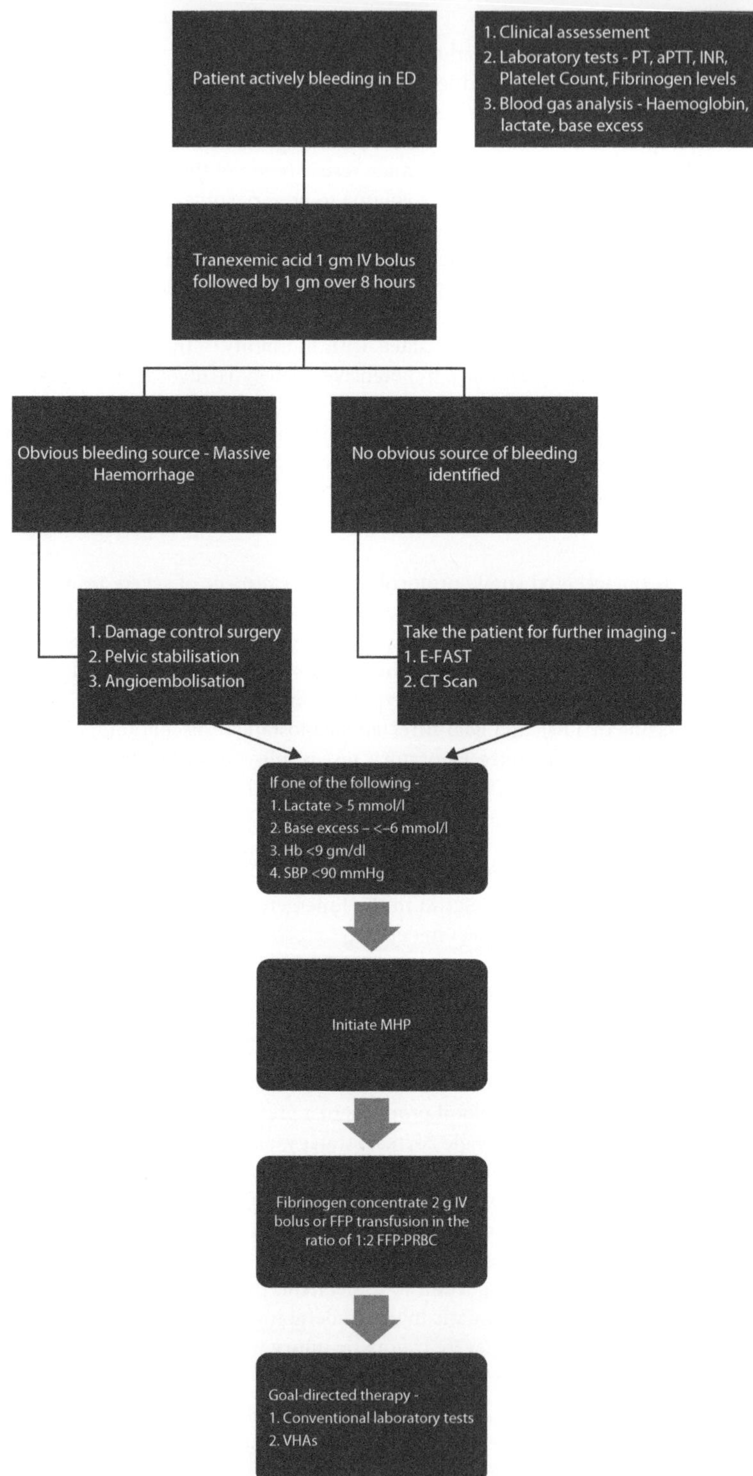

Figure 7.1.1 Management of actively bleeding patients in the emergency department.

plasma (FFP) for correction of TIC.[13,14] Cryoprecipitate or fibrinogen and platelets should be administered if the patient requires >4 units of RBCs before laboratory results are available.[15] A significant concern with the use of large volumes of blood products is the potential for transfusion-associated circulatory overload and transfusion-related acute lung injury.

GOAL-DIRECTED TRANSFUSION

The heterogeneous nature of trauma necessitates treatment that is targeted to the individual patient's needs. Theoretically, an approach tailored for each patient theoretically guides may be more beneficial in contrast to a universal transfusion protocol. Goal-directed therapy is a Grade 1B recommendation in the recent European guidelines. Studies have shown that a change in approach by means of using a goal-directed transfusion with the help of point of care tests has improved patient outcomes. The interim analysis of the Strategy of Transfusion in Trauma (STATA) trial, which compared a fixed ratio transfusion (1:1:1) to a thromboelastography (TEG)-guided administration of coagulation factor concentrates and fibrinogen in patients with major trauma, revealed no difference in mortality.[9,16]

TRANEXAMIC ACID

The CRASH-2[17] trial demonstrated that the use of TXA in adult trauma victims was associated with a reduction in all-cause mortality. Subsequent analysis also revealed that use beyond 3 hours was associated with increased risk of death due to bleeding. International guidelines recommend its use within the first 3 hours following trauma. However, the recently concluded Prehospital Tranexamic Acid for Severe Trauma (PATCH) trial did not find any difference in the number of patients surviving with a favourable functional outcome at the end of 6 months.[18,19] Use of TXA is associated with the potential risk of venous thromboembolism (VTE) and studies have suggested an association with increased VTE rates. Theoretically, TXA, as an antifibrinolytic drug, could increase the incidence of post-injury fibrinolysis shutdown. TXA should be administered early and probably not to patients with evidence of fibrinolysis shutdown. Studies on the administration of TXA to non-trauma haemorrhage have indicated a significant increase in VTE over 24 hours. By contrast, the CRASH-2 and CRASH-3 trials done on trauma patients fail to report any increase in the incidence of VTE. These trials, however, have been criticised for reporting lower VTE, which is probably due to the low rate of patients who actually required transfusion and lack of VTE screening. Although their findings are also resonated by the PATCH trial, where the incidence of venoocclusive disease did not differ between the TXA group and the placebo group. On the other hand, STAAMP and Prehospital TXA for TBI trials had substantially higher VTE rates.[13,14,19]

USE OF BICARBONATE

Bicarbonate should be given only if severe acidosis persists despite resuscitation, as bicarbonate therapy is ineffective or rather harmful, owing to excess HCO3-derived CO_2, which is highly soluble across cell membranes, causing a cellular respiratory acidosis not reflected in arterial pH or $PaCO_2$ measurements.

COAGULATION FACTOR CONCENTRATES

The use of coagulation factor concentrates as first-line therapy enables faster correction and reduces the volume of blood products transfused, with a potential for fewer side effects from plasma administration.

FIBRINOGEN CONCENTRATE

Early use of fibrinogen concentrate has been explored in the fibrinogen in the initial resuscitation of severe trauma (FiiRST) trial. This randomised, placebo-controlled feasibility study of 50 hypotensive trauma patients showed increased plasma fibrinogen levels in the fibrinogen concentrate group, with 96% of subjects receiving the intervention within

1 hour.[20] The Reversal of Trauma-Induced Coagulopathy (RETIC) trial compared the use of FFP with fibrinogen concentrate. The study included adult patients with major trauma who had coagulopathy identified using rotational thromboelastometry (ROTEM). The harmful effect of massive transfusion in the plasma arm led to early termination of the trial. However, in both trials, targeted use of fibrinogen concentrates was associated with earlier correction of coagulopathy, reduced transfusion of blood products and decreased rate of massive transfusion.[21,22] In the Fibrinogen Early in Severe Trauma study (FEISTY), it was found that the administration of fibrinogen concentrate helped in achieving the appropriate fibrinogen levels much faster than the group which received cryoprecipitate. Although the level was reached faster, the ultimate values were equal for both the groups, and thus further studies are warranted for same.[23] The CRYOSTAT-2 trial studied the role of cryoprecipitate administration in trauma patients requiring activation of MHP and found that there was no role of empirical high-dose cryoprecipitate administration in reducing the 28-day mortality.[24]

SPECIAL CONSIDERATIONS

Trauma patients who present with occult bleeding but are otherwise compensated pose a different challenge in resuscitation. A common source for bleeding in trauma victims is injury to the solid abdominal organs. Targeted resuscitation of these patients is an important approach, as most transition to a hypercoagulable state by 24–48 hours. TBI poses unique challenges in the management of coagulation. Skull being a fixed space warrants a more aggressive approach to obtain timely haemostasis to avoid intracranial hypertension. The CRASH-3 study identified a survival benefit of early TXA administration in patients with mild-to-moderate but not severe TBI.[13] One major challenge in TBI-associated TIC is the use of pharmacological prophylaxis against VTE. The transition to hypercoagulability after injury poses a major clinical threat, with high VTE rates noted in patients who have TBI. The decision to initiate anticoagulation to prevent post-injury clotting and thrombotic complications needs to be weighed against the risk of exacerbating bleeding.

FURTHER AND UPCOMING RESEARCH

A lot of research is being conducted in the field of trauma to minimise bleeding and its associated problems. CRASH-4 trial is presently underway in mild TBI patients to understand the role of TXA administration in these patients.[23] FEISTY Junior[24] is a study being undertaken for paediatric patients with severe trauma to analyse the effects of the administration of fibrinogen concentrate early to trauma victims. More investigations are needed into the role of inflammation, the mechanisms of hypercoagulability and organ dysfunction during late TIC. A better understanding of the complex and dynamic pathophysiology of TIC may help reduce potentially preventable deaths due to trauma-induced shock and organ dysfunction in the future.

THERAPEUTIC TARGETS EMERGING FROM PATHOPHYSIOLOGY

Improved understanding of TIC has identified several promising molecular and cellular pathways for therapeutic intervention.

PROTECTION OF THE ENDOTHELIAL GLYCOCALYX

The endothelial glycocalyx plays a crucial role in vascular permeability and coagulation regulation. Damage to this structure contributes significantly to TIC pathogenesis. Emerging therapies focus on preserving glycocalyx integrity:

i. *Ascorbic Acid:* A randomised controlled trial has shown that high-dose intravenous vitamin C reduces glycocalyx degradation and improves microvascular perfusion in septic shock patients by lowering the perfused boundary region, a marker of glycocalyx shedding.[25]

ii. *Hydrocortisone:* Animal models of acute pancreatitis demonstrated that hydrocortisone preserves intestinal capillary endothelial glycocalyx, maintaining vascular barrier function and reducing tissue edema.[26,27]

iii. *Albumin:* Acting as a colloid and molecular carrier, albumin supports oncotic pressure and scavenges reactive oxygen species, thereby stabilising glycocalyx structure and enhancing microcirculatory flow.[28]

iv. *Plasma-based Resuscitation:* Compared to crystalloids, plasma infusion has shown superior endothelial protection in a pneumosepsis model, likely due to reduced fluid overload and preserved glycocalyx composition.[29,30]

MODULATION OF THE PROTEIN C PATHWAY

Thrombomodulin and protein C are central to anticoagulant and anti-inflammatory processes. Targeting this axis offers dual benefits in TIC:

i. *Recombinant Thrombomodulin (rTM):* Clinical use of rTM combined with antithrombin has demonstrated efficacy in lowering mortality in sepsis-associated disseminated intravascular coagulation (DIC) without increasing bleeding risk.[31]

ii. *Solulin (a thrombomodulin analogue):* In preclinical stroke models, Solulin improved reperfusion and reduced infarct size, supporting its therapeutic potential in thrombotic settings.[32]

iii. *VhH Anti-Thrombomodulin Antibodies:* These agents inhibit thrombin-activatable fibrinolysis inhibitor (TAFI) activation and enhance fibrinolysis under flow conditions *in vitro*, offering a novel, targeted strategy to rebalance coagulation in TIC.[33]

Targeting Neutrophil Extracellular Traps (NETs) and Damage-Associated Molecular Patterns (DAMPs): Both NETs and DAMPs contribute to immune-thrombotic complications in TIC:

i. *NET Inhibition:* NET formation has been implicated in deep vein thrombosis and systemic inflammatory injury. Therapeutic approaches aiming to inhibit NETosis or enhance NET clearance may reduce thrombotic burden.[34,35]

ii. *DAMP Modulation:* DAMPs activate innate immune pathways via Toll-like receptors (TLRs), perpetuating systemic inflammation and coagulopathy. Intervening in these signalling cascades may attenuate endothelial and coagulation disturbances.[36]

Complement Pathway Inhibition: Excessive activation of the complement system, particularly the C5a–C5aR1 axis, plays a key role in immunothrombosis:

i. *C5a Blockade:* C5a enhances NET formation by inhibiting mitochondrial STAT3, promoting thrombosis. Inhibition of C5a may reduce microvascular thrombus formation and improve organ perfusion in critical illness.[37]

ii. *C5aR1 Targeting:* Clinical studies show that blocking the interaction between C5a and its receptor reduces platelet aggregation and endothelial injury in disorders such as atypical hemolytic uremic syndrome (aHUS) and COVID-19–related coagulopathy.[38,39]

Collectively, these targeted strategies offer promising avenues for improving outcomes in TIC by modulating core pathophysiological processes such as endothelial dysfunction, thromboinflammation, and dysregulated fibrinolysis.

FUTURE DIRECTIONS: PERSONALISED COAGULOPATHY MANAGEMENT

Emerging technologies promise to take TIC management into the era of precision medicine:

i. Point of care genomics and proteomics to rapidly profile coagulation and inflammatory status.

ii. Artificial intelligence models integrating trauma severity, labs, and viscoelastic data to guide therapy in real time.

iii. Nanotechnology-based diagnostics for earlier detection of endothelial injury or DAMP release.

Ultimately, the future lies in early identification, continuous monitoring, and adaptive treatment algorithms based on evolving patient-specific data, improving outcomes through timely and personalised interventions.

CONCLUSION

A greater understanding of TIC, coupled with advances in point-of-care coagulation testing and availability of coagulation factors and fibrinogen concentrates, allows the clinician to employ a goal-directed approach to massive transfusion, as opposed to traditional fixed-ratio approaches. However, to achieve the best outcomes, hospitals need to tailor their approaches according to available resources, provide adequate training and establish local guidelines or algorithms.

TAKE-HOME MESSAGE

Managing trauma-induced coagulopathy works best when resuscitation is balanced and guided by real-time coagulation testing. Using blood and blood products in fixed ratios, along with cryoprecipitate or factor concentrates when viscoelastic assays indicate a need, helps restore clotting effectively. Early TXA use has been shown to improve outcomes in bleeding trauma patients and should be given as soon as possible when indicated.

REFERENCES

1. O'Donovan S, van den Heuvel C, Baldock M, Byard RW. Causes of fatalities in motor vehicle occupants: An overview. Forensic Sci Med Pathol. 2022;18(4):511–5.

2. Pfeifer R, Tarkin IS, Rocos B, Pape H-C. Patterns of mortality and causes of death in polytrauma patients—Has anything changed? Injury. 2009;40(9):907–11.

3. Brohi K, Cohen MJ, Ganter MT, Schultz MJ, Levi M, Mackersie RC, Pittet JF. Acute coagulopathy of trauma: Hypoperfusion induces systemic anticoagulation and hyperfibrinolysis. J Trauma. 2008 May;64(5):1211–7. doi: 10.1097/TA.0b013e318169cd3c; discussion 1217

4. Roberts I. Tranexamic acid in trauma: How should we use it? J Thromb Haemost. 2015;13:S195–9.

5. Kudo D, Yoshida Y, Kushimoto S. Permissive hypotension/hypotensive resuscitation and restricted/controlled resuscitation in patients with severe trauma. J Intensive Care. 2017;5(1):11.

6. Gaski IA, Naess PA, Baksaas-Aasen K, Skaga NO, Gaarder C. Achieving balanced transfusion early in critically bleeding trauma patients: An observational study exploring the effect of attending trauma surgical presence during resuscitation. Trauma Surg Acute Care Open. 2023;8(1):e001160.

7. Kleinveld DJB, Hamada SR, Sandroni C. Trauma-Induced coagulopathy. Intensive Care Med. 2022;48(11):1642–5.

8. Polderman KH. Hypothermia and coagulation. Crit Care. 2012;16(Suppl 2):A20. doi:10.1186/cc11278

9. Rossaint R, Afshari A, Bouillon B, Cerny V, Cimpoesu D, Curry N. The European guideline on management of major bleeding and coagulopathy following trauma : Sixth edition. Crit Care. 2023;1–45.

10. Coccolini F, Pizzilli G, Corbella D, Sartelli M, Agnoletti V, Agostini V, et al. Pre-hospital plasma in haemorrhagic shock management: Current opinion and meta-analysis of randomized trials. World J Emerg Surg. 2019;14:6.

11. Guyette FX, Sperry JL, Peitzman AB, Billiar TR, Daley BJ, Miller RS, et al. Prehospital blood product and crystalloid resuscitation in the severely injured patient: A secondary analysis of the prehospital air medical plasma trial. Ann Surg. 2021 Feb 1;273(2):358–64.

12. Rauch S, Marzolo M, Cappello TD, Ströhle M, Mair P, Pietsch U, et al. Severe traumatic brain injury and hypotension is a frequent and lethal combination in multiple trauma patients in mountain areas - An analysis of the prospective international alpine trauma registry. Scand J Trauma Resusc Emerg Med. 2021 Apr 30;29(1):61.

13. Guyette FX, Brown JB, Zenati MS, Early-Young BJ, Adams PW, Eastridge BJ, et al. Tranexamic acid during prehospital transport in patients at risk for hemorrhage after injury: A double-blind, placebo-controlled, randomized clinical trial. JAMA Surg. 2021 Jan 1;156(1):11–20.

14. Nascimento B, Callum J, Tien H, Peng H, Rizoli S, Karanicolas P, et al. Fibrinogen in the initial resuscitation of severe trauma (FiiRST): A randomized feasibility trial. Br J Anaesth. 2016 Dec;117(6):775–82.

15. Nunns GR, Moore EE, Stettler GR, Moore HB, Ghasabyan A, Cohen M, et al. Empiric transfusion strategies during life-threatening hemorrhage. Surgery. 2018 Aug;164(2):306–11.

16. Dos Reis Rodrigues R, Oliveira R, Lucena L, Paiva H, Cordeiro V, Carmona MJ, et al. STATA - Strategy of transfusion in trauma patients: A randomized. Trial. J Clin Trials. 2016;06(05).

17. Roberts I, Shakur H, Coats T, Hunt B, Balogun E, Barnetson L, et al. The CRASH-2 trial: A randomised controlled trial and economic evaluation of the effects of tranexamic acid on death, vascular occlusive events and transfusion requirement in bleeding trauma patients. Health Technol Assess. 2013;17(10):1–79. doi:10.3310/hta17100

18. PATCH-Trauma Investigators and the ANZICS Clinical Trials Group, Gruen RL, Mitra B, et al. Prehospital tranexamic acid for severe trauma. N Engl J Med. 2023;389(2): 127–36. doi:10.1056/NEJMoa2215457

19. CRASH-3 Trial Collaborators. Effects of tranexamic acid on death, disability, vascular occlusive events and other morbidities in patients with acute traumatic brain injury (CRASH-3): A randomised, placebo-controlled trial. Lancet. 2019;394(10210):1713–23. doi:10.1016/S0140-6736(19)32233-0

20. Innerhofer P, Fries D, Mittermayr M, Innerhofer N, von Langen D, Hell T, et al. Reversal of trauma-induced coagulopathy using first-line coagulation factor concentrates or fresh frozen plasma (RETIC): A single-centre, parallel-group, open-label, randomised trial. Lancet Haematol. 2017 Jun;4(6):e258–71.

21. Winearls J, Wullschleger M, Wake E, McQuilten Z, Reade M, Hurn C, *et al.* Fibrinogen early in severe trauma study (FEISTY): Results from an Australian multicentre randomised controlled pilot trial. Crit Care Resusc. 2021 Mar;23(1):32–46.

22. Davenport R, Curry N, Fox EE, Thomas H, Lucas J, Evans A, *et al.* Early and empirical high-dose cryoprecipitate for hemorrhage after traumatic injury: The CRYOSTAT-2 randomized clinical trial. JAMA. 2023 Nov 21;330(19):1882–91.

23. Protocol_C4_v1.1_04Nov20_Final. CRASH-4 protocol v1.1 [Internet]. London: London School of Hygiene & Tropical Medicine; 2020 [cited 2025 Feb 11]. Available from: https://crash4.lshtm.ac.uk/wp-content/uploads/2021/01/Protocol_C4_v1.1_04Nov20_Final.pdf

24. George S, Wake E, Jansen M, Roy J, Maconachie S, Paasilahti A, *et al.* Fibrinogen early in severe paediatric trauma studY (FEISTY junior): Protocol for a randomised controlled trial. BMJ Open. 2022;12(5):e057780. doi:10.1136/bmjopen-2021-057780. Published 2022 May 4.

25. Belousoviene E, Pranskuniene Z, Vaitkaitiene E, Pilvinis V, Pranskunas A. Effect of high-dose intravenous ascorbic acid on microcirculation and endothelial glycocalyx during sepsis and septic shock: A double-blind, randomized, placebo-controlled study. BMC Anesthesiol. 2023;23(1):309. doi:10.1186/s12871-023-02265-z. Published 2023 Sep 12.

26. Gao SL, Zhang Y, Zhang SY, Liang ZY, Yu WQ, Liang TB. The hydrocortisone protection of glycocalyx on the intestinal capillary endothelium during severe acute pancreatitis. Shock. 2015;43(5):512–7. doi:10.1097/SHK.0000000000000326

27. Chappell D, Jacob M, Hofmann-Kiefer K, Bruegger D, Rehm M, Conzen P, *et al.* Hydrocortisone preserves the vascular barrier by protecting the endothelial glycocalyx. Anesthesiology. 2007;107(5):776–84. doi:10.1097/01.anes.0000286984.39328.96

28. Aldecoa C, Llau JV, Nuvials X, Artigas A. Role of albumin in the preservation of endothelial glycocalyx integrity and the microcirculation: A review. Ann Intensive Care. 2020;10(1):85. doi:10.1186/s13613-020-00697-1. Published 2020 Jun 22.

29. van den Brink DP, Kleinveld DJB, Polet CA, Veltman H, Roelofs JJTH, Weber NC, *et al.* Plasma attenuates endothelial injury compared to crystalloids in a ventilated rat pneumosepsis model. PLoS One. 2025;20(2):e0319272. doi:10.1371/journal.pone.0319272. Published 2025 Feb 25.

30. Milford EM, Reade MC. Resuscitation fluid choices to preserve the endothelial glycocalyx. Crit Care. 2019;23(1):77. doi:10.1186/s13054-019-2369-x. Published 2019 Mar 9.

31. Su EJ, Geyer M, Wahl M, Mann K, Ginsburg D, Brohmann H, *et al.* The thrombomodulin analog solulin promotes reperfusion and reduces infarct volume in a thrombotic stroke model. J Thromb Haemost. 2011;9(6):1174–82. doi:10.1111/j.1538-7836.2011.04269.x

32. Iba T, Hagiwara A, Saitoh D, Anan H, Ueki Y, Sato K, *et al.* Effects of combination therapy using antithrombin and thrombomodulin for sepsis-associated disseminated intravascular coagulation. Ann Intensive Care. 2017;7(1):110. doi:10.1186/s13613-017-0332-z. Published 2017 Nov 2.

33. van Moorsel MVA, Poolen GC, Koekman CA, Verhoef S, de Maat S, Barendrecht A, *et al.* VhH anti-thrombomodulin clone 1 inhibits TAFI activation and enhances fibrinolysis in human whole blood under flow. J Thromb Haemost. 2022;20(5):1213–22. doi:10.1111/jth.15674

34. Yao M, Ma J, Wu D, Fang C, Wang Z, Guo T, *et al.* Neutrophil extracellular traps mediate deep vein thrombosis: From mechanism to therapy. Front Immunol. 2023;14:1198952. doi:10.3389/fimmu.2023.1198952. Published 2023 Aug 23.

35. Retter A, Singer M, Annane D. "The NET effect": Neutrophil extracellular traps-a potential key component of the dysregulated host immune response in sepsis. Crit Care. 2025;29(1):59. doi:10.1186/s13054-025-05283-0. Published 2025 Feb 4.

36. Piccinini AM, Midwood KS. DAMPening inflammation by modulating TLR signalling. Mediators Inflamm. 2010;2010:672395. doi:10.1155/2010/672395

37. Li J, Liu B. The roles and potential therapeutic implications of C5a in the pathogenesis of COVID-19-associated coagulopathy. Cytokine Growth Factor Rev. 2021;58:75–81. doi:10.1016/j.cytogfr.2020.12.001

38. Aiello S, Gastoldi S, Galbusera M, Ruggenenti P, Portalupi V, Rota S, et al. C5a and C5aR1 are key drivers of microvascular platelet aggregation in clinical entities spanning from aHUS to COVID-19. Blood Adv. 2022;6(3):866–81. doi:10.1182/bloodadvances.2021005246. Erratum in: Blood Adv. 2022 May 10;6(9):2812. doi: 10.1182/bloodadvances.2022007722]

39. Chen Y, Li X, Lin X, Liang H, Liu X, Zhang X, et al. Complement C5a induces the generation of neutrophil extracellular traps by inhibiting mitochondrial STAT3 to promote the development of arterial thrombosis. Thromb J. 2022;20(1):24. doi:10.1186/s12959-022-00384-0. Published 2022 Apr 29.

Chapter 7.2: Transfusion Management

Aparna Krishna, Venencia Albert, and Arulselvi Subramanian

INTRODUCTION

Mortality following traumatic injury is a major global health burden, and uncontrolled hemorrhage is one of the most preventable causes of death in these patients.[1] Patients with major hemorrhage present with coagulopathy at the time of presentation to the emergency.

There are several causes for worsening coagulopathy in trauma patients presenting with massive hemorrhage:

i. Consumption of coagulation factors and platelets for clot formation to prevent blood loss

ii. Dilution due to resuscitation with normal saline, crystalloids, and red blood cell transfusion

iii. Hormonal changes like an increase in vasopressin and adrenaline and increased generation of cytokines

iv. Hypoxia, acidosis, and hypothermia predispose to hemostatic defects by impairing the functional ability of platelets, coagulation proteases fall in thrombin generation, and accelerating fibrinolysis.

There has been a significant change in the transfusion support in coagulopathic patients over the last decade, and the recent guidelines and literature suggest early use of high ratios of plasma and platelet components along with red blood cells and limiting colloids and crystalloids, which is known as hemostatic resuscitation.[2] Severely injured patients are more prone to coagulopathy. They present with hemorrhagic shock and require transfusions and are at risk of coagulopathy, which increases their mortality. Early identification of those patients in coagulopathy will prevent the vicious cycle of hypothermia, acidosis, and bleeding.

HEMOSTATIC RESUSCITATION

The aim of component-based hemostatic resuscitation is to correct coagulopathy, reduce bleeding and clinical complications, and improve overall survival.

LIMITING CRYSTALLOID THERAPY

The latest recommendation is that fluid therapy with 0.9% normal saline or balanced crystalloid solution may be started in hypotensive bleeding trauma patients, and the use of colloids should be restricted as they are known to have adverse effects on hemostasis. Hypotonic solutions like Ringer's lactate may be avoided in patients with severe head trauma to minimize the fluid shift into damaged cerebral tissue.[3]

PACKED RED BLOOD CELL TRANSFUSION

Packed red blood cell (PRBC) transfusion improves arterial oxygen-carrying capacity and restores adequate circulating volume in hemorrhagic shock resuscitation in patients presenting with hemorrhagic shock. The latest European guidelines recommend a hemoglobin of 7–9 g/dl in trauma patients.[4] There is a risk of acute ischemia in traumatic brain injury (TBI) patients with acute anemia. Recent meta-analysis shows that neurological outcome is better in those with a hemoglobin threshold 7 g/dl when compared to 10 g/dl. When blood loss is massive and there is no time for pretransfusion testing, which involves blood grouping and crossmatching, O red blood cells (RBCs) and AB plasma products are issued until the blood group of the patient is known. Women of childbearing age should receive D-negative PRBCs if their blood type is not known or if they are D-negative. Men and older women may receive D-positive PRBCs if D-negative PRBCs are not available or if the inventory is low.

FRESH FROZEN PLASMA TRANSFUSION

In the initial management of patients with massive hemorrhage, fresh frozen plasma (FFP) or pathogen-inactivated FFP in an FFP/PRBC ratio of at least 1:2 is recommended. According to the PROPPR trial, early FFP, platelets, and PRBCs in a 1:1:1 ratio improved hemostasis and decreased 24-hour and 30-day mortality.[5,6] Many studies are in favor of considering transfusion of FFP early and in equal or high ratios to PRBC. FFP transfusion should be guided by viscoelastic testing or prothrombin time/activated partial thromboplastin time (PT/aPTT) values >1.5 times normal control.[7] Recent literature comparing PRBC-to-FFP ratios suggests that a general increase in FFP transfusion is beneficial, but the data are not completely reliable due to survivorship bias, where the patients who survive longer are likely to receive more FFP and lag in the delivery of FFP as it requires thawing. Increased fibrinolysis and low fibrinogen levels are seen in TIC. FFPs are used to replenish the fibrinogen and coagulation factors, but the amount of fibrinogen is variable in different plasma preparations. Pathogen-inactivated plasma has a higher content of fibrinogen and can prevent adverse effects like transfusion-associated acute lung injury (TRALI) and other infections.[8] AB plasma is widely used as a part of massive hemorrhagic protocols (MHPs) to cater to the early requirements of plasma. Due to the limited availability of AB plasma, the use of A-group plasma for trauma patients of unknown blood group is being studied. A study at our own center demonstrated that high FFP-to-PRBC and platelet (PLT)-to-PRBC ratios reduced 24-hour mortality but not overall in-hospital mortality in severely injured patients.[9]

PLATELET TRANSFUSION

Recent studies recommend using higher platelet-to-PRBC ratios. The groups that have received higher platelet-to-PRBC ratios showed improved survival.[9-11] The latest European guidelines suggest a platelet count of more than $50 \times 10^9/L$ in trauma patients with ongoing bleeding and a cutoff above $100 \times 10^9/L$ in patients with traumatic brain injury. An initial dose of 4–8 random donor platelets or one apheresis pack is recommended, which is expected to deliver a dose of $3–4 \times 10^{11}$ and increase the platelet count by $>30 \times 10^9$.[4] Platelet counts are usually normal at the time of admission, but they decline after 2 hours of hemostatic resuscitation and continuously thereafter. Data from systematic reviews suggests that higher platelet-to-PRBC ratios decrease 24-hour 30-day mortality and lower ICU stay.[10]

TRIGGERS OF TRANSFUSION

The decision to initiate transfusion of blood components following major trauma is guided by triggers. The triggers combine clinical signs like bleeding, shock, laboratory or viscoelastic tests, and contextual factors like hypothermia, acidosis, and dilution. The triggers of transfusion for each component—PRBCs, FFP, platelets, and cryoprecipitate—were studied in severely injured patients at our center.[12] According to this study, inferior extremity injury, deranged PT, and blood loss of more than 900 ml were identified as triggers for FFP and cryoprecipitate transfusion. The trauma resuscitation algorithms, which incorporate various triggers, should be designed for each center. Base deficit, lactate, deranged PT, aPTT, shock index, low fibrinogen level, thrombocytopenia, etc., are triggers for early component therapy.

FRESH WHOLE BLOOD

Fresh whole blood (FWB) is an optimum transfusion product in trauma patients, as all the blood constituents are transfused in physiological quantities. The FWB is commonly used in military settings. The main challenge is virological safety, which restricts its use outside military settings.[13]

REPLACEMENT OF FIBRINOGEN

Fibrinogen is essential for thrombosis. In the coagulation cascade, thrombin activates fibrinogen to form insoluble fibrin strands, and fibrinogen is the ligand for platelet aggregation. It has been found that the fibrinogen levels fall first in massive hemorrhage. The cutoff trigger for supplementing fibrinogen is 1.5 g/L. The data from observational studies suggest improved survival in high fibrinogen ratios.[14,15] The main source of fibrinogen is either cryoprecipitate or fibrinogen concentrate. Cryoprecipitate is rich in factors VIII, XIII, vWF, fibrinogen, and fibronectin. Cryoprecipitate may have additional benefits due to other coagulation factors but has a risk of viral transmission, whereas fibrinogen concentrate is available in standardized vials, where the concentration is known, can be stored at room temperature, has no viral transmission risk, and can be reconstituted at the bedside, but there is an increased risk of thromboembolism. The latest European guidelines suggest that an initial fibrinogen supplementation of 3–4 g, which is equivalent to 15–20 single donor units of cryoprecipitate or 3–4 g of fibrinogen concentrate, may be required. The repeat doses should be guided by viscoelastic monitoring and laboratory assessment of fibrinogen levels.[4]

PROTHROMBIN COMPLEX CONCENTRATES

Three- or four-factor prothrombin complex concentrates (PCCs) can be considered for use in traumatic coagulopathy. Vitamin K_1 (phytomenadione) is co-administered with PCC to activate the production of vitamin K-dependent factors. Studies have demonstrated that PCCs reduced the requirement of transfusion, but there was no improvement in mortality, while there is a higher risk for venous and thrombotic complications.

OTHER HEMOSTATIC AGENTS

ANTIFIBRINOLYTIC AGENTS—TRANEXAMIC ACID

Tranexamic acid (TXA) has become one of the integral parts of treatment in the initial management of coagulation and bleeding. The latest guidelines recommend TXA should be administered to a trauma patient who is bleeding or at risk of significant bleeding as early as possible and within 3 hours after injury. A loading dose of 1g is infused over 10 minutes, followed by an IV infusion of 1 g over 8 hours. The guidelines recommend that for administration of TXA, there is no need to wait for the results of viscoelastic tests.[4] The evidence was from the CRASH-2 trial, which showed reduction in mortality and bleeding deaths.[16] Another study in TBI patients, CRASH-3, concluded that early treatment with TXA was shown to reduce death in mild and moderate injury but not in severe head injury.[17]

RECOMBINANT ACTIVATED COAGULATION FACTOR VII

Recombinant activated factor VII (rFVIIa) is not often recommended as a first-line treatment. It is suggested only when the bleeding and traumatic coagulopathy cannot be controlled by all other measures. In patients with isolated head injury, no positive effect has been demonstrated. Also, in severely bleeding patients, rFVIIa has not been shown to improve survival while it increases thromboembolic complications and hence needs to be used with caution.[18]

MASSIVE TRANSFUSION PROTOCOLS AND COMPONENT THERAPY

MHPs are structured approaches to the management of severe hemorrhage in trauma patients. They typically involve the rapid administration of PRBCs, FFP, and platelets in fixed ratios, along with the use of adjunctive therapies such as TXA and fibrinogen replacement.

Components of MHPs: MHPs are designed to deliver blood components in a balanced ratio (e.g., 1:1:1) to restore hemostasis and prevent dilutional coagulopathy. The protocol is usually activated in response to criteria such as the need for multiple transfusions within a short time or the presence of significant hemodynamic instability.

Goals of MHPs: The primary goals of MHPs are to rapidly correct coagulopathy, restore blood volume and oxygen-carrying capacity, and minimize the risk of adverse outcomes associated with massive transfusion. Early activation and adherence to the protocol are critical for achieving these goals.

MASSIVE HEMORRHAGIC PROTOCOLS

Trauma is associated with TIC, which needs prompt management with appropriate and adequate blood component replacement. In an emergency, when a patient presents with massive hemorrhage, the preparedness of the blood bank with standard operating procedures for emergency blood release and massive transfusion protocols enables an effective response and increases the chance to salvage the patient. Early resuscitation with blood components restores the tissue oxygenation of vital organs in an exsanguinating patient and provides adequate coagulation factors that have been lost due to bleeding. The American College of Surgeons Trauma Quality Improvement program has framed best practice guidelines for massive transfusion that can be measured to determine if MHP is achieving the designed goals. Some examples of quality indicators are blood product turnaround time, wastage and utilization, transfusion and adverse events, patient mortality, and laboratory values. Initial resuscitation is provided for a patient with major hemorrhage, and as per the Advanced Trauma Life Support (ATLS) guidelines,[19] the blood loss is estimated and the Massive Transfusion Protocol (MTP) is activated. At various centers, there are individualized prediction scores and triggers for activation of MTP.[20,21] The MTP is activated by a call to the blood bank by the treating team. The blood components are organized and released in consecutive packs. These packs are prepared prior to a request and are requested by phone call, which reduces the delay in supply time. These packs ensure a balanced supply of blood products under emergency situations. The size and composition of the packs depend on the physical distance between the blood bank and the trauma bay and the availability of the blood products. A designated trauma center should have a 24-hour blood transfusion service with specific operating procedures for rapid delivery of blood components. Timely and precise communication between the treating team and blood bank is imperative. The MTP is outlined below (Figure 7.2.1).

The MTP should address the following:

i. Triggers for initiating massive transfusion in trauma

ii. Resuscitation in the trauma bay includes the following:
   (a) MTP product availability
   (b) MTP product delivery
   (c) MTP blood product transfusion

iii. Continuing MTP in the operating room, angio-suite, and intensive care unit

iv. Transfusion medicine processes for the delivery of blood products

v. Transfusion targets

vi. The use of adjuncts for massive transfusion patients

vii. Termination of MTP

viii. Performance improvement morning

On arrival to the emergency department, the patient's vital signs should be assessed immediately, and blood samples obtained for type and screen, complete blood count, PT, aPTT, blood gas analysis, and viscoelastic testing when available. If an urgent uncrossmatched transfusion is required, two units of group O Rh-positive RBCs for males or two units of group O Rh-negative RBCs for females, along with group AB FFP, should be issued. When there is no need for immediate uncrossmatched blood, transfusion should proceed according to the patient's blood type. Patients who remain unstable with ongoing hemorrhage should receive further transfusion guided by clinical status and fibrinogen levels. If massive transfusion becomes necessary, blood components should be delivered in predefined packs. Continuous

TRIGGERS

- Non-responder (SBP<90 mmHg) to 1–2 L IV fluids
- Exsanguinating patient in extremis, needing life-saving surgery

- Activated by Senior resident (Emergency medicine or Trauma Surgery) on duty
- *Done by phone or by sending a Manual transfusion request form with at least one patient identifier and term MHP should be mentioned at a prominent position *No plain papers/consultation form, hospital identification number and EDTA blood sample not mandatory

- 2nd batch
- 4 units of RBC, FFP, RDP
- RBC -Group specific (saline crossmatched)
- FFP: Group specific/compatible FFP
- RDP: Non-specific ABO Group
- TAT-15 minutes
    - Hospital attendant shall bring the requisition form and collect the units from the blood center in cold boxes
- EDTA blood sample should be sent when the second batch of blood components is issued

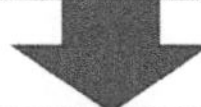

- 3rd batch
- 2 units of RBC, FFP, RDP
- RBC-Group specific (saline crossmatched)
- FFP: Group specific/compatible FFP
- RDP: Non-specific ABO Group
- TAT-15 minutes
    - Hospital attendant shall bring the requisition form and collect the units from the blood center in cold boxes
- Auto cut off or as per demand of MHP after release of the third batch of blood

Transport of blood by hospital attendant

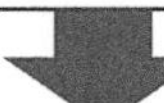

End points: Control of bleeding and normalizing hemodynamic status
If not bleeding, based on lab values

Laboratory-based cutoff

Laboratory-based cutoff	TEG-based cutoff
Hb >8 g/dl	R time <9 mins
PT<18 secs	K-time <4 mins
aPTT<35 secs	αangle >60°
Platelet >1lakh	MA >55 mm
Fibrinogen >1.0 mg/dl	LY30 <7.5%

- Discontinue MHP if further resuscitation is futile
- Termination of MHP at any time and return of unused blood components to blood bank within 30 min from time of release
- SR trauma surgery during activation of MHP shall be responsible for completing the documents with the blood center

Figure 7.2.1 Massive hemorrhagic protocol at a tertiary care trauma center.

reassessment is essential, and additional transfusion should follow either the massive transfusion packs or laboratory-guided correction until the patient stabilizes.

The criteria to terminate the protocol are very important to prevent wastage of resources. The ratio-based resuscitation may be discontinued, and goal-directed transfusion instituted based on laboratory values or radiographic evidence of ongoing bleeding. The endpoints for termination of MTP are as follows:

i. Hb ≥10 g/dL
ii. PT<18 seconds
iii. APTT<35 seconds
iv. Platelet count >150 × 10^9
v. Fibrinogen >180 g/L

The endpoints can be defined based on rapid thromboelastography (TEG) and rotational thromboelastometry (ROTEM) values, as well as according to availability.[22] The endpoints may vary across different centers.

CONCLUSION

TIC remains a major contributor to early mortality in severely injured patients, and its management requires rapid recognition and coordinated, protocol-driven care. Modern hemostatic resuscitation emphasizes early balanced transfusion of red cells, plasma, and platelets, supported by fibrinogen replacement and timely use of TXA. Viscoelastic assays, when available, help guide targeted correction of coagulation deficits, while conventional laboratory tests continue to play an important role, especially in resource-limited settings. Massive transfusion protocols provide a structured approach to delivering blood components efficiently, reduce delays, and standardize care during active hemorrhage. Continuous reassessment, clear communication between clinical teams and the blood bank, and timely protocol termination are all essential to avoid complications and conserve resources. By integrating early identification, balanced transfusion strategies, and evidence-based adjuncts, outcomes in TIC can be significantly improved.

TAKE-HOME MESSAGE

Early recognition and prompt treatment of TIC are essential in trauma care. Hemostatic resuscitation, focused on balanced use of plasma, platelets, and red blood cells, helps restore clotting in severely injured patients. Early use of fibrinogen and TXA, when indicated, also supports better bleeding control. Diagnosis should be guided by both standard coagulation tests and viscoelastic assays to target therapy more accurately. Reducing crystalloid use and following structured transfusion strategies are important steps that improve survival and reduce complications.

REFERENCES

1. Teixeira PGR, Inaba K, Hadjizacharia P, Brown C, Salim A, Rhee P, *et al.* preventable or potentially preventable mortality at a mature trauma center. J Trauma Inj Infect Crit Care. 2007 Dec;63(6):1338–47.

2. Curry NS, Davenport RA, Hunt BJ, Stanworth SJ. Transfusion strategies for traumatic coagulopathy. Blood Rev. 2012 Sep;26(5):223–32.

3. Edwards MJ, Lustik MB, Clark ME, Creamer KM, Tuggle D. The effects of balanced blood component resuscitation and crystalloid administration in pediatric trauma patients requiring transfusion in Afghanistan and Iraq 2002 to 2012. J Trauma Acute Care Surg. 2015 Feb;78(2):330–5.

4. Rossaint R, Afshari A, Bouillon B, Cerny V, Cimpoesu D, Curry N, *et al.* The European guideline on management of major bleeding and coagulopathy following trauma: Sixth edition. Crit Care. 2023 Mar 1;27(1):80.

5. Baraniuk S, Tilley BC, del Junco DJ, Fox EE, van Belle G, Wade CE, *et al.* Pragmatic randomized optimal platelet and plasma ratios (PROPPR) trial: Design, rationale and implementation. Injury. 2014 Sep;45(9):1287–95.

6. Beckermann J, Swartz H, Albright J, Street W, Martin S, Hagen C, *et al.* Achieving optimal massive transfusion ratios: The trauma white board, whole blood, and liquid plasma. Real world low-tech solutions for a high stakes issue. Injury. 2022 Sep; 53(9):2974–8.

7. Yuan S, Ferrell C, Chandler WL. Comparing the prothrombin time INR versus the APTT to evaluate the coagulopathy of acute trauma. Thromb Res. 2007 Jan;120(1):29–37.

8. Ishikura H, Kitamura T. Trauma-induced coagulopathy and critical bleeding: The role of plasma and platelet transfusion. J Intensive Care. 2017 Jan 20;5(1):2.

9. Krishna A, Subramanian A, Chaurasia R, Sinha T, Pandey S. Effect of high ratios of plasma and platelets to red blood cell transfusions during early resuscitation on the mortality of severely injured trauma patients. Asian J Transfus Sci.

10. Quintana MT, Zebley JA, Vincent A, Chang P, Estroff J, Sarani B, *et al.* Cresting mortality: Defining a plateau in ongoing massive transfusion. J Trauma Acute Care Surg. 2022;93(1):43–51.

11. Aichholz PK, Lee SA, Farr CK, Tsang HC, Vavilala MS, Stansbury LG, *et al.* Platelet transfusion and outcomes after massive transfusion protocol activation for major trauma: A retrospective cohort study. Anesth Analg. 2022 Aug;135(2):385–93.

12. Krishna A, Subramanian A, Chaurasia R, Sinha TP, Pandey S, Malhotra R. Transfusion practices in severely injured patients at a level 1 trauma center. J Emerg Trauma Shock. 2024;17:84–90.

13. Hanna K, Bible L, Chehab M, Asmar S, Douglas M, Ditillo M, *et al.* Nationwide analysis of whole blood hemostatic resuscitation in civilian trauma. J Trauma Acute Care Surg. 2020 Aug;89(2):329–35.

14. Nakamura Y, Ishikura H, Kushimoto S, Kiyomi F, Kato H, Sasaki J, *et al.* Fibrinogen level on admission is a predictor for massive transfusion in patients with severe blunt trauma: Analyses of a retrospective multicentre observational study. Injury. 2017 Mar;48(3):674–9.

15. Meizoso JP, Moore EE, Pieracci FM, Saberi RA, Ghasabyan A, Chandler J, *et al.* Role of fibrinogen in trauma-induced coagulopathy. J Am Coll Surg. 2022 Apr;234(4):465–73.

16. Roberts I, Prieto-Merino D, Manno D. Mechanism of action of tranexamic acid in bleeding trauma patients: An exploratory analysis of data from the CRASH-2 trial. Crit Care [Internet]. 2014 [cited 2019 Jun 19];18(6). Available from: https://www.ncbi.nlm.nih.gov/pmc/articles/PMC4277654/

17. CRASH-3 trial collaborators. Effects of tranexamic acid on death, disability, vascular occlusive events and other morbidities in patients with acute traumatic brain injury (CRASH-3): A randomised, placebo-controlled trial. Lancet. 2019 Nov;394 (10210):1713–23.

18. Lombardo S, Millar D, Jurkovich GJ, Coimbra R, Nirula R. Factor VIIa administration in traumatic brain injury: An AAST-MITC propensity score analysis. Trauma Surg

Acute Care Open. 2018;3(1):e000134. doi:10.1136/tsaco-2017-000134. Published 2018 Mar 22.

19. Mutschler M, Paffrath T, Wölfl C, Probst C, Nienaber U, Schipper IB, *et al.* The ATLS® classification of hypovolaemic shock: A well-established teaching tool on the edge? Injury. 2014 Oct;45:S35–8.

20. Nunez TC, Voskresensky IV, Dossett LA, Shinall R, Dutton WD, Cotton BA. Early prediction of massive transfusion in trauma: Simple as ABC (assessment of blood consumption)? J Trauma Inj Infect Crit Care. 2009 Feb;66(2):346–52.

21. Chico-Fernández M, García-Fuentes C, Alonso-Fernández MA, Toral-Vázquez D, Bermejo-Aznarez S, Alted-López E. Massive transfusion predictive scores in trauma. Experience of a transfusion registry. Med Intensiva Engl Ed. 2011 Dec;35(9):546–51.

22. Camazine MN, Hemmila MR, Leonard JC, Jacobs RA, Horst JA, Kozar RA, *et al.* Massive transfusion policies at trauma centers participating in the American College of Surgeons Trauma Quality Improvement Program. J Trauma Acute Care Surg. 2015 Jun;78(6):S48–53.

Chapter 8

IMPACT OF TRAUMA-INDUCED COAGULOPATHY ON CLINICAL OUTCOMES

Abhishek Singh, Nistha Malik, Hemant Choudhary, and Nishtha Chawla

DOI: 10.1201/9781003711070-8

INTRODUCTION

Trauma-induced coagulopathy (TIC) is a complex and life-threatening condition that emerges early following traumatic injury and significantly contributes to increased morbidity and mortality in trauma patients.[1] Unlike traditional models that attribute coagulopathy solely to haemodilution and hypothermia, TIC is now recognized as an endogenous response to trauma and shock, involving the interplay of inflammation, tissue injury, endothelial dysfunction, and fibrinolysis.[2] The prevalence of TIC among severely injured patients ranges from 25% to 35% upon hospital admission, underscoring its clinical significance and the urgency for early recognition and intervention.[3] The presence of TIC has been independently associated with poor clinical outcomes, including increased transfusion requirements, longer intensive care unit stays, higher incidence of multiple organ failure, and a greater risk of death.[4] Recent advancements in diagnostic techniques, such as viscoelastic assays, have facilitated a better understanding of the pathophysiology of TIC and helped tailor more effective, individualized treatment strategies.[5] Early goal-directed therapy, including the use of balanced transfusion protocols, tranexamic acid, and point-of-care coagulation monitoring, has shown promise in mitigating the adverse outcomes associated with TIC.[6] This chapter explores the underlying mechanisms of TIC, its impact on clinical outcomes, and the evolving strategies aimed at improving the prognosis of trauma patients. By understanding the intricate relationship between trauma, coagulation, and systemic response, clinicians can enhance their approach to managing one of the most challenging aspects of trauma care.

COMPLICATIONS ASSOCIATED WITH TIC

INCREASED RATES OF TRANSFUSION

Patients with TIC get significantly more blood product transfusions than non-coagulopathic patients,[7] which increases the risk of other associated complications such as acute respiratory distress syndrome (ARDS), systemic inflammatory response syndrome, and mortality after injury.[8] Since there is no consensus on optimal resuscitation ratios; however, various studies have shown that low crystalloid and overall blood product usage and lower packed red blood cells-to-fresh frozen plasma (PRBC:FFP) ratios, have shown survival benefit in trauma patients requiring massive transfusion.[9] The use of massive blood transfusion has significantly reduced the mortality of severely injured trauma patients but can be associated with several complications. The list of complications appears in Table 8.1.

INFECTION RATES

In humans, allogeneic blood transfusions cause immunosuppression.[10] The exact mechanisms underlying transfusion-related immunomodulation (TRIM) are unknown, but they include transfusion-associated microchimerism (TA-MC), which occurs when small populations of donor allogeneic leukocytes from the blood donor engraft in the transfusion recipient and survive for years or decades. In transfusion recipients, the donor's hematopoietic stem cells engraft, resulting in microchimerism. TRIM may raise the risk of cancer recurrence after potentially curative surgery,[11] as well as the incidence of postoperative bacterial infections.[12] A meta-analysis explored the association between blood transfusions and postoperative bacterial infections. It reported that patients who received transfusions had an odds ratio of 3.45 for developing such infections compared to those who did not. In trauma patients, the odds ratio increased to 5.263. These results provide strong evidence that transfusions are significantly linked to a higher risk of postoperative infections, particularly among trauma patients.[13] Multiple studies conducted at individual institutions have demonstrated a dose dependent relationship between blood transfusions and infection rates in trauma

Table 8.1 Complications of massive blood transfusion and their mechanisms

Complication category	Complication	Mechanism
Thermal	Hypothermia	Infusion of cold blood products and IV fluids; surgical exposure; impaired thermoregulation; reduced metabolic heat production
Electrolyte disturbances	Hyperkalaemia	Potassium release from haemolysed stored RBCs; increased risk in renal impairment and crush injuries
	Hypokalaemia	Stress-induced catecholamine surge causing intracellular shift; potassium uptake by transfused RBCs; metabolic alkalosis
	Hypocalcaemia	Citrate in stored blood binds ionized calcium; worsens in liver dysfunction due to reduced citrate metabolism
	Hypomagnesemia	Large volumes of magnesium-poor fluids; citrate chelation of magnesium
Acid base imbalance	Metabolic acidosis	Tissue hypoperfusion; anaerobic metabolism; impaired clearance of lactate and citrate
	Metabolic alkalosis	Metabolism of citrate to bicarbonate; hypokalaemia contributing to alkalosis
Coagulation abnormalities	Dilutional coagulopathy and thrombocytopenia	Dilution of clotting factors and platelets by RBC transfusion, lacking these components
	Disseminated intravascular coagulation (DIC)	Trauma- or transfusion-triggered consumptive coagulopathy causing depletion of clotting factors and platelets
Pulmonary complications	TRALI (transfusion-related acute lung injury)	Immune and non-immune pathways causing neutrophil activation → endothelial injury → non-cardiogenic pulmonary edema
	TACO (transfusion-associated circulatory overload)	Rapid transfusion causes circulatory overload; higher risk in the elderly, infants, and cardiac patients
Immune-mediated effects	TRIM (transfusion-related immunomodulation)	Reduced IL-2, impaired macrophage and NK function, altered CD4/CD8 ratio
	TA-GVHD (transfusion-associated graft vs. host disease)	Donor T lymphocytes attack host tissues, especially in immunocompromised recipients
	Post-transfusion purpura	Anti–HPA-1a antibodies cause severe platelet destruction
Hemolytic reaction	Immediate haemolytic reaction	ABO-incompatible transfusion → antigen–antibody complexes → complement activation → intravascular haemolysis

patients.[14-16] A prospective study of 1,172 trauma patients admitted to an intensive care unit over two years found that receiving blood products was linked to significantly higher rates of infection and mortality. Multivariate analysis indicated that each unit of PRBCs transfused increased the infection risk by 5%. This study confirmed a dose-dependent correlation between transfusion volume and negative clinical outcomes in trauma patients.[17]

VENOUS THROMBOEMBOLISM

Patients with traumatic injuries are at the highest risk for venous thromboembolism (VTE) among all hospitalized patients. The "true" incidence of VTE after injury and the clinical relevance of asymptomatic or "silent" VTE are mostly debated. Modifiable and non-modifiable risk factors, usage of thromboprophylaxis, and screening all have a role in determining whether individuals develop VTE and whether it is detected. Symptomatic VTEs are only the "tip of the iceberg." The prevalence of asymptomatic DVT and clinically silent pulmonary embolism (PE) makes it difficult to determine the true incidence of VTE. The majority of deep vein thrombosis (DVT) cases are asymptomatic; hence, objective diagnostic imaging is crucial for precisely assessing the incidence of DVT. Trauma patients have a "perfect storm" of variables that contribute to thrombogenesis, including injury, immobilization, and hypercoagulability. The risk of VTE following trauma is raised for at least 3 months after the injury and appears to normalize after 1 year. Several theories have been presented to explain why trauma patients exhibit hypercoagulability following injury. This includes decreased antithrombotic function (e.g., antithrombin III) and increased prothrombotic expression (e.g., prothrombin, tissue factor). Platelets play a crucial function, and resistance to activated protein C has also been identified.[18] Without thromboprophylaxis, the risk of DVT and PE is around 50% and 1%, respectively. However, the likelihood of getting VTE following trauma varies across trauma patients. The research identifies several risk variables associated with post-injury VTE. This list included patients over 45 years old who required bed rest for more than 3 days, had a history of VTE, had a spine fracture without neurological deficits, were in coma with a GCS score <7, had quadriplegia or paraplegia, had a pelvic fracture, a lower extremity fracture, had a lower extremity venous injury, or had complex lower limb wounds. Trauma patients should undergo VTE prophylaxis. There are several techniques for preventing VTE following trauma. Chemical thromboprophylaxis involves administering either low-molecular-weight heparin or unfractionated or mechanical thromboprophylaxis is often performed by intermittent pneumatic compression devices. A meta-analysis indicated that trauma patients who received thromboprophylaxis had a considerably lower incidence of DVT compared to those who did not receive any prophylaxis.[19] Combining mechanical and chemical thromboprophylaxis has been shown to lower the risk of DVT compared to chemical prophylaxis alone.[19] To reduce the risk of VTE, it's important to start thromboprophylaxis as soon as feasible. Delaying treatment beyond 72 hours raises the risk.[20] Missing thromboprophylaxis doses have been linked to DVT formation;[21] thus, it's important not to stop the therapy. IVC filters are indicated as thromboprophylaxis following trauma for people who cannot use chemical thromboprophylaxis.[22-24] The usage of inferior vena cava (IVC) filters for this indication has increased dramatically.[25] Haut *et al.* conducted a meta-analysis and showed that placing an IVC filter reduced PE and fatal PE in trauma patients, but had no effect on mortality from DVT.[26] The use of IVC filters for PE prophylaxis is still contentious due to a lack of strong evidence.[27] More prospective clinical trials are needed to better understand the mechanism of VTE in previously coagulopathic trauma patients and to discover possible targets for prevention and treatment.

ACUTE LUNG INJURY (ALI) AND ACUTE RESPIRATORY DISTRESS SYNDROME (ARDS)

ARDS was initially described in 1967 by Ashbaugh and Levine.[28] Despite advancements in its diagnosis and treatment, ARDS continues to be a major cause of morbidity among trauma patients.[29] Long-term outcomes for ARDS survivors remain concerning, with reduced physical functioning and suboptimal health-related quality of life persisting even two years post-discharge.[30] ARDS typically presents with early symptoms like breathlessness and low oxygen levels, followed by radiographic lung infiltrates (Figure 8.1).[31] It may result from direct pulmonary insults (e.g., inhalation injuries, lung contusions, pneumonia) or indirect injuries (e.g., severe infections, extensive transfusions, pancreatitis).[31]

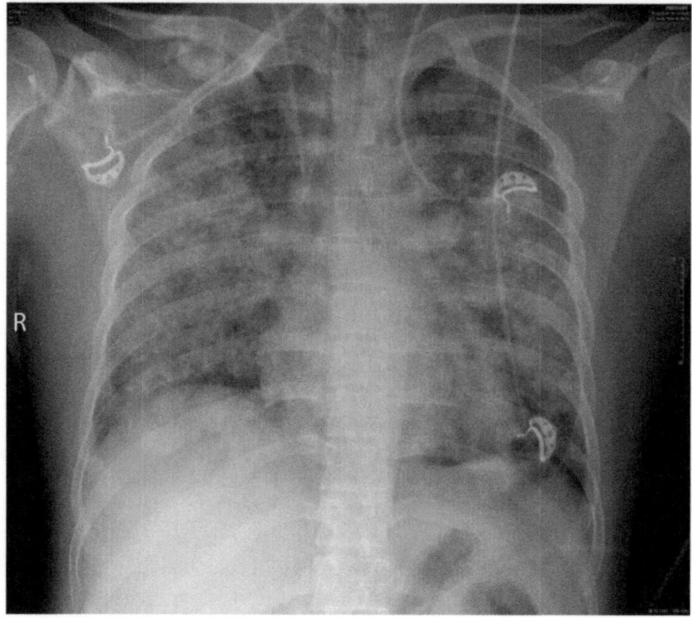

Figure 8.1 Chest X-ray showing bilateral infiltrates in a patient with trauma-induced acute respiratory distress syndrome (ARDS).

The underlying pathology involves damage to alveoli and accumulation of protein-rich fluid and debris, contributing to elevated pulmonary vascular resistance.[32] Multiple factors, including endothelial disruption, neutrophilic and cytokine-mediated injury, oxidative stress, ventilator-associated trauma, and coagulation-fibrinolysis imbalance, play a role in ARDS progression.[31,32] Severe trauma triggers a pronounced inflammatory response, making ARDS more prevalent in such patients. Trauma victims requiring blood transfusions are particularly vulnerable. Early transfusion of PRBCs has emerged as a strong, independent risk factor for ARDS, with risk correlating to the volume transfused.[33,34] While administration of FFP is also linked to an increased ARDS risk, platelets and cryoprecipitate are not.[35] To counteract transfusion-related inflammation, pre-storage leukoreduction has been introduced. Nevertheless, studies show no significant difference in ARDS incidence between patients receiving leukoreduced vs. standard PRBCs over 28 days.[36] Although acute lung injury (ALI) and ARDS are distinct, they share overlapping causes and pathways.[37] Trauma-related ARDS remains less thoroughly studied compared to sepsis-associated cases. There's a lack of robust evidence supporting ARDS management strategies tailored specifically to trauma patients. Interventions for ventilated ARDS patients should ideally focus on improving outcomes like shorter ventilation duration, ICU stay, and mortality.[38] Evidence-backed strategies, such as lung-protective ventilation using low tidal volumes (~6 ml/kg predicted body weight), moderate PEEP (5 cm H_2O), and plateau pressures ≤30 cm H_2O, align with general ARDS management guidelines.[39] Until more targeted research emerges, clinicians are encouraged to adhere to these proven methods. Investigating the role of coagulation in trauma-related ARDS presents challenges akin to broader ARDS research. Trauma-induced activation of coagulation pathways within lung tissue has been documented, yet the mechanisms remain complex and intertwined with inflammatory and reparative processes. Although several trials on coagulation-modulating therapies have been inconclusive, future research may identify patient subsets most likely to benefit from such treatments. Personalized medicine could hold promise for optimizing care in posttraumatic ARDS cases.

TIC ASSOCIATED MULTIPLE ORGAN FAILURE (MOF)

Despite improvements in trauma care, multiple organ failure (MOF) remains a leading cause of delayed mortality among trauma patients.[40,41] The incidence of MOF in critically injured individuals ranges from 15% to 40%,[41–45] with associated mortality rates between 24% and 51%.[45] Although MOF-related deaths have declined in recent years,[41,45] patients who develop MOF still experience mortality rates up to ten times higher than those without MOF.[43,44] In the setting of severe trauma, early hypo coagulopathy is recognized as a risk factor for MOF linked to TIC, while thromboembolic complications arising later in the clinical course are also associated with the development of MOF. Contributing transfusion-related risk factors include the volume of fluids and red blood cells administered, the storage duration of transfused red cells, and high ratios of FFP to red blood cells, particularly FFP: RBC ratios equal to or exceeding 1:1. Hemorrhagic shock combined with early coagulopathy increases the likelihood of MOF, while later occurrences of thromboembolism (at least 24 hours post-admission) also raise the risk. These patterns suggest that the coagulation profile evolves in MOF development. A proposed explanation is that trauma patients may transition from an initial hypocoagulable state upon arrival to a later hypercoagulable condition during hospitalization, which may predispose them to MOF. This shift may be driven by the activation of protein C in response to tissue injury through thrombomodulin and extracellular histone complexes. Activated protein C inhibits coagulation factors Va and VII, promoting hypocoagulopathy and increased fibrinolysis.[46–49] However, excessive consumption of protein C and subsequent failure to regulate these factors can lead to a hypercoagulable state. This may result in the formation of vascular thrombi, causing organ tissue damage and ultimately contributing to MOF. Further investigation is needed to validate this model. Early identification of patients at elevated risk for MOF could support targeted monitoring and preventive strategies. Recognizing early shock and hypocoagulopathy as predictors of TIC-associated MOF, and acknowledging the significance of late-stage hypercoagulability and thromboembolic events, will be crucial. Prospective studies are necessary to better understand the influence of TIC and transfusion practices on late-stage trauma outcomes.

BOX A: RISK FACTORS FOR TIC-ASSOCIATED MOF

i. Hypocoagulation on admission to the emergency department
ii. High activated protein C levels on admission to the emergency department
iii. High extracellular histone levels on admission to the emergency department
iv. Depleted protein C levels during hospital stay
v. Thromboembolic events, e.g., DIC and DVT, during hospital stay

---

NEUROCOGNITIVE IMPAIRMENTS

TIC in traumatic brain injury (TBI) can result in various complications, including both short- and long-term neurocognitive impairments. Common in moderate to severe TBI, TIC can even cause platelet dysfunction in cases of minor TBI.[50] TIC can result in a range of neurocognitive impairments, including the following:[50–52]

i. Short-term issues such as loss of consciousness, altered consciousness, and post-traumatic amnesia.

ii. The "talk and die" phenomenon, where mild TBI patients experience delayed neurological decline, potentially increasing mortality.

iii. Long-term effects include disturbances in attention, memory, language, processing speed, and executive functions, as well as an elevated risk of post-traumatic seizures, Parkinsonism, and dementia.

While direct causative links between coagulopathy, TBI, and neurocognitive impairments have not been firmly established, several hypotheses suggest potential connections. We will discuss some of these below. Although the trauma itself directly causes neurocognitive impairments, TIC exacerbates the damage. Potential molecular mechanisms for neurocognitive impairments directly related to trauma include disruption of dopaminergic neurons due to cell loss in the substantia nigra and caudate nucleus following cortical injury, axonal injury, neuronal cell death, inflammation, excitotoxicity from calcium and glutamate, mitochondrial oxidative stress, and amyloid-beta (Aβ) production.[8,9,53,54] Mechanisms by which TIC contributes to neurocognitive impairments include the following: High doses of thrombin can trigger reactive astrocytes and microglia to produce reactive oxygen species and inflammatory cytokines such as tumour necrosis factor α (TNFα) and interleukin 1β (IL-1β), which can lead to cell death and disruption of the blood-brain barrier. Additionally, activation of proteinase-activated receptors (PAR1 and PAR2) can escalate the production of inflammatory cytokines, impair N-methyl-D-aspartate (NMDA) receptor function, and disrupt neuronal plasticity, particularly in the hippocampus, striatum, and cerebral cortex. Increased levels of matrix metalloproteinase 9 and Aβ42 also play a role in these impairments.[10,55] In addition to these factors, various psychological and social elements, such as premorbid functioning, social support, and comorbid psychiatric disorders, also affect neurocognitive outcomes following TIC in TBI. Existing literature indicates that neurocognitive impairments significantly affect both short- and long-term outcomes in TBI patients. In the short term, TIC is associated with lower Glasgow Coma Scale (GCS) scores and higher mortality rates.[56] A study by Abdelmalik *et al.*, using data from the Citicoline Brain Injury Treatment Trial (COBRIT), found that patients exhibited worse functional and cognitive outcomes, specifically in memory and language, at 180 days post-TBI.[57] Long-term poor functional outcomes are influenced by factors such as premorbid functioning, social support, and age, and may include difficulties with daily activities, reduced employability, dependence on others, and a diminished quality of life. There is also an increased risk of comorbid conditions, including depression, post-traumatic stress disorder, dementia, seizure disorders, and parkinsonism, which further exacerbate disability and negatively impact outcomes. Neurocognitive impairments, whether short- or long-term, contribute to higher morbidity and mortality in TBI patients. Given that TIC is prevalent in severe injuries and often leads to neurocognitive sequelae, timely intervention and support are crucial to improving outcomes and reducing associated mortality and morbidity. Early involvement of mental health professionals may be a key step in addressing these challenges. In conclusion, the impact of TIC on neurocognitive function in TBI is profound and multifaceted. While TIC exacerbates both short- and long-term neurocognitive impairments, it also intertwines with various psychological and social factors that influence overall patient outcomes. As research continues to uncover the complex mechanisms underlying these impairments, it is essential to focus on early detection, comprehensive management, and multidisciplinary support. By integrating timely interventions and mental health care, we can better address the challenges posed by TIC and improve the quality of life and functional recovery for TBI patients.

MORTALITY AND PROGNOSIS

TIC is a critical determinant of both early and late outcomes in trauma patients. Its presence on admission has been consistently associated with a significant increase in mortality, independent of injury severity and physiological derangements. Early recognition and management of TIC are therefore essential to improving prognosis.

Table 8.2 Trauma-induced coagulopathy incidence and mortality in traumatic brain injury across studies

Study	TIC incidence (%)	Mortality (%)
Rani et al.[58]	62	35.4
Albert et al.[59]	41.6	44
Chhabra et al.[61]	46	51
Kulkarni et al.[62]	56.3	71.43

INCREASED EARLY MORTALITY

TIC is strongly associated with early deaths within the first 24 hours, primarily due to uncontrolled haemorrhage. Studies have shown a 2- to 4-fold increase in mortality in patients with coagulopathy compared to those without (Table 8.2). Rani et al.[58] reported a mortality rate of 53.8% in TIC-positive TBI patients, compared to 23.5% in those without TIC. Albert et al.[59] found that prolonged prothrombin time (PT) and activated partial thromboplastin time (aPTT), along with low fibrinogen (<150 mg/dL), were independent predictors of in-hospital death. Chhabra et al.[60] highlighted that hypofibrinogenemia was associated with a 4.5-fold increased risk of mortality in TBI.

WORSENED PROGNOSIS DESPITE STANDARD RESUSCITATION

Even with aggressive fluid resuscitation and surgical control of bleeding, TIC remains an independent predictor of poor outcomes, including a higher risk of multi-organ failure. Chhabra et al.[61] demonstrated that coagulopathy on admission served as an independent prognostic marker for unfavourable neurological outcomes and death in patients with acute TBI. Kulkarni et al.[62] further emphasized that abnormalities in coagulation profiles (such as prothrombin time [PT], activated partial thromboplastin time (aPTT), and international normalized ratio [INR]) in trauma admissions correlate with increased ICU requirement and mortality.

CORRELATION WITH INJURY SEVERITY

TIC is more prevalent in patients with severe traumatic brain injury, polytrauma, and major vascular injury, which correlates with higher Injury Severity Scores (ISSs) and worse prognosis.

LONG-TERM OUTCOMES

Patients who survive the initial haemorrhagic phase but present with TIC often face prolonged ICU stays, increased ventilator days, and a higher risk of nosocomial infections and organ dysfunction, adversely affecting long-term recovery and rehabilitation. Addressing TIC effectively requires prompt recognition and management in trauma care. Strategies may include early administration of blood products, use of pro-coagulant agents, and close monitoring to address coagulopathy and its effects swiftly. Implementing these measures can help mitigate the impact of TIC and improve survival rates in trauma patients.

CHRONIC COMPLICATIONS OF TIC

Chronic complications of TIC can significantly impact a patient's long-term health and quality of life. Repeated or severe bleeding into joints and muscles can lead to chronic pain, stiffness, and decreased range of motion. Over time, this can result in joint deformities or muscle atrophy. Severe bleeding may cause damage to internal organs. Chronic diseases of the vital organ can arise from these injuries, including liver dysfunction, kidney damage, or gastrointestinal problems. The trauma associated with severe injury and the stress of managing chronic complications can lead to post-traumatic stress disorder (PTSD), anxiety, depression, or other mental health conditions. Persistent pain due to tissue damage, joint damage, or ongoing bleeding issues can significantly affect daily life and functional abilities. Long-term effects can include decreased mobility and functional limitations, impacting the ability to perform daily activities and affecting the overall well-being of the patient. Chronic coagulopathy can lead to prolonged or problematic wound healing, increasing the risk of infections and complications from injuries. Long-term use of medications or interventions to manage TIC (like anticoagulants or clotting factor concentrates) may also lead to additional complications or side effects. Chronic immobilization or reduced physical activity due to pain or joint issues can contribute to bone density loss and increased risk of fractures. Effective management of these complications typically involves a multidisciplinary approach, including ongoing medical care, physical therapy, mental health support, and lifestyle adjustments to address and mitigate the long-term effects of TIC.

IMPACT OF TIC ON REHABILITATION AND QUALITY OF LIFE

TIC can significantly impact rehabilitation processes, influencing both the approach and outcomes of recovery. TIC can lead to bleeding complications or internal bleeding, making rehabilitation exercises and activities more hazardous. Therapists must carefully design and monitor activities to avoid exacerbating these risks. Due to bleeding or clotting issues, healing times may be extended, leading to longer periods of immobilization or reduced physical activity. This can impact muscle strength, joint mobility, and overall function. Chronic pain or discomfort from trauma or coagulopathy can hinder participation in rehabilitation. Managing pain effectively is crucial to ensure patients can engage in therapy. If TIC results in joint damage, muscle weakness, or reduced mobility, rehabilitation programs need to be adapted to address these limitations while still promoting functional recovery. The stress and trauma associated with severe injuries and their complications can lead to psychological challenges. Mental health support, including counselling or therapy, can be an essential part of the rehabilitation process. Rehabilitation must be individualized, taking into account the specific complications and needs related to TIC. This might involve tailored exercise programs, specialized equipment, and close monitoring of progress. Several investigations have assessed the long-term outcomes of patients with TIC exhibiting a hypocoagulable profile. The Trauma Recovery Project (TRP) analysed quality of life (QOL), functionality, and psychological wellbeing in injured individuals without severe neurotrauma. Findings at 12- and 18-months post-injury showed that over 75% of adults continued to experience functional impairments.[63] Similarly, the CONTROL multicentre randomized controlled trial on activated factor VII, involving severely injured adults with persistent bleeding (excluding severe head injuries), revealed that survivors had markedly low QOL at three months post-injury. More than 70% faced moderate to severe limitations in routine tasks, mobility, and experienced pain or discomfort, while over 50% reported difficulties with self-care, anxiety, or depression.[64] A longitudinal study tracking 156 paediatric patients with blunt trauma (without spinal cord or brain injuries) found their physical health scores remained below those of healthy peers at the six-month follow-up.[65] On the other hand, the hypercoagulable end of TIC, often seen in those who survive initial resuscitation, has been connected to multiple organ dysfunction, ARDS, and thrombotic complications such as VTE, all contributing to prolonged hospital stays.[66] Patients needing prolonged ICU care often progress to a state of chronic critical illness, which has been associated with poor long-term outcomes in trauma patients without TBI.[66] A study evaluating long-term effects following acute pulmonary embolism noted that over half of the patients experienced shortness of breath and decreased physical capacity, with chronic thromboembolic pulmonary hypertension developing in up to 3.8% within two years.[67,68] Post-thrombotic syndrome has been reported in 20–50% of cases, even with optimal treatment.[69] Nevertheless, with appropriate medical intervention, rehabilitation, and comprehensive support, many patients with TIC can regain a satisfactory quality of life. Recovery paths vary individually, and outcomes are often improved through a multidisciplinary care approach.

CONCLUSION

TIC is a condition that occurs after severe trauma, where the body's ability to achieve homeostasis is disrupted. TIC is triggered by factors such as severe blood loss, tissue injury, shock, hypothermia, acidosis, and the body's inflammatory response. These factors cause a complex interaction that impairs the normal clotting process, often resulting in hyperfibrinolysis and consumption of clotting factors. TIC impacts clinical outcomes, leading to increased bleeding, transfusion requirements, multiorgan failure, and mortality. Therefore, Early recognition of TIC is crucial. Management strategies to mitigate the impact of TIC include early administration of blood products, coagulation factors, and antifibrinolytic agents like tranexamic acid. The goal is to restore normal clotting function, control bleeding, and improve the chances of survival and on long-term recovery, functional outcomes, and quality of life in trauma patients. Future trials should be based on improving the understanding of TIC, developing better diagnostic tools, and optimizing treatment protocols to enhance patient outcomes.

TAKE-HOME MESSAGE

TIC is a complex, multifactorial condition that occurs rapidly after severe trauma and significantly increases the risk of bleeding, organ failure, and death. TIC is characterized by impaired clot formation, hyperfibrinolysis and endothelial dysfunction. Early recognition and targeted treatment, such as the use of blood products, tranexamic acid, and minimizing the use of crystalloids, are critical in improving outcomes. Prompt and effective management is essential to reduce mortality and improve recovery in trauma patients.

REFERENCES

1. Brohi K, Singh J, Heron M, Coats T. Acute traumatic coagulopathy. Journal of Trauma and Acute Care Surgery. 2003;54(6):1127–30.

2. Maegele M. Coagulopathy after traumatic brain injury: Incidence, pathogenesis, and treatment options. Transfusion. 2013;53(Suppl 1):28S–37S.

3. Frith D, Goslings JC, Gaarder C, Maegele M, Cohen MJ, Allard S, et al. Definition and drivers of acute traumatic coagulopathy: Clinical and experimental investigations. Journal of Thrombosis and Haemostasis. 2010;8(9):1919–25.

4. Levy JH, Dutton RP, Hemphill III JC, Shander A, Cooper D, Paidas MJ, et al. Multidisciplinary approach to the challenge of hemostasis. Anesthesia & Analgesia. 2010;110(2):354–64.

5. Schöchl H, Solomon C, Traintinger S, Nienaber U, Tacacs-Tolnai A, Windhofer C, *et al.* Thromboelastometric (ROTEM) findings in patients suffering from isolated severe traumatic brain injury. Journal of Neurotrauma. 2011;28(10):2033–41.

6. Crash-2 Collaborators. The importance of early treatment with tranexamic acid in bleeding trauma patients: An exploratory analysis of the CRASH-2 randomised controlled trial. The Lancet. 2011;377(9771):1096–101.

7. Brohi K, Cohen MJ, Ganter MT, Matthay MA, Mackersie RC, Pittet JF. Acute traumatic coagulopathy: Initiated by hypoperfusion: Modulated through the protein C pathway? Annals of surgery. 2007;245(5):812–8.

8. Charles A, Shaikh A, Walters M, Huehl S, Pomerantz R. Blood transfusion is an independent predictor of mortality after blunt trauma. The American surgeon. 2007;73(1):1–5.

9. Kutcher ME, Kornblith LZ, Narayan R, Curd V, Daley AT, Redick BJ, *et al.* A paradigm shift in trauma resuscitation: Evaluation of evolving massive transfusion practices. JAMA Surgery. 2013;148(9):834–40.

10. Buddeberg F, Schimmer BB, Spahn DR. Transfusion-transmissible infections and transfusion-related immunomodulation. Best Practice & Research Clinical anaesthesiology. 2008;22(3):503–17.

11. Lapierre V, Aupérin A, Tiberghien P. Transfusion-induced immunomodulation following cancer surgery: Fact or fiction? JNCI: Journal of the National Cancer Institute. 1998;90(8):573–80.

12. Dunne JR, Malone D, Tracy JK, Gannon C, Napolitano LM. Perioperative anemia: An independent risk factor for infection, mortality, and resource utilization in surgery. Journal of Surgical Research. 2002;102(2):237–44.

13. Hill GE, Frawley WH, Griffith KE, Forestner JE, Minei JP. Allogeneic blood transfusion increases the risk of postoperative bacterial infection: A meta-analysis. Journal of Trauma and Acute Care Surgery. 2003;54(5):908–14.

14. Claridge JA, Sawyer RG, Schulman AM, McLemore EC, Young JS. Blood transfusions correlate with infections in trauma patients in a dose-dependent manner. The American surgeon. 2002;68(7):566–72.

15. Bochicchio GV, Napolitano L, Joshi M, Bochicchio K, Shih D, Meyer W, Scalea TM. Blood product transfusion and ventilator-associated pneumonia in trauma patients. Surgical Infections. 2008;9(4):415–22.

16. Dunne JR, Riddle MS, Danko J, Hayden R, Petersen K. Blood transfusion is associated with infection and increased resource utilization in combat casualties. The American Surgeon. 2006;72(7):619–26.

17. Bochicchio GV, Napolitano L, Joshi M, Bochicchio K, Meyer W, Scalea TM. Outcome analysis of blood product transfusion in trauma patients: A prospective, risk-adjusted study. World Journal of Surgery. 2008;32:2185–9.

18. Harr JN, Moore EE, Chin TL, Ghasabyan A, Gonzalez E, Wohlauer MV, *et al.* Platelets are dominant contributors to hypercoagulability after injury. Journal of Trauma and Acute Care Surgery. 2013;74(3):756–62.

19. Barrera LM, Perel P, Ker K, Cirocchi R, Farinella E, Morales Uribe CH. Thromboprophylaxis for trauma patients. Cochrane Database of Systematic Reviews. 2013;3:CD008303.

20. Nathens AB, McMurray MK, Cuschieri J, Durr EA, Moore EE, Bankey PE, *et al.* The practice of venous thromboembolism prophylaxis in the major trauma patient. Journal of Trauma and Acute Care Surgery. 2007;62(3):557–63.

21. Louis SG, Sato M, Geraci T, Anderson R, Cho SD, Van PY, *et al.* Correlation of missed doses of enoxaparin with increased incidence of deep vein thrombosis in trauma and general surgery patients. JAMA Surgery. 2014;149(4):365–70.

22. Rogers FB, Shackford SR, Wilson J, Ricci MA, Morris CS. Prophylactic vena cava filter insertion in severely injured trauma patients: Indications and preliminary results. The Journal of Trauma. 1993;35(4):637–41.

23. Rogers FB, Shackford SR, Ricci MA, Wilson JT, Parsons S. Routine prophylactic vena cava filter insertion in severely injured trauma patients decreases the incidence of pulmonary embolism. Journal of the American College of Surgeons. 1995;180(6): 641–7.

24. Comes RF, Mismetti P, Afshari A, Force EVGT. European guidelines on perioperative venous thromboembolism prophylaxis: Inferior vena cava filters. European Journal of Anaesthesiology. 2018;35(2):108–11.

25. Shackford SR, Cook A, Rogers FB, Littenberg B, Osler T. The increasing use of vena cava filters in adult trauma victims: Data from the American College of Surgeons National Trauma Data Bank. The Journal of Trauma. 2007;63(4):764–9.

26. Haut ER, Garcia LJ, Shihab HM, Brotman DJ, Stevens KA, Sharma R, *et al.* The effectiveness of prophylactic inferior vena cava filters in trauma patients: A systematic review and meta-analysis. JAMA Surgery. 2014;149(2):194–202.

27. Bandle J, Shackford SR, Sise CB, Knudson MM, Group CS. Variability is the standard: The management of venous thromboembolidisease following trauma. The Journal of Trauma and Acute Care Surgery. 2014;76(1):213–6.

28. Ashbaugh DG, Bigelow DB, Petty TL, Levine BE. Acute respiratory distress in adults. Lancet. 1967;2(7511):319–23.

29. Vincent JL, Zambon M. Why do patients who have acute lung injury/acute respiratory distress syndrome die from multiple organ dysfunction syndrome? Implications for management. Clinics in Chest Medicine. 2006;27(4):725–31. 10.1016/j.ccm.2006. 06.010.

30. Cheung AM, Tansey CM, Tomlinson G, Diaz-Granados N, Matte A, Barr A, *et al.* Two-year outcomes, health care use, and costs of survivors of acute respiratory distress syndrome. American Journal of Respiratory and Critical Care. 2006;174(5): 538–44.

31. Ware LB. Pathophysiology of acute lung injury and the acute respiratory distress syndrome. Seminars in Respiratory and Critical Care Medicine. 2006;27(4):337–49. 10.1055/s-2006-948288.

32. Ware LB, Matthay MA. The acute respiratory distress syndrome. The New England Journal of Medicine. 2000;342(18):1334–49.

33. Chaiwat O, Lang JD, Vavilala MS, Wang J, MacKenzie EJ, Jurkovich GJ, Rivara FP. Early packed red blood cell transfusion and acute respiratory distress syndrome after trauma. Anesthesiology. 2009;110(2):351–60.

34. Silverboard H, Aisiku I, Martin GS, Adams M, Rozycki G, Moss M. The role of acute blood transfusion in the development of acute respiratory distress syndrome in patients with severe trauma. The Journal of Trauma. 2005;59(3):717–23.

35. Watson GA, Sperry JL, Rosengart MR, Minei JP, Harbrecht BG, Moore EE, *et al.* Inflammation and the Host Response to Injury Investigators. Fresh frozen plasma is independently associated with a higher risk of multiple organ failure and acute respiratory distress syndrome. Journal of Trauma and Acute Care Surgery. 2009;67(2):221–30.

36. Watkins TR, Rubenfeld GD, Martin TR, Nester TA, Caldwell E, Billgren J, *et al.* Effects of leukoreduced blood on acute lung injury after trauma: A randomized controlled trial. Critical Care Medicine. 2008;36(5):1493–9.

37. Willson DF, Notter RH. The future of exogenous surfactant therapy. Respir Care. 2011;56(9):1369–86. 10.4187/respcare.01306.

38. Raoof S, Goulet K, Esan A, Hess DR, Sessler CN. Severe hypoxemic respiratory failure: Part 2–nonventilatory strategies. Chest. 2010;137(6):1437–48. 10.1378/chest.09-2416.

39. Bakowitz M, Bruns B, McCunn M. Acute lung injury and the acute respiratory distress syndrome in the injured patient. Scandinavian Journal of Trauma, Resuscitation and Emergency Medicine. 2012;20:54.

40. Sauaia A, Moore FA, Moore EE, Moser KS, Brennan R, Read RA, Pons PT. Epidemiology of trauma deaths: A reassessment. Journal of Trauma and Acute Care Surgery. 1995;38(2):185–93.

41. Soreide K, Kruger AJ, Vardal AL, Ellingsen CL, Soreide E, Lossius HM. Epidemiology and contemporary patterns of trauma deaths: Changing place, similar pace, older face. World Journal of Surgery. 2007;31(11):2092–103.

42. Dewar DC, Tarrant SM, King KL, Balogh ZJ. Changes in the epidemiology and prediction of multiple-organ failure after injury. The Journal of Trauma and Acute Care Surgery. 2013;74(3):774–9.

43. Nast-Kolb D, Aufmkolk M, Rucholtz S, Obertacke U, Waydhas C. Multiple organ failure still a major cause of morbidity but not mortality in blunt multiple trauma. The Journal of Trauma. 2001;51(5):835–41.

44. Brattstrom O, Granath F, Rossi P, Oldner A. Early predictors of morbidity and mortality in trauma patients treated in the intensive care unit. Acta Anaesthesiologica Scandinavica. 2010;54(8):1007–17.

45. Ciesla DJ, Moore EE, Johnson JL, Burch JM, Cothren CC, Sauaia A. A 12-year prospective study of postinjury multiple organ failure: Has anything changed? Archives of Surgery. 2005;140(5):432–8.

46. Gando S, Nakanishi Y, Kameue T, Nanzaki S. Soluble thrombomodulin increases in patients with disseminated intravascular coagulation and in those with multiple organ dysfunction syndrome after trauma: Role of neutrophil elastase. The Journal of Trauma. 1995;39(4):660–4.

47. Kutcher ME, Xu J, Vilardi RF, Ho C, Esmon CT, Cohen MJ. Extracellular histone release in response to traumatic injury: Implications for a compensatory role of activated protein C. The Journal of Trauma and Acute Care Surgery. 2012;73(6): 1389–94.

48. Floccard B, Rugeri L, Faure A, Saint Denis M, Boyle EM, Peguet O, Levrat A, Guillaume C, Marcotte G, Vulliez A, Hautin E. Early coagulopathy in trauma patients: An on-scene and hospital admission study. Injury. 2012;43(1):26–32.

49. Raza I, Davenport R, Rourke C, Platton S, Manson J, Spoors C, *et al.* The incidence and magnitude of fibrinolytic activation in trauma patients. Journal of Thrombosis and Haemostasis. 2013;11(2):307–14.

50. Herbert J, Guillotte A, Hammer R, Litofsky N. Coagulopathy in the setting of mild traumatic brain injury: Truths and consequences. Brain Science. 2017;7(7):92.

51. Ali MFA, Ghoul AMF, Refaat MI. The effect of serum D-dimer levels on the cognitive outcome of patients with moderate traumatic brain injury. Egyptian Journal of Neurosurgery. 2021;36(1):10.

52. Abdelmalik PA, Boorman DW, Tracy J, Jallo J, Rincon F. Acute traumatic coagulopathy accompanying isolated traumatic brain injury is associated with worse long-term functional and cognitive outcomes. Neurocrit Care. 2016;24(3):361–70.

53. Walker KR, Tesco G. Molecular mechanisms of cognitive dysfunction following traumatic brain injury. Frontiers in Aging Neuroscience. 2013;5:29.

54. Jenkins PO, De Simoni S, Bourke NJ, Fleminger J, Scott G, Towey DJ, Svensson W, Khan S, Patel MC, Greenwood R, Friedland D. Stratifying drug treatment of cognitive impairments after traumatic brain injury using neuroimaging. Brain. 2019;142(8): 2367–79.

55. De Luca C, Virtuoso A, Maggio N, Papa M. Neuro-coagulopathy: Blood coagulation factors in central nervous system diseases. The International Journal of Molecular Sciences. 2017;18(10):2128.

56. Harhangi BS, Kompanje EJO, Leebeek FWG, Maas AIR. Coagulation disorders after traumatic brain injury. Acta Neurochir (Wien). 2008;150(2):165–75.

57. Abdelmalik P, Jallo J, Rincon F. Acute traumatic coagulopathy accompanying traumatic brain injury is associated with worse long term cognitive and functional outcomes: A retrospective analysis of the COBRIT data. (S27. 005). Neurology. 2015; 84(14_supplement):S27–005.

58. Rani P, Panda N, Hazarika A, Ahluwalia J, Chhabra R. Trauma-induced coagulopathy: Incidence and outcome in patients with isolated traumatic brain injury in a level I trauma care center in India. Asian journal of neurosurgery. 2019;14(04):1175–80.

59. Albert V, Arulselvi S, Agrawal D, Pati HP, Pandey RM. Early posttraumatic changes in coagulation and fibrinolysis systems in isolated severe traumatic brain injury patients and its influence on immediate outcome. Hematology/oncology and stem cell therapy. 2019;12(1):32–43.

60. Chhabra G, Rangarajan K, Subramanian A, Agrawal D, Sharma S, Mukhopadhayay AK. Hypofibrinogenemia in isolated traumatic brain injury in Indian patients. Neurology India. 2010;58(5):756–7.

61. Chhabra G, Sharma S, Subramanian A, Agrawal D, Sinha S, Mukhopadhyay AK. Coagulopathy as prognostic marker in acute traumatic brain injury. Journal of emergencies, trauma, and shock. 2013;6(3):180–5.

62. Kulkarni KK, Bhandari AP, Rathod P. Study of coagulation profile in patients admitted to a trauma center in a tertiary care hospital. Journal of Applied Hematology. 2021;12(1):26–30.

63. Holbrook TL, Anderson JP, Sieber WJ, Browner D, Hoyt DB. Outcome after major trauma: 12-month and 18-month follow-up results from the trauma recovery project. J. Trauma. 1999;46;765–71.

64. Christensen MC, Banner C, Lefering R, Vallejo-Torres L, Morris S. Quality of life after severe trauma: Results from the global trauma trial with recombinant factor VII. The Journal of Trauma. 2011;70:1524–31.

65. Winthrop AL, Brasel KJ, Stahovic L, Paulson J, Schneeberger B, Kuhn EM. Quality of life and functional outcome after pediatric trauma. Journal of Trauma and Acute Care Surgery. 2005;58(3):468–74.

66. Moore EE, Moore HB, Kornblith LZ, Neal MD, Hoffman M, Mutch NJ, Schöchl H, Hunt BJ, Sauaia A. Trauma-induced coagulopathy. Nature Reviews Disease Primers. 2021;7(1):30.

67. Klok FA, Van Der Hulle T, Den Exter PL, Lankeit M, Huisman MV, Konstantinides S. The post-PE syndrome: A new concept for chronic complications of pulmonary embolism. Blood reviews. 2014;28(6):221–6.

68. Pengo V, Lensing AW, Prins MH, Marchiori A, Davidson BL, Tiozzo F, *et al.* Incidence of chronic thromboembolic pulmonary hypertension after pulmonary embolism. New England Journal of Medicine. 2004;350(22):2257–64.

69. Anderson DR, Morgano GP, Bennett C, Dentali F, Francis CW, Garcia DA, *et al.* American society of hematology 2019 guidelines for management of venous thromboembolism: Prevention of venous thromboembolism in surgical hospitalized patients. Blood advances. 2019;3(23):3898–944.

Chapter 9

FUTURE DIRECTIONS IN TRAUMA-INDUCED COAGULOPATHY

Richa Chauhan and Jasmita Dass

DOI: 10.1201/9781003711070-9

INTRODUCTION

Management of trauma is time-bound navigation of the interplay of endogenous factors like shock, hypoperfusion, metabolic acidosis, endothelial injury, dysregulated fibrinolysis, coagulopathy, trauma-induced brain injury, and iatrogenic factors like massive blood transfusions, hypocalcemia, and surgical interventions. Quick judgment of the type and extent of trauma, rapid transport of the patient to the appropriate trauma care facility, and volume management are the baseline factors that determine the crucial next 24 hours for the patient.[1] It is pertinent to control bleeding and identify early trauma-induced coagulopathy (TIC) through clinical, biochemical, and hematological factors triggering massive transfusion protocol (MTP).[2] Research and advancements in trauma care focus on investigating early markers of TIC and on testing based algorithms or artificial intelligence (AI)-based scoring systems to administer the right blood product at the right time,[3] supplementing existing guidelines.[4,5] Moreover, early TIC transitions to a procoagulant phenotype, and the management needs to be changed accordingly. Inflammation takes center stage, and many novel treatments attempt to mitigate these effects to reduce TIC. In this chapter, we aim to cover the developments in diagnostic strategies, current guidelines, scope for improvement, future directions, and advanced research in TIC.

ENHANCED DIAGNOSTIC CAPABILITIES

The use of advanced diagnostic tools and point-of-care testing (POCT) aids in diagnosing TIC.[5-9] Various point-of-care (POC) devices used in TIC are detailed in Table 9.1. A representative overview of commonly used point-of-care and bedside diagnostic devices in acute and critical care settings is shown in Figure 9.1.

CONVENTIONAL VEM-BASED TRAUMA GUIDELINES

Conventional viscoelastic methods (VEMs) of clot dynamics generate real-time coagulation parameters like reaction time (RT), rate of clot formation angle (alpha angle), time for 2 mm to 20 mm tracing amplitude (k time), maximum amplitude (MA), clot strength (G), and clot lysis at 30 minutes (Ly30). A randomized clinical trial conducted at a Level 1 academic trauma center compared thromboelastography (TEG)-guided MTP in trauma patients with conventional coagulation assays (CCAs). It revealed a statistically significant decrease in mortality when using less plasma and platelet blood products, with VEM-based decision algorithms triggering transfusions.[20] Pragmatic algorithms for VEM-guided transfusion management are outlined by Gonzalez, Moore, et al.[21] The utility of VEM extends to the detection of distinct patterns of TBI associated with a hypercoagulable state lacking fibrinolysis.[22]

ADVANCED TECHNOLOGIES

Sonorheometry (sonic estimation of elasticity via resonance [SEER]) is a novel next-generation hemostasis analyzer that employs sonic estimation of elasticity via resonance (SEER) to measure the developing clot stiffness (CS). This reduces interference by mechanical clot formation and increases accuracy. However, more studies are needed for validation and future use.[23] Rapid microfluidics thromboelastography (μ-TEG) is a recently described viscoelastic method to study oscillatory flow of whole blood in circular tubes and generate TEG-equivalent results. High shear rates ranging from 1.2 to 20 s^{-1} move blood back and forth in tubes, and a pressure sensor monitors the movements. High shear rates accelerate

Table 9.1 Various POCTs in trauma settings

POCT	Devices	Technique	Sample requirement	Parameters	Advantages/limitations
Non-invasive Hb/Hct monitoring, POC blood lactate, POC ultrasound, capnometer					
Noninvasive continuous hemoglobin monitoring[10,11]	Masimo sensor (Masimo Rainbow Disposable Adhesive Sensor) and monitor (Masimo Radical-7, Masimo Corp, Irvine, California, USA).	Co-oxymetry	The device uses a pulse oximeter probe applied to the third or fourth digit of the left hand.	Spectromphotometric-Hb (Sp-Hb)	Larger validation studies needed to prove its accuracy in predicting transfusion requirement especially pediatric trauma patients. Bias reported at low levels.
Prehospital blood lactate[12]	Stat Strip Xpress (SSX) (Nova Biomedical, Waltham, MA, USA)	Measures the size of the electrical current produced due to the chemical reaction between lactate in the blood and the enzyme lactate oxidase in the test strip.	0.6 mL capillary sample; analysis time 13 seconds	Whole blood lactate; [measurement range: 0.3–20.0 mmol/L; Operational temperature span: 15–40°C].	Concordance with standard measurements and reproducibility demonstrated in previous studies; negative bias in higher concentration
Pre-hospital US (PHUS)[13,14]	-Extended Focused Assessment with Sonography for Trauma (eFAST) -Transthoracic echocardiography -Lung ultrasound/Bilateral Lung Ultrasound in Emergency (BLUE) protocol	Portable ultrasound devices		Point of care US (POCUS)	Concerns regarding feasibility, education, and quality assurance

(*Continued*)

Table 9.1 (*Continued*)

POCT	Devices	Technique	Sample requirement	Parameters	Advantages/limitations
Capnometry[15]	Capnometer	A unique CO_2 sensor to measure its absorption in the infrared spectrum, from which the CO_2 concentration is calculated	Patients inhale and exhale normally into a handheld device with nasal prongs/ under CPAP mask, for a short period of time (<60 seconds).	Provides breath-to-breath ventilation data End tidal CO_2 ($ETCO_2$).	Capnography provides feedback on the quality of compressions and when a compressor change is needed. An $ETCO_2$ <10 mmHg indicates that compressions are not fast or deep enough. If circulation is restored, a spike in $ETCO_2$ often appears before a pulse is detected
Plethysmography	Pulse oximeter	Measures pulsatile changes in blood volume and gas trapped based on the transmittance or absorbance of light	Pulses of red and infrared LED to pick up the peaks and troughs of pulse waves over several hundred times per second are converted to an electrical signal and pulse waveforms.	Perfusion index (PI) [ratio of pulsatile on non-pulsatile light absorbance or reflectance expressed as %]	Together with PI it is useful for non-invasive peripheral perfusion assessment, e.g., MightySat Rx (Masimo Corp, Irvine, California, USA).

PT/INR- PT-ratio (PT-r)[9,16]					
POC PT-r	CoaguChek XS (Roche, Mannheim, Germany) CoaguChek XS Plus/ Pro (Roche, Mannheim, Germany) Coag-Sense (CoaguSense Inc, Fremont, California) Hemochron Signature Elite (Werfen, New Jersey, USA) i-STAT (Abbott Point of Care, New Jersey, USA) ProTime and ProTime III (ITC, New Jersey, USA)	Electrochemical cleavage (amperometric) Optical/mechanical (microfluidics flow) Electrochemical cleavage	Capillary or venous WB (native or citrated) Whole blood, non-citrated	PT/INR ratio	Calibration, ISI for POC INR instrument thromboplastins is assigned by the manufacturers. Typically, 3–5% of the coefficient of variation (CV). Most devices are CLIA approved QC available
Viscoelastic methods (VEMs)					
Rapid VEM[9]					
ROTEM at 5 minutes (ROTEM 5)[17]	ROTEM® [Werfen (Tem Innovations GmbH), Munich, Germany]	Viscoelastic method	Whole blood (WB); citrated	Clot firmness in EXTEM at 5 minutes -A5(17)	Cutoff values <35 mm have been proposed however, cutoff as low as 30 mm and 25 mm have been defined for triggering transfusion. Still not used as an independent parameter for decision-making.

(Continued)

Table 9.1 (*Continued*)

POCT	Devices	Technique	Sample requirement	Parameters	Advantages/limitations
Rapid TEG (rTEG)[18]	TEG6s (Haemonetics Corp., Boston, USA) TEG-5000 (Haemonetics Corp., Boston, USA)	Resonance technology Automated cartridge-based system Laser light scattering is collected in reflection and/or transmission mode and the fluctuations of laser speckle intensity is processed to derive parameters of coagulation and fibrinolysis	Whole blood (WB); citrated Non-anticoagulated whole blood, a few drops	CK.R CFF.MA CK.Ly30 CRT.MA Blood viscoelasticity index, G $\lvert G^*(\omega)\rvert$	Smallest cartridge-based VEM Comparative studies with the demonstration of linearity with conventional TEG available. Validation studies required
QStat[19]	Multi-channel cartridge that provides semi-quantitative indications of the coagulation and clot lysis state of a 3.2% citrated venous whole blood sample using the Quantra® Hemostasis Analyzer (Hemosonics, North Carolina, USA).	Viscoelastic properties of whole blood	Whole blood (WB); citrated	CT: Clot time (Results in ~ 5 minutes) CS: Clot stiffness PCS: Platelet contribution to clot stiffness FCS: Fibrinogen contribution to clot stiffness (~12.5 minutes) CSL: Clot stability to lysis (44 ± 10 minutes)	Validation studies are required

Abbreviations: *CPAP: continuous positive airway pressure; POC: point-of-care; PT/INR: prothrombin time/international standardized ratio; ISI: International Sensitivity Index; CLIA: Clinical Laboratory Improvement Amendments; ROTEM: rotational thromboelastometry; TEG: thromboelastography.*

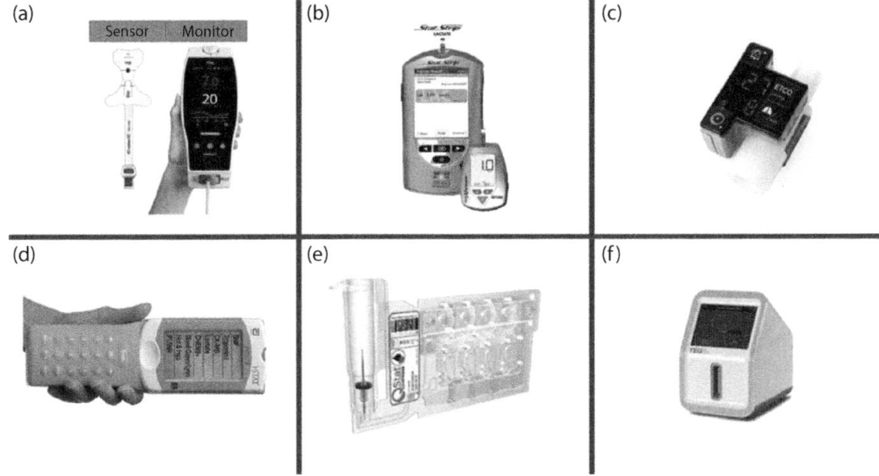

Figure 9.1 Representative point-of-care and bedside diagnostic devices used in acute and critical care: (A) pulse oximetry sensor and monitor, (B) handheld blood glucose analyzer, (C) portable capnometer, (D) handheld blood gas and electrolyte analyzer, (E) viscoelastic hemostasis assay cartridge, and (F) automated thromboelastography system. (The figure is an author-created composite illustration using representative device images for academic and educational purposes and is not reproduced from a single published source.)

fibrin polymerization and, hence, yield rapid results. The results are available in 10 minutes. Wang *et al.* demonstrated a good agreement with the conventional TEG.[24]

EDUCATION AND AWARENESS

Raising awareness about TIC and promoting preventive measures and pre-hospital management.

i. It is important to recognize that the management of TIC can be improved if measures are started in the pre-hospital phase. An example is the multidisciplinary collaborative chain management model. Multidisciplinary collaborative chain management models in which the team comprises the emergency department, operating room, anesthesiology, radiology, laboratory, and specialists from various surgical departments. The teams are trained in their respective job responsibilities. The multidisciplinary collaborative chain model has enabled speedier interventions and control of complications among trauma patients.[25]

ii. Another formal way is remote damage control resuscitation (RDCR), which has been formally inducted by military forces to reduce the incidence of TIC. In this method, the concept of damage control resuscitation is applied in pre-hospital and austere care settings. It aims to achieve early management of compressible bleeds, avoid crystalloid and colloid infusion, balance volume resuscitation, and prevent coagulopathy and its aggravators, such as acidosis, hypothermia, and hypocalcemia.[26] Adoption of this approach led to remarkable benefits in Israel, both for the military and civilian trauma. However, they note that applying the RDCR approach requires continuous evidence-based education and training, as well as a bottom-up approach.[27]

FUTURE DIRECTIONS AND INNOVATIONS

NOVEL THERAPEUTIC TARGETS FOR TRAUMA COAGULOPATHY
DEVELOPMENT OF DRUGS TARGETING SPECIFIC PATHWAYS INVOLVED IN TIC

Gosselin *et al.* used rheometry, turbidity, and confocal microscopy to study the influence of individual and combined factors on fibrin clot dynamics during TIC using a plasma model of a simulated TIC (STIC). They propose that this can help to develop targeted therapies in TIC.[28] A Hungarian study group recruited 117 bleeding trauma patients for evaluation by high-resolution fluororespirometry of isolated platelets to study mitochondrial respiration. Upon arrival, the platelet oxyphosphorylation capacity was correlated with rotational thromboelastometry (ROTEM) parameters. The pathophysiology of platelet mitochondrial dysfunction may reveal new therapeutic targets soon.[29] Early sex hormone milieu post-trauma influences initial outcomes in trauma patients. A prospective study on 288 trauma patients revealed increased testosterone levels at 6 hours after trauma and its positive correlation with multiorgan failure, while after 24 hours, estrogen elevation increased the chances of multiorgan failure.[30] Li C *et al.* studied calcitonin gene-related peptide (CGRP) expression and its protective effect on TBI in rat models. They have postulated that CGRP's differential sex-based expression can be a novel option in drug targeting in TBI.[31] Severe trauma induces emergency myelopoiesis;[32,33] three important events occur—an expansion of myeloid-derived suppressor cells (MDSCs), lymphocyte dysfunction and lymphopenia, and inadequate stress erythropoiesis. Studies to develop targeted therapy to rectify these events are ongoing. Beta-adrenergic blockade,[34] recombinant erythropoietin,[35] blocking lymphocyte apoptosis, and abrogating MDSCs response by reducing PD-L1 expression have been or are being investigated.[33] Mechanisms of *enhanced hyperfibrinolysis* include activation of protein C, reduced activity of coagulation factors, increased tPA activity, fibrinogen oxidation, degradation, hemodilution, and acidosis. Subsequent *fibrinolysis shutdown* sets in TIC.[36] Understanding the pathophysiology of the hemostatic effects of damaged or activated endothelium via anticoagulant and antifibrinolytic systems will further help build therapeutic targets.[37] *Endogenous or primary factors*, including genetics, medications, comorbidities, and innate immune defects, can hamper the primary response in TIC. Similarly, *secondary factors* of acidosis, hypothermia, and dilution can modify outcomes of primary coagulopathy. *Ischemia reperfusion events* after resuscitation lead to sustained activation of coagulation pathways and fibrinolysis inhibition during late phases of TIC, which can result in organ damage due to systemic inflammatory response syndrome.[37] Thus, the degree of resuscitation and its response may also predict mortality, forming an area for further research.

GENOMIC AND BIOMARKER-BASED STRATEGIES

In a large genome-wide association study (GWAS) and transcriptome-wide association study (TWAS) of genetic effects on TBI, an estimate of heritability for the impact of outcome variations among patients with TBI was 26%. Though the researchers did not find any statistically significant association with a particular set of genes/transcriptomes, they identified areas of research with plausible genes and transcriptomes.[38] Biomarker research to predict coagulopathy in trauma remains in its infancy. Among patients with TBI, a 2022 systematic review included only 12 studies and found that Copeptin had the highest sensitivity and S100A12 had the highest specificity for predicting coagulopathy. For progressive hemorrhagic injury, IL-33 had the best sensitivity, while Galectin-3 had the best specificity.[39] A study exploring POCT iSTAT showed that high levels of glial fibrillary acidic protein (GFAP) were predictive of higher Rotterdam scores on initial scans and TBI progression.[40] Another study in mice showed elevated plasma concentrations of the damage molecule high-mobility group box-1 (HMGB-1) post-trauma. The investigators demonstrated they could correct the ROTEM-EXTEM profile by adding an anti-HMGB-1 monoclonal antibody, and the results improved further when recombinant thrombomodulin was also supplemented.[41]

Table 9.2 Impact of genes/factors on TIC in patients with traumatic brain injury[42–46]

Name of the gene/factor	Impact
FVL, PT, MTHFR, LA, Factor VIII, Hcy	Increased rate of venous thromboembolism
Syndecan-1	Marker of glycocalyx degradation leading to hypocoagulability, Increased transfusion requirement, worse outcomes
Activated protein C	Increased transfusion requirement, worse outcomes, multi-organ failure
Inherited bleeding, thrombotic, and platelet disorders (BPDs) genes	High throughput sequencing platform to detect the genetic variants in BPD genes available
PROS1 (protein S encoding gene)	Heterozygous mutations create transient thrombotic risk

IDENTIFICATION OF GENETIC MARKERS AND MOLECULAR TARGETS FOR PERSONALIZED THERAPY

Christopher David *et al.* have reviewed the idea of precision medicine in trauma care. They found a relative scarcity of genomic studies in TIC and pharmacology compared to TBI and trauma-related sepsis. Further, there is a need for more data utilizing genomics in clinical decision-making, thus a potential research area.[42] Inherited and acquired predispositions to thrombophilia are listed in Table 9.2.

ADVANCED RESEARCH IN TRAUMA COAGULOPATHY
ROLE OF HEMOGLOBIN AND A-GLOBIN IN TIC

Systemic hyperfibrinolysis during the early phase of TIC contributes to morbidity and mortality in trauma patients. Hyperfibrinolysis occurs in ~25% of TIC patients. Proteomics-based *in vitro* research in hyperfibrinolysis has revealed the role of fibrinolysis augmentation by releasing hemoglobin and alpha globins from injured cells.[36,47] Further, *in vitro* studies showed only α-globin shortened R time and increased Ly30 for citrated native TEG. In addition, α-globin augmented tPA-induced plasmin activity.[36]

USAGE OF FACTOR V IN ADDITION TO PROTHROMBIN COMPLEX CONCENTRATE (PCC) AS A REVERSAL STRATEGY FOR THE MANAGEMENT OF BLEEDING COMPLICATIONS, ESPECIALLY IN PATIENTS ON NEWER ORAL ANTICOAGULANTS (NOACS)

It is pertinent to note the history of prior bleeding tendencies, whether inherited or acquired in trauma patients, from either accompanying informants or personal identification cards. Patients on vitamin K antagonists or NOACs like factor Xa inhibitors and direct thrombin inhibitors (DTIs) require reversal of anticoagulant effect as soon as possible to control exsanguination. In patients not on NOACs, a meta-analysis examined the use of PCC with fresh frozen plasma (FFP) in TIC, an off-label use. They found that the PCC+FFP combination was associated with faster international normalized ratio (INR) corrections and a reduced requirement for red blood cell (RBC) and plasma transfusions. At the same time, there was no impact on platelet transfusions or the development of deep vein thrombosis.[48] Even with these improvements, PCC had no overall impact on mortality.[49] PCC at doses of 25-30 IU/Kg is given, and therapy is tailored to reduce INR to <1.4 in 15 minutes; otherwise, a repeat dose can be administered.[50] Among patients on NOACs, antidotes are idaracizumab for the direct thrombin inhibitor (DTI) dabigatran and andexanet alpha for anti-Xa inhibitors. However, these are not available at many centers across the world, and PCC can be used to mitigate the coagulopathy of trauma in patients on NOACs. For PCC in *in vitro* experiments simulating coagulopathy of NOAC, PCC supplementation alone increased the thrombin generated. Moreover, adding factor V to PCC corrected fibrin production under flow and partially corrected clotting time in static conditions.[51]

ENGINEERED FACTOR V FOR PREVENTION AND TREATMENT OF ACUTE TRAUMATIC COAGULOPATHY

An engineered active factor V, called SuperFVa, has been manufactured; it is resistant to the effects of APC and has a stabilizing disulfide bond in the A2–A3 domain. SuperFVA was tested in mice with acute TIC and led to normalization of the activated partial thromboplastin time (APTT), factor V, and factor VIII levels. Upon treatment, the mice also showed reduced thrombin-antithrombin complexes (TAT). Further, mice were given a liver laceration, and transfusion of superFVa could mitigate bleeding, prevent prolongation of APTT, prevent generation of APC, and prevent a reduction in levels of factor V and factor VIII. Thus, it prevented the development of coagulopathy of acute trauma.[52]

IMPLICATION OF IMMUNE CELL INFLAMMATION IN THE PATHOPHYSIOLOGY OF TIC

IL-6 MEDIATED MONOCYTE ACTIVATION LEADING TO FIBRINOGEN OXIDATION AND DEGRADATION

The role of leukocyte activation cannot be undermined in TIC. Tissue injury releases cytokines like Interleukin-6 (IL-6) and tumor necrosis factor-alpha (TNF-α), generating mitochondrial superoxides from neutrophils and monocytes. These cytokines activate myeloperoxidase-derived reactive oxygen species (ROS) from neutrophils and nitric oxide (NO) from monocytes and lymphocytes. Their target for oxidation includes fibrinogen, a central protein in coagulation pathways.[53] Oxidative denaturation of fibrinogen occurs in the first hour of severe trauma, thus producing a state of hypocoagulability and contributing to exsanguination. After 3 hours, Lipopolysaccharide-induced inflammation causes degradation of fibrinogen. Thus, with the hypothesis that fibrinogen can be saved from oxidative destruction by quenching with antioxidants, the researchers used rat models to study cytokine levels at various stages of leukocyte activation and the resultant effect on coagulation.[53]

THERAPEUTIC TARGETS

Tranexamic acid (TXA) helps control bleeding as part of standard care in polytrauma during the initial 3 hours when priming of inflammation and fibrinogen oxidation before its degradation begins. During this time, aggressive fibrinogen replacement along with TXA is useful. Based on a rat-model study by Han *et al.*, the timing of cocktails of anti-inflammatory and antioxidant drugs–high-dose vitamin C, thiamine, N-acetyl cysteine (NAC), and hydrocortisone—during the initial 3 hours can protect fibrinogen destruction, especially its Aα chain, which is not protected from lysis by plasminogen by using TXA alone.[53] Suppression of inflammation by the melanocortin pathway using a novel drug, melanocortin fusion protein (AQB-565), given in the initial hours, can potentially protect against fibrinogen oxidation and subsequent degradation.[54]

NOVEL ANTI-INFLAMMATORY MELANOCORTIN FUSION PROTEIN (AQB-565) INHIBITS FIBRIN

DEGRADATION AND PREVENTS TIC

The 'Glue Grant' research program, which focused on inflammation and genetic pathways activated in leukocytes post-polytrauma, indicated that >80% of the genome of leukocytes was activated, with the most significant changes in inflammation and innate immunity genes within the first 12 hours of injury.[55] Also, functional fibrinogen is rapidly depleted after trauma, which is accompanied by its selective oxidization. Melanocortins are known to protect against ischemia and reperfusion injury, but no peptide alone interacts with all five receptors, causing a lack of widespread anti-inflammatory effects. Aequs Biopharma developed a linear polypeptide, AQB-565, composed of adrenocorticotropic hormone (ACTH) and α-melanocyte-stimulating hormone (α-MSH). AQB-565 given immediately post-trauma could attenuate cytokine increase, restore prothrombin time and fibrinogen levels, and reduce oxidation of fibrinogen with hemorrhagic shock post-trauma in rats. In addition, it reduced the intracellular $TNF\alpha$ expression, reduced NFκb translocation, and inhibited ROS and mitochondrial superoxide and NO generation in monocytes.[54] Hence, suppressing inflammation by activating melanocortin pathways may be a novel approach for preventing and treating trauma-induced coagulopathy. However, no clinical trials have yet been registered for the use of AQB-565.

TRAUMA-INDUCED MYOSIN [SKELETAL MUSCLE MYOSIN (SkM)] AND COAGULOPATHY

Skeletal muscle myosin (SkM) is released into the circulation post-traumatic injury. Interaction of blood with SkM activates thrombin via the myosin–factor Va–factor Xa complex and suppresses fibrinolysis by activating thrombin-activatable fibrinolysis inhibitor (TAFI), thereby promoting procoagulant effects. SkM also has an anticoagulant effect, mediated by an increased activated protein C (APC) system.[56] Coleman *et al.* demonstrated that higher SkM levels in trauma patients led to better viscoelastic test results, including a higher α-angle, higher maximal amplitude (MA), and lower fibrinolysis at 30 minutes (Ly30). Patients with higher SkM levels required fewer red cell and FFP transfusions in the first 6 hours post-trauma. Penetrating trauma patients had higher levels of SkM than patients with blunt trauma. The results elucidated that full-SkM deficiency is associated with hypocoagulability and hyperfibrinolysis, leading to higher bleeding.[57] In the future, there might be a possibility of supplementing full-SkM in trauma patients.

OMICS CHARACTERIZATION (METABOLOMICS AND PROTEOMICS ALTERATIONS) IN TRAUMA-INDUCED COAGULOPATHY AND THE EFFECT OF TRANSFUSION STRATEGIES

SomaLogic proteomic analysis in the study by Moore *et al.* in 2022 showed that TIC defined based on conventional coagulation tests (CCTs), VEMs, and clinical scoring failed to identify patients at risk of MTP. The SOMAscan assay uses aptamers (~40-mer oligonucleotide strands with proprietary side chains) selected for binding to human plasma proteins and protein complexes, enabling the quantification of >1300 protein levels in parallel. The v. 1.3k assay measures a broad range of secreted proteins, including markers of cell death, hormones, growth factors, cytokines, and more. The assay signal is expressed as relative fluorescence units (RFUs). In addition to the RFU data, SomaLogic also performed a normalization using internal standard samples and provided normalized data. The proteins that differed significantly in patients with the TIC criteria were compared with those that differed significantly in patients according to massive transfusion status. Apolipoprotein 1, bone morphogenetic protein 1, growth hormone receptor, and complement C5b-C6 complex were all downregulated in TIC, as defined by INR, TEG, clinical score, and MTP requirement. The MTP-defined TIC group had many dysregulated proteins compared to each of INR-TIC, TEG-TIC, or Clin-TIC.[58] For example, APC is associated with massive bleeding and not necessarily associated with a prolonged INR, which supports the controversy that APC is not the central driver of TIC. Damage-associated molecular patterns (DAMPs) like HMGB-1 and histones are associated with platelet activation and TIC. Complement activation is also associated with INR-TIC and TEG-TIC. In the Control of Major Bleeding After Trauma (COMBAT) study, the samples were studied for differential metabolomics and proteomics among trauma patients with or without platelet transfusions within the first 24 hours. The patients who required platelet transfusions had higher levels of tranexamic acid, inflammatory proteins, carnitines, and polyamines.[59] A parallel study in the COMBAT study on patients who received red cell transfusions showed they were associated with lower levels of markers of hypoxia, such as lactic acid, succinate, spermidine, and other polyamines, while levels of additives like mannitol, phosphate, and plasticizers were higher. Arginine metabolite levels also change, indicating an impact on NO metabolism.[60]

ROLE OF ARTIFICIAL INTELLIGENCE (AI) AND PREDICTIVE MODELING IN COAGULOPATHY PREDICTION

AI IN DIAGNOSTICS AND PROGNOSTICS
IMPLEMENTATION OF AI TOOLS FOR EARLY DETECTION AND PREDICTION OF TIC

The standard diagnostic techniques have the limitation of taking ample time to yield results that compromise the crucial decision-making in the first hour post-injury. Hence, predictive models based on machine learning (ML) can provide valuable adjuncts for immediate decision-making and triaging. AI models that predict the likelihood of TIC or TBI in patients can substantially improve resource utilization and optimal allocation of therapeutic products to patients in need. Perkins *et al.* employed a Bayesian network-based ML model trained using data from the Activation of Coagulation and Inflammation in Trauma (ACIT) study. They validated the 14-predictor model in a large cohort for early prediction of TIC.[61] Similarly, Kaiyuan *et al.* published their findings on ML models based on traditional and newer testing results to predict the likelihood of acute traumatic coagulopathy.[62]

PREDICTIVE MODELING
USE OF MACHINE LEARNING MODELS TO ANTICIPATE TIC DEVELOPMENT AND OUTCOMES

A recent review by Henry T. Peng *et al.* collected 89 studies over the years that have employed AI in various aspects of trauma care research. Broad categories where AI is used are prediction of outcome, risk assessment for triage, prediction of transfusions, detection of hemorrhage, and prediction of coagulopathy.[3] Predictions of survival based on linear statistical models were built in 2001 and are known as Trauma and Injury Severity Score (TRISS); these are universally used.[64] Thereafter, advanced ML techniques such as deep neural networks, fuzzy logic inference systems, XGBoost, artificial neural networks, Bayesian networks, and natural language processing, have been used in various studies for predicting survival, mortality, triaging, risk calculation of hemorrhagic shock, and detection of intracranial hemorrhage. This means feeding multipronged exhaustive data of clinical, laboratory, and anatomic features from hospital registries, trial data, and registries into these ML networks and subsequently validating these algorithms on a prospective basis. Age, gender, systolic pressure, Glasgow Coma Scale, heart rate, respiratory rate, SpO_2, temperature, injury severity score, shock index, and type of injury were the most frequently used parameters in model development. Recently, Benjamin Andrew in 2022 studied early prediction of MTP for patients with traumatic hemorrhage using an ML model.[63] However, not all models can be used universally in pre-hospital settings for clinical triage of patients; hence, the output may not be available when 'needed' in the golden hour of trauma care.[3]

COLLABORATIVE EFFORTS AND GLOBAL INITIATIVES IN TRAUMA CARE

INTERNATIONAL GUIDELINES AND CONSENSUS STATEMENTS

Collaborative efforts are underway among leading trauma and coagulation experts worldwide to create standardized guidelines. Readers are referred to the following guidelines:

i. Advanced Trauma Life Support (ATLS) guidelines by the American College of Surgeons[4]

ii. European guidelines on the management of major bleeding and coagulopathy following trauma[5]

INTERNATIONAL RESEARCH CONSORTIA

The formation of consortia to conduct large-scale studies on TIC and improve evidence-based practices has led to multicenter trials that have refined practices and increased educational activities. A few such consortia and their goals are listed in Table 9.3. Table 9.4 lists the important clinical trials over the last decade or so on trauma outcomes, including TIC.

Table 9.3 International trauma networks

Consortium	Main goals	Website details
TACTIC: Trans-Agency Consortium for Trauma-Induced Coagulopathy[64]	(i) Basic science groundwork for future therapeutic candidates; (ii) development of acute coagulopathy scoring systems; (iii) coagulation factor composition-based computational analysis; (iv) characterization of novel analytes including tissue factor, polyphosphates, histones, meizothrombin and a-thrombin–antithrombin complexes, factor XIa, platelet and endothelial markers of activation, signatures of protein C activation and fibrinolysis markers; and (v) assessment of viscoelastic tests and new point-of-care methods.	https://tacticproject.org/
Trans-Agency Blood–Brain Interface Program (TBBIP)[65]	(1) blood sciences; (2) exosome therapeutics; (3) next generation *in vitro* blood–brain barrier (BBB) models; and (4) BBB delivery and targeting.	https://grants.nih.gov/grants/guide/rfa-files/RFA-HL-20-021.html
International Trauma Research Network (INTRN)[66]	Develop fundamental, translational and clinical research programs that span the complete breadth of Trauma disciplines. Support educational programs to ensure rapid translation of research into clinical practice Key projects: 2008: Activation of Coagulation and Inflammation in Trauma (ACIT) 2013-2019: Targeted Action for Curing Trauma-Induced Coagulopathy (TACTIC) CRYOSTAT-1: Feasibility of delivering early cryoprecipitate in patients at two major trauma centers	https://www.c4ts.qmul.ac.uk/intrn/intrn

Table 9.4 Important clinical trials in progress in TIC.

Trial	Premise/aim	Key findings
Pre-hospital Antifibrinolytics for Traumatic Coagulopathy and Hemorrhage (PATCH-Trauma) trial, 2023[67] and ongoing trials [NCT ID: NCT01990768]	Prehospital administration of TXA increases the likelihood of survival with a favorable functional outcome among patients with major trauma and suspected trauma-induced coagulopathy	Prehospital administration of TXA followed by an infusion over 8 hours did not result in a greater number of patients surviving with a favorable functional outcome at 6 months than placebo. Mayo clinical trials aim to study two dosing regimens for TXA in reducing TBI.
Fluid in resuscitation of severe trauma (FIRST) trial[68]	0.9% saline vs. hydroxyethyl starch (HES) in severe trauma to study impact on resuscitation, fluid volume, gastrointestinal recovery, renal function, and blood product requirement	In penetrating trauma, HES provided significantly better lactate clearance and less renal injury than saline. No firm conclusions could be drawn for blunt trauma.
Fibrinogen in the initial resuscitation of severe trauma (FiiRST) trial[69]	Feasibility study of randomization to either 6 g fibrinogen concentrate (FC) or placebo amongst 50 hypotensive adult trauma patients	Early infusion of FC (within 1 hour of hospital arrival) is feasible and safe; and it increases fibrinogen concentration during early hours of trauma care.
The Connect Trial [NCT ID: NCT02088099][70]	It will test the effectiveness of using modern technologies, such as phone consultation and other telehealth communication systems, to deliver specialized brain rehabilitation resources remotely to patients.	Using electronic technology in management of TBI to patients with minimal access to specialized care in trauma care.
Randomized TrauCC trial [NCT02750150][71]	Role of freeze dried plasma in TIC that can be administered within 6 minutes of reconstitution without cross matching.	Drastic reduction in time to treatment studied in this French trial.
TrICI trial [NCT03128658][72]	A 5-day demographic, physiological, clinical variables and lab data will be collected	Computational model will be developed to predict occurrence of life threatening TIC, inflammation and multi organ failure in trauma patients.

IMPORTANCE OF ONGOING RESEARCH, EDUCATION, AND QUALITY IMPROVEMENT IN TIC MANAGEMENT

CONTINUOUS EDUCATION AND TRAINING
DEVELOPMENT OF TRAINING PROGRAMS FOR HEALTHCARE PROVIDERS IN LOW- AND MIDDLE-INCOME COUNTRIES (LMIC)

Continuing professional development (CPD) in low- and middle-income countries (LMICs) is required to strengthen trauma care and improve mortality rates. These courses can be made mandatory for employment and recertification every few years to ensure improved trauma

Table 9.5   International organizations providing trauma courses and the intended beneficiaries

Course	Directed to	International organizer (country)
Advanced Trauma Life Support (ATLS)	Doctors	American College of Surgeons
AO trauma courses	Trauma surgeons and orthopedic surgeons	AO Foundation
Primary Trauma Care (PTC)	Anesthetists, doctors, nurses, physician assistants, others	Primary Trauma Care Foundation
Trauma Evaluation and Management (TEAM)	Doctors, medical students, nurses	American College of Surgeons
Advanced Trauma Management (Live virtual course)	Clinicians (physicians, nurses, NPs, APPs)	Harvard Medical School (Offered by Beth Israel Deaconess Medical Center)
Individual local courses	Variable	
Advanced Trauma Operative Management (ATOM) course	Senior surgical residents, trauma fellows, military surgeons and general surgeons	American College of Surgeons
Advanced Surgical Skills for Exposure in Trauma (ASSET)	Doctors	American College of Surgeons
Definitive Surgical Trauma Care (DSTC) course	Surgeons, anesthesiologists, operating room nurses	American College of Surgeons

care and keep physicians abreast of developments. Table 9.5[62,73] details a few such courses. In addition, various nursing associations provide access to continuous education activities.[74]

IMPLEMENTATION OF BEST PRACTICES AND PROTOCOLS TO ENHANCE PATIENT CARE
TELEMEDICINE PLATFORMS TO PROVIDE REAL-TIME EXPERT CONSULTATION IN REMOTE OR RESOURCE-LIMITED SETTINGS

The use of telemedicine for trauma management at rural centers is reported as early as 2008 across seven hospitals in Mississippi. Telemedicine virtual consults led to the management of 412/463 trauma patients, while only 51 were called to the trauma center. This improvement was massive considering the pre-telemedicine era, when 351 patients were referred to the trauma center, and led to markedly reduced hospital costs compared to the pre-telemedicine era.[75] Telemedicine requires two-way audio-video communication between a resource-limited and an expert trauma care facility. Telehealth is the need of the hour to ensure that Level I and II trauma centers are not overloaded, and at the same time, patients requiring urgent interventions are treated partially at the point of contact, enabling successful transfer to the trauma center.[76]

ENCOURAGING INNOVATION AND RESEARCH TO ADDRESS GAPS IN TIC MANAGEMENT
USE OF MOBILE APPS AND DIGITAL TOOLS FOR RAPID DIAGNOSIS AND MANAGEMENT OF TIC

The American College of Surgeons (ACS) Committee on Trauma (COT) has a mobile application, the MyATLS App, through which users can access the 10th edition of the Advanced Trauma Life Support (ATLS) program.[77] Educational video games (EVGs) to triage trauma patients were compared to didactic training methods (MyATLS app and Trauma Life Support MCQ Review). EVG training led to fewer patients being under-triaged at 6 months compared to didactic methods.[78] In addition, mobile applications for patient education for trauma patients were also developed,[79] but their use is not widely reported.

FUTURE DIRECTION FOR INDIA

India's geopolitical status makes its trauma scenario unique. Apart from road traffic accidents (RTAs), the country has a history of various natural disasters, agricultural-related trauma, armed civilian conflicts, and terrorist attacks.[80] India can address its gap by establishing a formalized trauma care system for prevention and management. Measures to improve road safety, engineering techniques, traffic calming measures, the rectification of 'black spots', and law enforcement will further strengthen the system.[81] Government schemes can include the provision of Unique Disability Identification (UDID) for citizens where patients with bleeding or thrombotic tendencies, primary or acquired immune defects, or drug history are readily available. The country can strengthen grassroots-level basic life support and advanced trauma care training across schools, medical schools, and nursing colleges, and extend it to non-medical graduate programs. India can strengthen its digital registry of trauma care to ensure multicentric data is available for advanced research and the development of a robust database. Rapid-action trauma care ambulances equipped with advanced diagnostics and emergency trauma care can be deployed on national highways or in accident-prone areas (as available from RTA records). Human resources and facilities are limited at the primary healthcare level and can be augmented through telemedicine. India should focus on the availability of pre-hospital trauma care, transfusion facilities, including component therapy, and dedicated teams of pre-hospital trauma care professionals with a reasonable coverage area to provide 'in-time' hemorrhage control and identify early TIC. The Institute of National Importance (INI), with research facilities in collaboration with Indian trauma care societies, can widen its research to integrate Indian genomics data and newer therapeutics in early bleeding, coagulopathy, and inflammation with existing tools of trauma care in India.

TAKE-HOME MESSAGE

Through this chapter, we have highlighted the current and future diagnostic techniques that enable quick and real-time checks of patient vitals pertinent to TIC and TBI. Comprehensive medical and paramedical staff training in the management of trauma and a dedicated multidisciplinary team approach for trauma care are the keys to appropriate trauma care. More insights from molecular biology that play a role in initial hemorrhage and later coagulopathy and concordant therapeutic trials for their targets will keep adding to the evolving practice in trauma care. With the artificial intelligence boom, we expect streamlining of the initial management of trauma patients that can buy time before life-threatening changes set in.

Figure Credits: Figure 9.1 is a composite created from non-copyrighted product images taken from manufacturers' websites for different POC equipment.

REFERENCES

1. Moore EE, Moore HB, Kornblith LZ, Neal MD, Hoffman M, Mutch NJ, *et al*. Trauma-induced coagulopathy. Nat Rev Dis Primer. 2021;7(1):30.

2. Baksaas-Aasen K, Gall LS, Stensballe J, Juffermans NP, Curry N, Maegele M, Brooks A, *et al*. Viscoelastic haemostatic assay augmented protocols for major trauma haemorrhage (ITACTIC): A randomized, controlled trial. Intensive Care Med. 2021;47(1):49–59.

3. Peng HT, Siddiqui MM, Rhind SG, Zhang J, da Luz LT, Beckett A, *et al.* Artificial intelligence and machine learning for hemorrhagic trauma care. Mil Med Res. 2023; 10(6):6.

4. Galvagno SM, Nahmias JT, Young DA. Advanced trauma life support® update 2019: Management and applications for adults and special populations. Anesthesiol Clin. 2019;37(1):13–32.

5. Rossaint R, Afshari A, Bouillon B, Cerny V, Cimpoesu D, Curry N, *et al.* The European guideline on management of major bleeding and coagulopathy following trauma: Sixth edition. Crit Care Lond Engl. 2023;27(1):80.

6. Stojek L, Bieler D, Neubert A, Ahnert T, Imach S, *et al.* The potential of point-of-care diagnostics to optimise prehospital trauma triage: A systematic review of literature. Eur J Trauma Emerg Surg. 2023;49(4):1727–39.

7. Goodman MD, Makley AT, Hanseman DJ, Pritts TA, Robinson BR, *et al.* All the bang without the bucks: Defining essential point-of-care testing for traumatic coagulopathy. J Trauma Acute Care Surg. 2015;79(1):117–24.

8. Dirkmann D, Britten MW, Frey UH. Point-of-care testing in trauma patients— methods and evidence. AINS. 2018;53(6):440–57.

9. Stein P, Kaserer A, Spahn GH, Spahn DR. Point-of-care coagulation monitoring in trauma patients. Semin Thromb Hemost. 2017;43(4):367–74.

10. Romanelli A, De Rosa RC. Continuous non-invasive hemoglobin monitoring in pediatric trauma setting. World J Pediatr Surg. 2023;6(4):e000614.

11. Gamal M, Abdelhamid B, Zakaria D, Dayem OAE, Rady A, Fawzy M, *et al.* Evaluation of noninvasive hemoglobin monitoring in trauma patients with low hemoglobin levels. Shock Augusta Ga. 2018;49(2):150–3.

12. Magnusson C, Herlitz J, Axelsson C, Höglind R, Lökholm E, Hörnfeldt TH, *et al.* Added predictive value of prehospital measurement of point-of-care lactate in an adult general EMS population in Sweden: A multi-centre observational study. Scand J Trauma Resusc Emerg Med. 2024;32(1):72.

13. Amaral CB, Ralston DC, Becker TK. Prehospital point-of-care ultrasound: A transformative technology. SAGE Open Med. 2020;8:2050312120932706.

14. van der Weide L, Popal Z, Terra M, Schwarte LA, Ket JCF, Kooij FO, *et al.* Prehospital ultrasound in the management of trauma patients: Systematic review of the literature. Injury. 2019;50(12):2167–75.

15. Conway A, Chang K, Goudarzi Rad M, Mafeld S, Parotto M, *et al.* Smart capnometry: Personalising the diagnosis and management of respiratory disease. Clin Med. 2019;19(Suppl 2):94.

16. Wool GD. Benefits and pitfalls of point-of-care coagulation testing for anticoagulation management: An ACLPS critical review. Am J Clin Pathol. 2019;151(1):1–17.

17. Kelly JM, Rizoli S, Veigas P, Hollands S, Min A, *et al.* Using rotational thromboelastometry clot firmness at 5 minutes (ROTEM® EXTEM A5) to predict massive transfusion and in-hospital mortality in trauma: A retrospective analysis of 1146 patients. Anaesthesia. 2018;73(9):1103–9.

18. Neal MD, Moore EE, Walsh M, Thomas S, Callcut RA, Kornblith LZ, *et al.* A comparison between the TEG 6s and TEG 5000 analyzers to assess coagulation in trauma patients. J Trauma Acute Care Surg. 2020;88(2):279–85.

19. Michelson EA, Cripps MW, Ray B, Winegar DA, Viola F. Initial clinical experience with the Quantra QStat System in adult trauma patients. Trauma Surg Acute Care Open. 2020;5(1):e000581.

20. Gonzalez E, Moore EE, Moore HB, Chapman MP, Chin TL, Ghasabyan A, *et al.* Goal-directed hemostatic resuscitation of trauma-induced coagulopathy: A pragmatic randomized clinical trial comparing a viscoelastic assay to conventional coagulation assays. Ann Surg. 2016;263(6):1051–9.

21. Gonzalez E, Moore EE, Moore HB. Management of trauma-induced coagulopathy with thrombelastography. Crit Care Clin. 2017;33(1):119–34.

22. Samuels JM, Moore EE, Silliman CC, Banerjee A, Cohen MJ, Ghasabyan A, *et al.* Severe traumatic brain injury is associated with a unique coagulopathy phenotype. J Trauma Acute Care Surg. 2019;86(4):686–93.

23. Rossetto A, Wohlgemut JM, Brohi K, Davenport R. Sonorheometry versus rotational thromboelastometry in trauma: A comparison of diagnostic and prognostic performance. J Thromb Haemost JTH. 2023;21(8):2114–25.

24. Wang J, Choi CU, Shin S. Rapid microfluidic-thromboelastography (μ-TEG) for evaluating whole blood coagulation and fibrinolysis at elevated shear rates. Sens Actuators B Chem. 2023;390:133873.

25. Xiang S, Tang W, Shang X, Ni H. Practice of multidisciplinary collaborative chain management model in constructing nursing path for acute trauma treatment. Emerg Med Int. 2022;2022:1342773.

26. Gerhardt RT, Strandenes G, Cap AP, Rentas FJ, Glassberg E, Mott J, *et al.* Remote damage control resuscitation and the Solstrand Conference: Defining the need, the language, and a way forward. Transfusion (Paris). 2013;53 (Suppl 1):9S–16S.

27. Talmy T, Mitchnik IY, Malkin M, Avital G, Benov A, Glassberg E, *et al.* Adopting a culture of remote damage control resuscitation in the military: Insights from the Israel defense forces decade of experience. Transfusion (Paris). 2023;63 (Suppl 3): S83–95.

28. Gosselin AR, White NJ, Bargoud CG, Hanna JS, Tutwiler V, *et al.* Hyperfibrinolysis drives mechanical instabilities in a simulated model of trauma induced coagulopathy. Thromb Res. 2022;220:131–40.

29. Jávor P, Rárosi F, Horváth T, Török L, Hartmann P, *et al.* Mitochondrial dysfunction in trauma-related coagulopathy: Is there causality? Study protocol for a prospective observational study. Eur Surg Res Eur Chir Forsch Rech Chir Eur. 2023;64(2):304–9.

30. Zolin SJ, Vodovotz Y, Forsythe RM, Rosengart MR, Namas R, Brown JB, *et al.* The early evolving sex hormone environment is associated with significant outcome and inflammatory response differences after injury. J Trauma Acute Care Surg. 2015; 78(3):451–7.

31. Li C, Ajmal E, Alok K, Powell K, Wadolowski S, Tambo W, *et al.* CGRP as a potential mediator for the sexually dimorphic responses to traumatic brain injury. Biol Sex Differ. 2024;15(1):44.

32. Fuchs A, Monlish DA, Ghosh S, Chang SW, Bochicchio GV, Schuettpelz LG, *et al.* Trauma induces emergency hematopoiesis through IL-1/MyD88-dependent production of G-CSF. J Immunol Baltim Md. 2019;202(10):3020–32.

33. Loftus TJ, Mohr AM, Moldawer LL. Dysregulated myelopoiesis and hematopoietic function following acute physiologic insult. Curr Opin Hematol. 2018;25(1):37–43.

34. Bible LE, Pasupuleti LV, Alzate WD, Gore AV, Song KJ, Sifri ZC, *et al.* Early propranolol administration to severely injured patients can improve bone marrow dysfunction. J Trauma Acute Care Surg. 2014;77(1):54–60.

35. Corwin HL, Gettinger A, Rodriguez RM, Pearl RG, Gubler KD, Enny C, *et al.* Efficacy of recombinant human erythropoietin in the critically ill patient: A randomized, double-blind, placebo-controlled trial. Crit Care Med. 1999;27(11):2346–50.

36. Morton AP, Hadley JB, Ghasabyan A, Kelher MR, Moore EE, Bevers S, *et al.* The α-globin chain of hemoglobin potentiates tissue plasminogen activator induced hyperfibrinolysis in vitro. J Trauma Acute Care Surg. 2022;92(1):159–66.

37. Moore HB, Gando S, Iba T, Kim PY, Yeh CH, Brohi K, *et al.* Defining trauma-induced coagulopathy with respect to future implications for patient management: Communication from the SSC of the ISTH. J Thromb Haemost JTH. 2020;18(3):740–7.

38. Kals M, Kunzmann K, Parodi L, Radmanesh F, Wilson L, Izzy S, *et al.* A genome-wide association study of outcome from traumatic brain injury. EBioMedicine. 2022;77:103933.

39. Sperry JL, Luther JF, Okonkwo DO, Vincent LE, Agarwal V, Cotton BA, *et al.* Blood biomarkers for predicting coagulopathy occurrence in patients with traumatic brain injury: A systematic review. Biomark Med. 2022;16(12):935–45.

40. Sperry JL, Luther JF, Okonkwo DO, Vincent LE, Agarwal V, Cotton BA, *et al.* Early GFAP and UCH-L1 point-of-care biomarker measurements for the prediction of traumatic brain injury and progression in patients with polytrauma and hemorrhagic shock. J Neurosurg. 2024;10;1–10.

41. Sloos PH, Maas MAW, Meijers JCM, Nieuwland R, Roelofs JJTH, Juffermans NP, *et al.* Anti-high-mobility group box-1 treatment strategies improve trauma-induced coagulopathy in a mouse model of trauma and shock. Br J Anaesth. 2023;130(6):687–97.

42. Davis CS, Wilkinson KH, Lin E, *et al.* Precision medicine in trauma: A transformational frontier in patient care, education, and research. Eur J Trauma Emerg Surg Off Publ Eur Trauma Soc. 2022;48(4):2607–12.

43. Rubin-Asher D, Zeilig G, Ratner A, Asher I, Zivelin A, Seligsohn U, *et al.* Risk factors for failure of heparin thromboprophylaxis in patients with acute traumatic spinal cord injury. Thromb Res. 2010;125(6):501–4.

44. Ostrowski SR, Johansson PI. Endothelial glycocalyx degradation induces endogenous heparinization in patients with severe injury and early traumatic coagulopathy. J Trauma Acute Care Surg. 2012;73(1):60–6.

45. Simeoni I, Stephens JC, Hu F, Deevi SV, Megy K, Bariana TK, *et al.* A high-throughput sequencing test for diagnosing inherited bleeding, thrombotic, and platelet disorders. Blood. 2016;127(23):2791–803.

46. Cohen MJ, Call M, Nelson M, Calfee CS, Esmon CT, Brohi K, Pittet JF, *et al.* Critical role of activated protein C in early coagulopathy and later organ failure, infection and death in trauma patients. Ann Surg. 2012;255(2):379–85.

47. Morton AP, Moore EE, Moore HB, Gonzalez E, Chapman MP, Peltz E, *et al.* Hemoglobin-based oxygen carriers promote systemic hyperfibrinolysis that is both dependent and independent of plasmin. J Surg Res. 2017;213:166–70.

48. Kao TW, Lee YC, Chang HT. Prothrombin complex concentrate for trauma induced coagulopathy: A systematic review and meta-analysis. J Acute Med. 2021;11(3):81–9.

49. Hannadjas I, James A, Davenport R, Lindsay C, Brohi K, Cole E. Prothrombin complex concentrate (PCC) for treatment of trauma-induced coagulopathy: Systematic review and meta-analyses. Crit Care Lond Engl. 2023;27(1):422.

50. Egea-Guerrero JJ, Quintana-Diaz M. Role of prothrombin complex concentrate in the severe trauma patient. Front Med. 2022;9:988919.

51. Brinkman HJM, Swieringa F, Zuurveld M, Veninga A, Brouns SLN, Heemskerk JWM, *et al.* Reversing direct factor Xa or thrombin inhibitors: Factor V addition to prothrombin complex concentrate is beneficial in vitro. Res Pract Thromb Haemost. 2022;6(3):e12699.

52. Joseph BC, Miyazawa BY, Esmon CT, Cohen MJ, von Drygalski A, Mosnier LO. An engineered activated factor V for the prevention and treatment of acute traumatic coagulopathy and bleeding in mice. Blood Adv. 2022;6(3):959–69.

53. Han CY, Pichon TJ, Wang X, Ringgold KM, St John AE, Stern SA, *et al.* Leukocyte activation primes fibrinogen for proteolysis by mitochondrial oxidative stress. Redox Biol. 2022 May;51:102263.

54. Han CY, Wang X, Ringgold KM, Bennett JC, St John AE, Berenson R, *et al.* A novel melanocortin fusion protein inhibits fibrinogen oxidation and degradation during trauma-induced coagulopathy. Blood. 2023;142(8):724–41.

55. Xiao W, Mindrinos MN, Seok J, Cuschieri J, Cuenca AG, Gao H, *et al.* A genomic storm in critically injured humans. J Exp Med. 2011;208(13):2581–90.

56. Battaglini D, Siwicka-Gieroba D, Rocco PR, Cruz FF, Silva PL, Dabrowski W, *et al.* Novel synthetic and natural therapies for traumatic brain injury. Curr Neuropharmacol. 2021;19(10):1661–87.

57. Coleman JR, Deguchi H, Deguchi TK, Cohen MJ, Moore EE, Griffin JH, Full-length plasma skeletal muscle myosin isoform deficiency is associated with coagulopathy in acutely injured patients. J Thromb Haemost JTH. 2022;20(6):1385–9.

58. Moore HB, Neal MD, Bertolet M, Joughin BA, Yaffe MB, Barrett CD, *et al.* Proteomics of coagulopathy following injury reveals limitations of using laboratory assessment to define trauma-induced coagulopathy to predict massive transfusion. Ann Surg Open Perspect Surg Hist Educ Clin Approaches. 2022;3(2):e167.

59. LaCroix IS, Cohen M, Moore EE, Dzieciatkowska M, Silliman CC, Hansen KC, *et al.* Omics markers of platelet transfusion in trauma patients. Transfusion (Paris). 2023; 63(8):1447–62.

60. LaCroix IS, Cohen M, Moore EE, Dzieciatkowska M, Nemkov T, Schaid TR Jr, *et al.* Omics markers of red blood cell transfusion in trauma. Int J Mol Sci. 2022;23(22): 13815.

61. Perkins ZB, Yet B, Marsden M, Glasgow S, Marsh W, Davenport R, *et al.* Early identification of trauma-induced coagulopathy: Development and validation of a multivariable risk prediction model. Ann Surg. 2021;274(6):e1119–28.

62. Li K, Wu H, Pan F, Chen L, Feng C, Liu Y, *et al.* A machine learning-based model to predict acute traumatic coagulopathy in trauma patients upon emergency hospitalization. Clin Appl Thromb Off J Int Acad Clin Appl Thromb. 2020;26:1076029619897827.

63. Benjamin AJ, Young AJ, Holcomb JB, Fox EE, Wade CE, Meador C, *et al.* Early prediction of massive transfusion for patients with traumatic hemorrhage: Development of a multivariable machine learning model. Ann Surg Open Perspect Surg Hist Educ Clin Approaches. 2023;4(3):e314.

64. Mann KG, Freeman K. TACTIC: Trans-agency consortium for trauma-induced coagulopathy. J Thromb Haemost JTH. 2015;13 Suppl 1(0 1):S63–71.

65. Ochocinska MJ, Zlokovic BV, Searson PC, Crowder AT, Kraig RP, Ljubimova JY, *et al.* NIH workshop report on the trans-agency blood-brain interface workshop 2016: Exploring key challenges and opportunities associated with the blood, brain and their interface. Fluids Barriers CNS. 2017;14(1):12.

66. Overview [Internet]. [cited 2025 Nov 18]. Available from: https://www.c4ts.qmul.ac.uk/intrn/intrn

67. PATCH-Trauma Investigators and the ANZICS Clinical Trials Group, Gruen RL, Mitra B, Bernard SA, *et al.* Prehospital tranexamic acid for severe trauma. N Engl J Med. 2023;389(2):127–36.

68. James MF, Michell WL, Joubert IA, Nicol AJ, Navsaria PH, Gillespie RS. Resuscitation with hydroxyethyl starch improves renal function and lactate clearance in penetrating trauma in a randomized controlled study: The FIRST trial (Fluids in Resuscitation of Severe Trauma). Br J Anaesth. 2011;107(5):693–702.

69. Nascimento B, Callum J, Tien H, Peng H, Rizoli S, Karanicolas P, *et al.* Fibrinogen in the initial resuscitation of severe trauma (FiiRST): A randomized feasibility trial. Br J Anaesth. 2016;117(6):775–82.

70. Brown A. The CONNECT Trial: A Randomized Pragmatic Clinical Trial Measuring the Effectiveness of a Remotely Provided Complex Brain Rehabilitation Intervention in Improving Participation Outcomes of Individuals With TBI, Their Families, and Local Primary Providers [Internet]. clinicaltrials.gov; 2019 Sep [cited 2025 Nov 18]. Report No.: NCT02088099. Available from: https://clinicaltrials.gov/study/NCT02088099

71. Garrigue D, Godier A, Glacet A, Labreuche J, Kipnis E, Paris C, *et al.* French lyophilized plasma versus fresh frozen plasma for the initial management of trauma-induced coagulopathy: A randomized open-label trial. J Thromb Haemost JTH. 2018;16(3):481–9.

72. University of Pennsylvania. Trauma Induced Coagulopathy and Inflammation [Internet]. clinicaltrials.gov; 2021 Mar [cited 2025 Nov 18]. Report No.: NCT03128658. Available from: https://clinicaltrials.gov/study/NCT03128658

73. Becalick DC, Coats TJ. Comparison of artificial intelligence techniques with UKTRISS for estimating probability of survival after trauma. UK Trauma and Injury Severity Score. J Trauma. 2001;51(1):123–33.

74. ATCN [Internet]. [cited 2025 Nov 18]. Available from: https://www.traumanurses.org/education/atcn

75. Duchesne JC, Kyle A, Simmons J, Islam S, Schmieg RE Jr, Olivier J, *et al.* Impact of telemedicine upon rural trauma care. J Trauma. 2008;64(1):92–7.

76. Hashmi ZG, Wallace EL, Kerby JD. Using telehealth to improve access to trauma care among injured rural patients in the US. JAMA Surg. 2023;158(11):1123–4.

77. MyATLS App | ACS [Internet]. [cited 2025 Nov 18]. Available from: https://www.facs.org/quality-programs/trauma/education/advanced-trauma-life-support/myatls-app/

78. Mohan D, Farris C, Fischhoff B, Rosengart MR, Angus DC, Yealy DM, *et al.* Efficacy of educational video game versus traditional educational apps at improving physician decision making in trauma triage: randomized controlled trial. BMJ. 2017;359:j5416.

79 Childs BR, Breslin MA, Nguyen MP, Simske NM, Whiting PS, Vasireddy A, *et al.* Implementation of a mobile app for trauma education: results from a multicenter study. Trauma Surg Acute Care Open. 2020;5(1):e000452.

80. Indian Society for Trauma & Acute Care (ISTAC)(R) [Internet]. [cited 2025 Nov 18]. Available from: https://www.traumaindia.org/

81. Babhulkar S, Apte A, Barick D, Hoogervorst P, Tian Y, Wang Y. Trauma care systems in India and China: A grim past and an evolving future. OTA Int Open Access J Orthop Trauma. 2019;2(Suppl 1):e017.

Chapter 10

CASE-BASED LEARNING IN TRAUMA-INDUCED COAGULOPATHY: NATIONAL AND INTERNATIONAL EXPERIENCES

DOI: 10.1201/9781003711070-10

Case 1: Navigating Coagulopathy in Trauma, Early Recognition and Intervention in Two Trauma Cases

Ajay Ambalakkatte

INTRODUCTION

Trauma-induced coagulopathy (TIC) is a complex phenomenon which significantly impacts patient outcomes after severe Injury. TIC exacerbates haemorrhage and increases mortality and morbidity associated with trauma, demanding prompt recognition and targeted haemostatic resuscitation. These two case reports from a level 1 trauma centre at AIIMS Nagpur highlights the utilization of predictors of TIC for early identification and prompt haemostatic resuscitation.

CASE 1

PATIENT INFORMATION

A 49-year-old female, a hospital worker, was brought within four hours of a road traffic incident where a pedestrian was hit by a two-wheeler.

CLINICAL FEATURES

She was triaged as Priority 1 due to her initial abnormal vital signs and dangerous mechanism of injury: Blood pressure (BP) of 90/64 mmHg, pulse rate (PR) of 93 bpm, Respiratory rate of 30 breaths per minute and oxygen saturation (SpO_2) of 98% on room air. Her temperature was 98.6° Fahrenheit. Upon primary survey, the patient had a patent and maintainable airway with no C-spine tenderness. There were no dilated neck veins, the trachea was central, and air entry was equal on both sides with normal vesicular breath sounds. Her chest compression test was negative. However, she presented with a significant source of haemorrhage from a right mangled extremity and a positive pelvic compression test. Her Glasgow Coma Scale (GCS) was 15/15 and pupils were equal and reacting to light on both sides. A high shock index (>1), extensive soft tissue injury of right upper limb (mangled extremity score 8) and class 4 haemorrhage were all predictive of TIC.

DIAGNOSTIC STUDIES

Baseline investigations, including coagulation parameters (using a Cobas T511 analyser), complete blood counts, renal function tests and blood group with cross matching was sent. A bedside Focused assessment by Sonography in Trauma (FAST) was done, which was negative for free fluid. A chest X-ray done was found to be normal and a pelvis X-ray showed an anteroposterior compression type 1 fracture. Arterial blood gas (ABG) analysis showed compensated metabolic acidosis and hyperlactatemia. Presence of base deficit of 8 mEq/L and lactate of more than 4mEq/L also was predictive of high risk for trauma-induced coagulopathy. The Trauma Associated Severe Haemorrhage (TASH) score of 20 calculated for this patient suggested a 65% risk of requiring a massive blood transfusion. Table 10.1 shows relevant blood investigations before and after haemostatic resuscitation.

THERAPEUTIC INTERVENTIONS

Initial interventions during primary assessment included administering 1 litre of warm balanced crystalloid solution maintaining permissive hypotension, applying a pelvic binder,

Table 10.1 Lab parameters

Parameter	Baseline	Value after haemostatic resuscitation and definitive management
Serum fibrinogen	<100	180
PT/INR (prothrombin time/ international normalized ratio)	27/ 2.1	14/1.0
TLC (total leucocyte count)	4500	3650
Hb	7.5	9.2
Platelet count	150,000	165,000

placing a pressure bandage with a tourniquet on the injured extremity for haemorrhage control and administration of 1 gram of tranexamic acid. In spite of these interventions, there was continuous bleeding from the extremity. Repeat FAST was negative.

A massive transfusion protocol (MTP) was initiated, and she was prepared for amputation of the right lower limb. She received 4 units of packed red blood cells (PRBCs), 4 units of fresh frozen plasma (FFP), and 6 units of random donor platelets. After the first bag of MTP, the patient was taken to the surgical suite for above elbow amputation with haemorrhage control. A second bag of MTP was transfused during the procedure.

OUTCOME

Following the surgical intervention to control bleeding and the comprehensive blood component therapy, her coagulation profile improved significantly, as evidenced by changes in her laboratory parameters, indicating a successful response to the aggressive management of her trauma-induced coagulopathy. She didn't have any complications in the post-operative period. She was sent home on the fifth day of surgical intervention.

CASE 2

PATIENT INFORMATION

A head-on collision with a truck led to the admission of a 47-year-old male engineer, who was the helmeted rider of a two-wheeler involved in the incident.

CLINICAL FEATURES

Upon arrival, he was triaged as Priority 1 with initial vital signs showing a BP of 110/79 mmHg, a heart rate of 160 bpm, SpO$_2$ of 78% on room air, and a respiratory rate of 30 breaths per minute. His airway was open (patent) and maintainable, with no cervical spine tenderness. There were no dilated neck veins, and his trachea was central. The patient showed decreased chest movements and reduced air entry on the right side, with a positive chest compression test on palpation and dullness on percussion over the right hemithorax. Additionally, he had a right upper extremity injury with active external bleeding. A pelvic compression test done was negative, and there were no signs of long bone fractures in his lower extremities. His neurological assessment revealed a GCS of 14/15 (confused), with pupils that were equal and reactive to light bilaterally. His temperature was 98°F. On analysing the clinical findings, he is having class 4 haemorrhage and a high shock index, which are high-risk factors for development of TIC.

DIAGNOSTIC STUDIES

A bedside extended Focused Assessment with Sonography in Trauma (eFAST) identified free fluid within the right hemithorax. This finding was further supported by a chest X-ray,

Table 10.2   Lab parameters

Parameter	Baseline	Post haemostatic resuscitation and haemorrhage control
Serum fibrinogen	150	260
PT/INR	30/2.5	19.4/1.40
TLC	12,000	9640
Hb	6.4	8.5
Platelet count	48,000	54,000

which showed layering throughout the right hemithorax, consistent with a haemothorax, and a non-homogenous opacity at the periphery of the mid-zone. The X-ray also revealed multiple right-sided rib fractures involving ribs 3 through 7, with segmental fractures of the 3rd and 4th ribs. Furthermore, a point-of-care lung ultrasound confirmed the presence of a pulmonary contusion by showing coalescing B-lines in Zone 2. A bedside pelvic X-ray was normal. ABG analysis indicated respiratory alkalosis with metabolic acidosis and Type 1 respiratory failure. Other initial laboratory investigations included complete blood counts, renal function tests, electrolytes, and blood for grouping and cross-matching. Relevant blood investigations are given in Table 10.2. Coagulation tests were performed using a Cobas T511 analyser. Chest X-ray showing pulmonary contusion and documented hypoxia were identified as risk factors for TIC. His TASH score was 15 which implied <50% chance for requirement of massive blood transfusion.

THERAPEUTIC INTERVENTIONS

As part of the primary survey, oxygen therapy was initiated at 15 litres/minute via a non-rebreathing mask to maintain oxygen saturation above 94%. A 28 Fr intercostal drainage tube was inserted into the right sixth intercostal space, which initially drained 500 ml of blood. A pressure dressing was applied to control external bleeding from the upper limb. The patient received 1 litre of warm balanced crystalloid solution at a maintenance rate and 1 gram of tranexamic acid.

While being transferred to the radiology suite for a contrast-enhanced computed tomography (CT) scan, the patient developed hemodynamic instability, with an increase in intercostal drain output and sustained bleeding from the right upper limb, highly suggestive of TIC. Consequently, haemostatic resuscitation was immediately commenced with blood products transfused in a 1:1:1 ratio. The patient was then planned for operative intervention, thoracotomy and possible amputation. After receiving 4 units of PRBCs, 4 units of FFP, and 6 units of random donor platelets (RDPs), the thoracic drain output decreased, though oozing persisted from the upper limb injury.

The upper extremity injury underwent debridement, and venous bleeding was controlled with ligation. Post-procedure, the patient was transferred to the ICU, where an additional 2 units of PRBCs and 2 units of FFP were administered.

OUTCOME

In the ICU, follow-up evaluations confirmed normalized coagulation parameters. The patient was discharged from the ICU after 24 hours and subsequently sent home safely on the 10th day following the removal of the intercostal drain. He was advised to return for a follow-up appointment in two weeks.

DISCUSSION

In both presented cases, several key predictors of TIC facilitated prompt identification and intervention. A high shock index (HR/SBP), especially notable in Case 2 despite an initial systolic blood pressure of 110 mmHg, served as an early warning sign of significant hemodynamic compromise and impending shock, even before overt hypotension. This highlights the shock index's utility as a sensitive, bedside tool for detecting occult shock and as a predictor of TIC.[1,2]

Beyond immediate vital signs, laboratory markers of hypoperfusion and acidosis were crucial indicators. In Case 1, the presence of compensated metabolic acidosis, hyperlactatemia, and a base deficit of 8 mEq/L signalled a high risk for TIC, emphasizing the cellular metabolic derangement.[3] Similarly, Case 2 presented with respiratory alkalosis and metabolic acidosis, reflecting both compensatory mechanisms and ongoing tissue hypoperfusion.[1] The identified pulmonary contusion and documented hypoxia in Case 2 further contributed to the risk factors for TIC, illustrating how multi-system injuries converge to predispose patients to coagulopathy.[4] Clinical findings such as the mangled extremities in both patients, the pelvic fracture in Case 1, and the haemothorax in Case 2 represented significant sources of ongoing blood loss, directly contributing to the development and severity of TIC.[5]

The prompt and aggressive haemostatic resuscitation initiated in both patients was instrumental in reversing the coagulopathy and achieving favourable outcomes. Despite initial interventions like crystalloid administration, pelvic binder application, and pressure dressings with tourniquets, persistent bleeding necessitated escalation to MTP. The 1:1:1 ratio transfusion of PRBCs, FFP, and platelets, alongside the early administration of tranexamic acid, reflects current best practices in resuscitation aimed at correcting the coagulopathy and restoring hemostasis.[6] The immediate transition to definitive surgical control of haemorrhage with amputation in Case 1 and vein ligation in the upper extremity in Case 2 underscore the principle that stopping the bleeding definitively is paramount to successful resuscitation.[6]

CONCLUSION

These cases highlight the critical role of a proactive and comprehensive approach in managing severely injured trauma patients. The positive outcomes, marked by normalized coagulation parameters, effective bleeding control, and swift, safe discharge, underscore the effectiveness of this strategy. Ultimately, these experiences reinforce that maintaining a high index of suspicion for TIC, driven by clinical predictors and laboratory markers, combined with rapid, balanced haemostatic resuscitation and definitive surgical intervention, is essential for improving survival and minimizing morbidity in this patient population.

TAKE-HOME MESSAGE

Early recognition of trauma-induced coagulopathy makes a major difference in outcomes. Simple bedside predictors like shock index, base deficit, lactate, active bleeding and the pattern of injuries can identify patients at high risk even before lab results are available. Starting haemostatic resuscitation early, giving tranexamic acid, and using a balanced 1:1:1 ratio of blood components helped correct coagulopathy in both cases. Quick surgical control of bleeding was equally important. These cases show that a structured approach, fast decision-making and coordinated teamwork can stabilize even severely injured patients and improve their chances of survival.

STATEMENT ON ETHICS AND CONSENT

This case report is based on retrospective data extracted from hospital medical records. No direct patient contact was involved. As the data were anonymized and analysed retrospectively, the requirement for informed patient consent was waived in accordance with institutional ethics guidelines.

REFERENCES

1. Bunch CM, Chang E, Moore EE, Moore HB, Kwaan HC, Miller JB, *et al.*, SHock-INduced Endotheliopathy (SHINE): A mechanistic justification for viscoelastography-guided resuscitation of traumatic and non-traumatic shock. Front Physiol. 2023;14:1094845.

2. Savioli G, Ceresa IF, Macedonio S, Gerosa S, Belliato M, Iotti GA, *et al.*, Trauma coagulopathy and its outcomes. Medicina. 2020;56(4):205.

3. Cohen MJ, Call M, Nelson M, Calfee CS, Esmon CT, Brohi K, *et al.*, Critical role of activated protein c in early coagulopathy and later organ failure, infection and death in trauma patients. Ann Sur. 2012;255(2):379–85.

4. Hess JR, Lindell AL, Stansbury LG, Dutton RP, Scalea TM. The prevalence of abnormal results of conventional coagulation tests on admission to a trauma center. Transfusion. 2009;49(1):34–9.

5. Niles SE, McLaughlin DF, Perkins JG, Wade CE, Li Y, Spinella PC, *et al.*, Increased mortality associated with the early coagulopathy of trauma in combat casualties. J Trauma. 2008;64(6):1459–65.

6. Rossaint R, Afshari A, Bouillon B, Cerny V, Cimpoesu D, Curry N, *et al.*, The European guideline on management of major bleeding and coagulopathy following trauma: Sixth edition. Crit Care. 2023; 27:80. doi:10.1186/s13054-023-04327-7

Case 2: Acquired Hemophilia A Mimicking Trauma-Induced Coagulopathy in a Young Polytrauma Patient

Andrea Capponi

INTRODUCTION

Trauma-induced coagulopathy (TIC) is a well-recognized, early complication in major trauma, occurring in ~25% of severely injured patients and associated with increased morbidity and mortality. TIC is characterized by a complex interplay of tissue injury, shock, endothelial dysfunction, and dysregulation of coagulation and fibrinolysis, leading to impaired hemostasis and a bleeding phenotype in the acute phase. Laboratory diagnosis of TIC often reveals abnormalities in conventional coagulation tests, including prolonged prothrombin time (PT) and activated partial thromboplastin time (aPTT), decreased fibrinogen, and platelet dysfunction.[1-4] A diagnostic challenge arises when aPTT is disproportionately prolonged relative to PT in a trauma patient. While TIC can cause mild to moderate prolongation of both PT and aPTT, a marked isolated or disproportionate prolongation of aPTT should prompt consideration of alternative etiologies, such as acquired hemophilia A. Acquired hemophilia A is a rare autoimmune disorder characterized by the development of autoantibodies against factor VIII, leading to severe bleeding and isolated aPTT prolongation,[5-9] which can mimic TIC in the trauma setting.[10] This case is unique because it describes a young, previously healthy patient who developed hemophilia A shortly after polytrauma, presenting with laboratory and clinical features that closely resemble TIC but requiring a fundamentally different treatment approach, namely, immunosuppression and bypassing agents rather than standard trauma resuscitation and hemostatic support. This case highlights the importance of maintaining a broad differential diagnosis for coagulopathy in the trauma intensive care unit, especially when laboratory findings are atypical for TIC, thereby increasing clinical awareness and promoting timely recognition and management of rare but critical conditions such as acquired hemophilia A.

CASE PRESENTATION

Background and emergency admission: A 20-year-old man without prior health issues was brought to the Emergency Department following a high-speed motorcycle crash. On arrival: Glasgow Coma Scale (GCS) 13, hypotension (blood pressure [BP] 80/40 mmHg), tachycardia, and signs of thoracoabdominal trauma. A positive exam triggered activation of a major trauma protocol. Initial management: Whole-body computed tomography (CT) revealed multiple rib fractures, bilateral pulmonary contusion, pelvic fracture, and grade IV liver injury. The patient received red blood cells, plasma, and platelets and underwent hepatic artery embolization. He was admitted to the ICU in critical condition.

Clinical progression: By day 2, stabilization occurred. However, on day 3, labs showed a dramatically prolonged aPTT (> 120 s), normal PT, stable platelet count, and fibrinogen. Clinically, he exhibited spontaneous bleeding from IV and drain sites. Conventional transfusions failed to correct coagulopathy.

DIAGNOSTIC ROTEM EVALUATION

ROTEM findings (Figure 10.1) revealed the following abnormalities:

ROTEM findings typically show a markedly prolonged INTEM coagulation time, reflecting intrinsic pathway dysfunction due to factor VIII inhibition, with normal or near-normal EXTEM parameters (reflecting preserved extrinsic pathway function) and reduced maximum clot firmness (MCF) if bleeding is severe or there is concomitant hypofibrinogenemia or thrombocytopenia. The FIBTEM MCF may be normal unless there is significant fibrinogen depletion, which is less likely in isolated acquired hemophilia A. This ROTEM pattern contrasts with classic TIC, where both EXTEM and INTEM may be affected, and hypofibrinogenemia is common. APTEM (aprotinin-modified ROTEM) results are critical in this context. In TIC with hyperfibrinolysis, EXTEM will show increased maximum lysis (ML), and APTEM will correct this by inhibiting fibrinolysis, normalizing the ML. In acquired hemophilia A, both EXTEM and APTEM will show prolonged coagulation time and impaired clot formation, but APTEM will not correct the abnormal parameters, confirming that coagulopathy is not due to hyperfibrinolysis but rather to a factor VIII inhibitor. This distinction is essential, as hyperfibrinolysis would prompt antifibrinolytic therapy, while acquired hemophilia A requires immunosuppression and bypassing agents. This case underscores the importance of integrating ROTEM, including APTEM, into the differential diagnosis of early post-trauma coagulopathy, as it can rapidly distinguish between TIC, hyperfibrinolysis, and rare acquired factor inhibitors, directly impacting management.

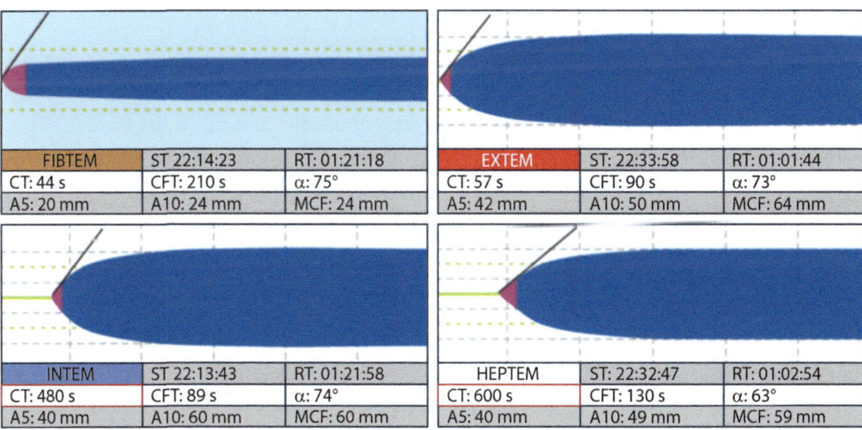

Figure 10.1 Rotational thermoelectrometry (ROTEM) Diagram. ST: start time; RT: run time; CT: coagulation time; CFT: clot formation time; Alpha: alpha angle in deg; A5: amplitude of clot firmness 5 mm after CT. A10: amplitude of clot firmness 10 mm after CT; MCF: maximum clot firmness; ML: maximum lysis during runtime. ROTEM pattern of acquired hemophilia A with inhibitors to factor VIII. Characteristic of acquired hemophilia, this ROTEM diagram shows a significantly prolonged INTEM and HEPTEM CT (480 seconds and 600 seconds, respectively), but short CTs in EXTEM and FIBTEM (57 seconds and 44 seconds, respectively), since the extrinsic and common pathways are not affected by this coagulopathy. The appropriate treatment is rFVIIa (recombinant activated factor VII) or activated PCC (Factor Eight Inhibitor Bypassing Activity [FEIBA]).

This pattern was highly suggestive of factor VIII inhibition. Subsequent assays confirmed:

i. Factor VIII activity < 1%

ii. Bethesda inhibitor titer > 5 BU Diagnosis: Acquired hemophilia A.

Treatment and outcome: Immediate treatment with bypassing agents (recombinant factor VIIa) was initiated, alongside immunosuppression with methylprednisolone and cyclophosphamide. Hemostasis improved rapidly, bleeding ceased, and coagulation parameters normalized. The patient continued ICU care for trauma-related injuries and was discharged to hematology follow-up on day 15, with full resolution of hemorrhage and progressing functional recovery.

DISCUSSION

TIC complicates major trauma through mechanisms such as endothelial activation, protein C mediated factor depletion, and hyperfibrinolysis. ROTEM is a valuable point of care (POC) tool enabling rapid identification of coagulopathy phenotypes, including early stage, trauma-induced abnormalities within minutes.[10] However, the isolated and severe prolongation of aPTT, as seen here, warrants investigation for acquired inhibitors, particularly factor VIII. International guidelines emphasize prompt use of bypassing agents (e.g., rFVIIa or prothrombin complex concentrate [PCC]) and immunosuppression. The emerging use of recombinant porcine factor VIII and even emicizumab shows promise in acquired hemophilia.[6-7]

CONCLUSION

This case illustrates the lifesaving potential of combining ROTEM diagnostics and early targeted therapy for unexpectedly acquired hemophilia A within trauma ICU settings. Early recognition and intervention can drastically reduce morbidity and mortality even in young, otherwise healthy patients.

TAKE-HOME MESSAGE

It is extremely rare for a young, previously healthy patient to develop acquired hemophilia A shortly after major polytrauma, presenting with clinical and laboratory features that mimic trauma-induced coagulopathy but are due to an immune mediated factor VIII inhibitor. The annual incidence of acquired hemophilia A in the general population is estimated at 0.2–1.48 cases per million, with a strong predilection for the elderly and those with underlying conditions such as malignancy, autoimmune disease, or the postpartum state; only about half of cases are idiopathic, and the occurrence in young, healthy individuals is exceptional. Acquired hemophilia A is rare but can present acutely post-trauma, mimicking TIC, and failing to recognize this immune-mediated coagulopathy can delay appropriate therapy, as management requires immunosuppression and bypassing agents rather than conventional trauma resuscitation.

STATEMENT ON ETHICS AND CONSENT

This case report is based on retrospective data extracted from hospital medical records. No direct patient contact was involved. As the data were anonymized and analyzed retrospectively, the requirement for informed patient consent was waived in accordance with institutional ethics guidelines.

REFERENCES

1. Brohi K, Cohen MJ, Davenport RA. Advances in the understanding of trauma-induced coagulopathy. Blood. 2016;128(8):1043–52.

2. Schöchl H, Solomon C, Traintinger S, Nienaber U, Tacacs-Tolnai A, Windhofer C, *et al.* Thromboelastometric (ROTEM) findings in patients suffering from isolated severe traumatic brain injury. J Neurotrauma. 2011 Oct;28(10):2033–41. doi: 10.1089/neu.2010.1744.

3. Iba T, Levy JH, Wada H, Thachil J. Mechanisms and management of coagulopathy of trauma and sepsis. J Thromb Haemost. 2023;21(12):3360–70.

4. Theusinger OM, Wanner GA, Emmert MY, Billeter A, Eismon J, Seifert B, *et al.* Hyperfibrinolysis diagnosed by ROTEM is associated with higher mortality in severe trauma. Anesth Analg. 2011;113(5):1003–12.

5. Tiede A, Collins P, Knoebl P, Teitel J, Kessler C, Shima M, *et al.* International recommendations for acquired hemophilia a management. Hamostaseologie. 2024;44(6):466–71.

6. Pfrepper C, Klamroth R, Oldenburg J, Holstein K, Eichler H, Hart C, Moehnle P, *et al.* Emicizumab for the Treatment of Acquired Hemophilia A: Consensus Recommendations from the GTH-AHA Working Group. Hamostaseologie. 2024 Dec; 44(6):466–471. doi: 10.1055/a-2197-9738. Epub 2023 Dec 4. PMID: 38049124.

7. Ellsworth P, Chen SL, Kasthuri RS, Key NS, Mooberry MJ, Ma AD. Recombinant porcine FVIII for bleed treatment in acquired hemophilia A: findings from a single-center, 18-patient cohort. Blood Adv. 2020 Dec 22;4(24):6240–6249. doi: 10.1182/bloodadvances.2020002977.

8. Chang R, Cardenas JC, Wade CE, Holcomb JB. Advances in the understanding of trauma-induced coagulopathy. Blood. 2016;128(8):1043–9.

9. Borro M, Tassara R, Paris L, Artom N, Brignone M, Rebella L, *et al.* Acquired hemophilia A treated with recombinant porcine factor VIII: Case report and literature review on its efficacy. Hematol Rep. 2023;15(1):17–22.

10. Webert KE. Pathophysiology and management of bleeding disorders in critical care. Semin Thromb Hemost. 2012;38(7):735–41.

Case 3: Massive Transfusion in Isolated Maxillofacial Trauma: A High-Acuity, Low-Occurrence Situation

Anukarthika S, Amrithanand V T, and Aparna Krishna

INTRODUCTION

Life-threatening bleeding associated with isolated maxillofacial trauma is rare. The midface is highly vascularised, primarily by branches of the external carotid artery including facial and maxillary arteries and connections to the internal carotid system, which can lead to rapid blood loss following severe injury. This case describes a young male with isolated facial trauma who developed sudden exsanguinating haemorrhage in the emergency department, requiring aggressive resuscitation and endovascular management. It highlights the importance of early teamwork, timely imaging, and targeted transfusion strategies in a high-acuity, low-occurrence situation.

PATIENT DEMOGRAPHICS

A young adult male was referred to our Emergency Department from a peripheral hospital following a two-wheeler road traffic injury. The mechanism of injury was unclear. He had no known pre-existing comorbidities or allergies.

CLINICAL PRESENTATION

Upon arrival, the primary survey revealed a secure airway with an endotracheal tube in place for airway protection. Breathing was supported by mechanical ventilation, with equal bilateral air entry. Circulation revealed tachycardia (heart rate [HR] 130 bpm), normotension (blood pressure [BP] 110/70 mmHg), shock index >1 and cold extremities. On disability assessment, the Glasgow Coma Scale (GCS) was E1VTM5, and the exposure only revealed bleeding from the maxillofacial zone (Figure 10.2). Shortly after arrival, the patient, who was initially compensating, suddenly deteriorated. His blood pressure plummeted to 50 mmHg, and he became increasingly unresponsive. Following Advanced Trauma Life Support (ATLS) principles, a rapid reassessment was performed.

We immediately noted active, profuse arterial bleeding from the nose and oral cavity, with blood on the floor (Figure 10.3). It prompted an urgent concern about the ongoing massive haemorrhage. Extended Focused Assessment with Sonography for Trauma (eFAST) remained negative, ruling out intrathoracic and intra-abdominal sources of bleeding.

There is no evidence of long bone or pelvic fractures, effectively excluding the "four more" sources.

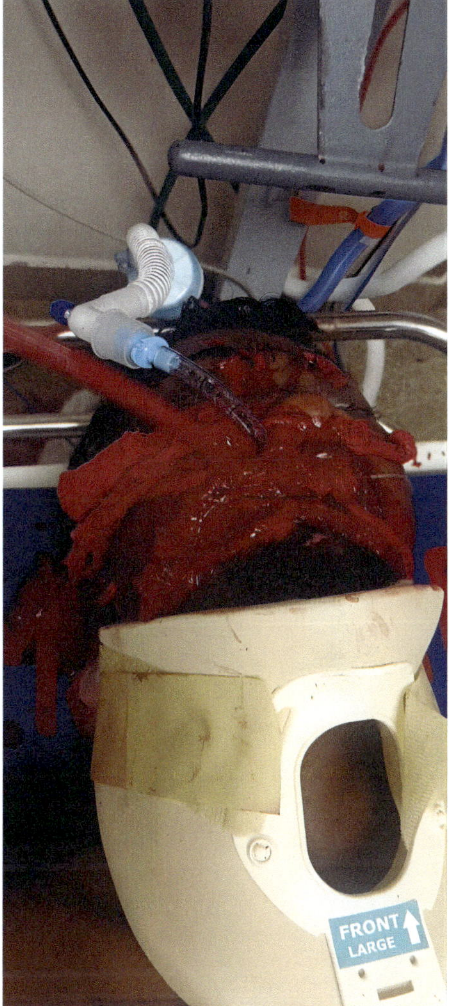

Figure 10.2 Patient with exsanguinating maxillofacial haemorrhage, showing airway secured with endotracheal tube and nasal packing *in situ*.

DIAGNOSTIC WORKUP

Adjuncts to the primary survey were promptly performed as part of the trauma assessment. Initial blood gas revealed high anion gap metabolic acidosis with a base excess of –20, consistent with Class IV haemorrhagic shock. Although initial laboratory parameters were within normal limits, including platelet count and international normalized ratio (INR), the thromboelastography (TEG) results showed a prolonged R-time, indicating delayed clot formation and a potential coagulopathy initially (Figure 10.4). However, following the episode of massive haemorrhage, only the serial blood investigations revealed a significant drop in haemoglobin from 10.2 g/dl to 7.0 g/dl, thrombocytopenia, and a prolonged INR, suggestive of evolving trauma-induced coagulopathy.

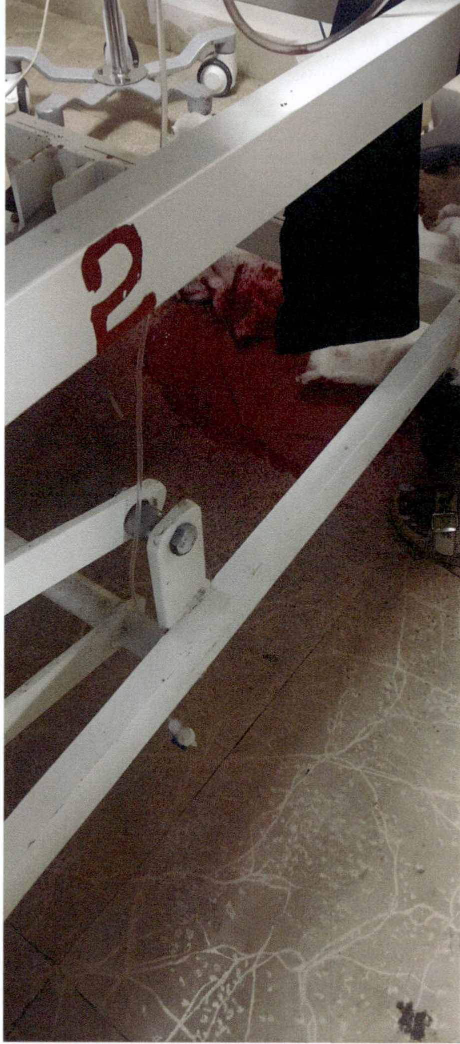

Figure 10.3   Primary survey revealing blood on the floor.

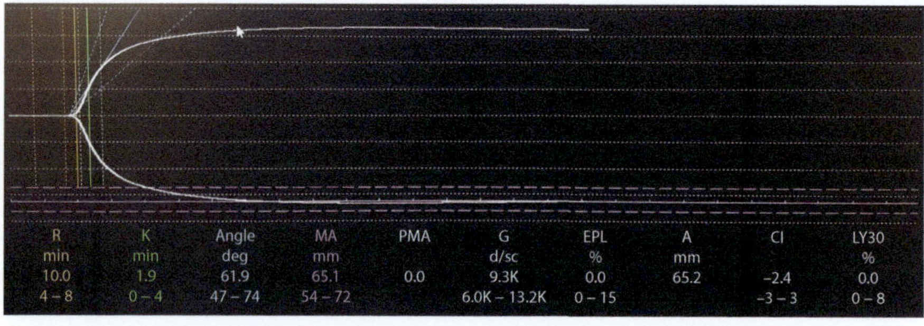

R min	K min	Angle deg	MA mm	PMA	G d/sc	EPL %	A mm	CI	LY30 %
10.0	1.9	61.9	65.1	0.0	9.3K	0.0	65.2	−2.4	0.0
4 – 8	0 – 4	47 – 74	54 – 72		6.0K – 13.2K	0 – 15		−3 – 3	0 – 8

Figure 10.4   Thromboelastography showing prolonged R time, indicating delay in clot formation.

Computed tomography (CT) angiography demonstrated active contrast extravasation from the lateral nasal wall near the sphenopalatine foramen, confirming rupture of the right sphenopalatine artery. Associated injuries included anterior and posterior table of frontal bone fracture, bilateral LeFort I, II fracture and left LeFort III fracture, comminuted type III naso-orbitoethmoid fracture, midpalatal fracture, mandibular symphysis fracture with bilateral condylar splaying. Thoracoabdominal injuries were ruled out on contrast-enhanced CT (CECT), confirming an isolated maxillofacial injury.

MANAGEMENT

Resuscitation followed ATLS principles. The presentation was consistent with exsanguination from a maxillofacial source, a rare but life-threatening scenario. Immediate resuscitation was escalated with activation of the Massive Haemorrhage Protocol (MHP), triggered by an Assessment of Blood Consumption (ABC) score $\geq$ 2. The MHP followed the "7 Ts" approach Trigger, Team preparation, Tranexamic acid, Test hourly, Transfuse, Temperature, and Termination of MTP ensuring structured and goal-directed resuscitation. Tranexamic acid was administered as an initial bolus of one gram, followed by an infusion of one gram over eight hours. Laboratory investigations, including a complete blood count and electrolyte levels, were within normal limits at baseline. Point-of-care TEG revealed a prolonged R-time, indicating coagulopathy. Eight units of packed red blood cells, six fresh-frozen plasma units, nine random donor platelet units, and eight cryoprecipitate units were transfused during resuscitation in the emergency department. To prevent citrate-induced hypocalcaemia, intravenous calcium gluconate was administered following the first round of transfusion. Forced-air warmers, warmed crystalloids, and core temperature monitoring were instituted to prevent hypothermia. Polyvinyl acetate nasal packs were inserted bilaterally; oral packing was also attempted to control the bleeding. With persistent bleeding, invasive arterial monitoring and multidisciplinary involvement were initiated. With stabilised hemodynamics and reduction of active haemorrhage, the MHP was discontinued. The lethal triad hypothermia, acidosis, and coagulopathy along with hypocalcaemia (the "lethal four") was proactively addressed throughout resuscitation.

CLINICAL COURSE AND OUTCOME

Following the transfusion of multiple blood products, the patient showed a prompt improvement in hemodynamics, with a rise in blood pressure and neurological recovery to a GCS of M6. This stabilisation enabled further definitive intervention. The patient was taken up for digital subtraction angiography (DSA), which revealed active extravasation from the right internal maxillary artery. Selective embolisation was successfully performed using polyvinyl alcohol (PVA) particles, achieving definitive haemorrhage control. Subsequently, given anticipated prolonged airway compromise and the need for surgical reconstruction, the patient underwent elective tracheostomy. He was taken up for open reduction and internal fixation (ORIF) of facial fractures, along with obliteration of the frontal sinus using autologous abdominal fat graft and tissue adhesive glue. During intensive care monitoring, the patient developed persistent cerebrospinal fluid (CSF) rhinorrhoea. A CT cisternography was performed to localise the leak site, followed by the placement of a lumbar drain for CSF diversion. Empirical broad-spectrum antibiotics were initiated and later tailored based on culture sensitivity, which revealed *Streptococcus agalactiae*. Due to continued CSF leakage, the patient was taken up by the otorhinolaryngology team for endoscopic endonasal repair of the skull base defect. Postoperatively, the patient remained hemodynamically stable, gradually weaned from ventilatory support, and demonstrated neurological recovery to full GCS. He was subsequently discharged in a stable condition with appropriate follow-up advice.

DISCUSSION

Massive haemorrhage secondary to maxillofacial trauma is rare but potentially catastrophic.[1] When it occurs, it poses significant diagnostic and therapeutic challenges due to the intricate vascular anatomy of the face and the urgent need for haemostasis before definitive imaging and intervention can be undertaken. In the acute trauma setting, the initial challenge lies in differentiating the source of bleeding, which can be obscured by profuse oronasal haemorrhage and soft tissue distortion.[2,3] Bleeding in facial trauma can arise from multiple arterial sources, including the sphenopalatine, internal maxillary, ethmoidal, or ophthalmic arteries.[3,4] While typically resilient due to collateral circulation, the richly vascularised midface region can become a liability when bleeding involves deep arterial branches. In such cases, conventional measures like nasal packing may prove insufficient, particularly when the source is posterior or within fractured bone compartments. Additionally, balloon tamponade must be used cautiously in the context of comminuted midfacial fractures, as it carries a risk of displacing bone fragments into adjacent vital structures.[5,6] A crucial step in management is the exclusion of more common life-threatening haemorrhagic sources such as intra-thoracic, intra-abdominal, pelvic, or long bone injuries. This necessitates imaging via CECT, which requires the patient to be sufficiently stabilised beforehand. This presents a therapeutic dilemma: the need to localise and treat the bleeding competes with the urgency to maintain hemodynamic stability in a rapidly deteriorating patient. Implementing an MHP is pivotal in this critical window. In the presented case, early activation of MHP enabled the prompt delivery of packed red blood cells, plasma, and platelets in balanced ratios, thereby preventing the progression to the lethal triad of hypothermia, acidosis, and coagulopathy.[7,8] Haemostatic resuscitation using MHP is not merely a volume replacement strategy it is an essential component of damage control resuscitation that mitigates trauma-induced coagulopathy, a multifactorial process influenced by tissue injury, shock, dilution, and systemic inflammation. Following MHP activation, the patient's hemodynamics improved significantly, and his neurological status progressed to a motor response of M6 on the GCS. This physiological stabilisation allowed for safe transfer to imaging and subsequent definitive intervention by angioembolization and stabilisation of the fracture.[9] MHP played a pivotal role in correcting early coagulopathy, restoring tissue perfusion, and preventing progression to the lethal triad of trauma. In trauma patients with ongoing arterial bleeding, especially from deep facial sources, MTP serves as a critical bridge to definitive haemorrhage control when immediate surgical or endovascular intervention is not feasible. Viscoelastic haemostatic assays, such as TEG, offer a real-time evaluation of coagulation dynamics and were particularly useful in this case. The prolonged reaction time (R-time) indicated impaired clot initiation, guiding targeted administration of fresh frozen plasma. This approach facilitated more precise correction of coagulopathy and minimised unnecessary transfusion, preserving resources and reducing the risk of transfusion-related complications.

CONCLUSION

Severe haemorrhage in isolated maxillofacial trauma demands fast decision-making and coordinated care. In this case the early activation of the MHP, prompt administration of balanced blood components, and use of tranexamic acid, to support the angioembolization provided effective control of the arterial bleed. This case reinforces that structured protocols, early recognition of coagulopathy, and rapid access to endovascular therapy can prevent deterioration and improve outcomes in rare but critical facial bleeding events.

TAKE-HOME MESSAGE

This case highlights the need for coordinated management and treatment approaches even in rare, high-acuity cases. Early recognition of major bleeding and trauma-induced coagulopathy is vital. A structured Massive Haemorrhage Protocol helps deliver balanced transfusion, guides targeted correction using laboratory and viscoelastic tests, and limits avoidable delays. Use of tranexamic acid as an early blood product support, along with close monitoring of temperature, calcium, and acid base status can help avert the lethal triad, and to stabilise the patient for surgical interventions.

STATEMENT ON ETHICS AND CONSENT

This case report is based on retrospective data extracted from hospital medical records. No direct patient contact was involved. As the data were anonymized and analysed retrospectively, the requirement for informed patient consent was waived in accordance with institutional ethics guidelines.

REFERENCES

1. Eastridge BJ, Holcomb JB, Shackelford S. Outcomes of traumatic hemorrhagic shock and the epidemiology of preventable death from injury. Transfusion. 2019;59:1423–8.

2. Jose A, Nagori SA, Agarwal B, Bhutia O, Roychoudhury A. Management of maxillofacial trauma in emergency: An update of challenges and controversies. J Emerg Trauma Shock. 2016;9:73–80.

3. Ardekian L, Samet N, Shoshani Y, Taicher S. Life-threatening bleeding following maxillofacial trauma. J Cranio-Maxillo-Fac Surg. 1993;21:336–8.

4. Duggan CA, Brylski JR. Angiographic demonstration of bleeding in intractable traumatic epistaxis. Radiology. 1970;97:605–6.

5. Perry M, Dancey A, Mireskandari K, Oakley P, Davies S, Cameron M. Emergency care in facial trauma: A maxillofacial and ophthalmic perspective. Injury. 2005;36:875–96.

6. Gwyn PP, Carraway JH, Horton CE, Adamson JE, Mladick RA. Facial fractures: Associated injuries and complications. Plast Reconstr Surg. 1971;47:225–30.

7. Consunji R, Elseed A, El-Menyar A, Sathian B, Rizoli S, Al-Thani H, et al. The effect of massive transfusion protocol implementation on the survival of trauma patients: A systematic review and meta-analysis. Blood Transfus. 2020;18:434–45.

8. Huber-Wagner S, Qvick M, Mussack T, Euler E, Kay MV, Mutschler W, et al. Massive blood transfusion and outcome in 1062 polytrauma patients: A prospective study based on the trauma registry of the German trauma society. Vox Sanguinis. 2007;92:69–78.

9. Bynoe RP, Kerwin AJ, Parker HHI, Nottingham JM, Bell RM, Yost MJ, et al. Maxillofacial injuries and life-threatening hemorrhage: Treatment with transcatheter arterial embolization. J Trauma Acute Care Surg. 2003;55:74.

Case 4: Use of Prothrombin Complex Concentrate in Paediatric Patients with TBI-Associated Coagulopathy

Venencia Albert, Arulselvi Subramanian, and Deepak Agrawal

INTRODUCTION

Trauma-induced coagulopathy (TIC) is a critical early complication in patients with severe traumatic brain injury (TBI). In children, TIC is reported present in up to 30% of TBI cases and is associated with higher mortality, worsened neurological outcomes, and increased transfusion requirements.[1,2] The underlying mechanisms include tissue trauma, systemic hypoperfusion, acidosis, and endothelial dysfunction, all of which initiate a cascade of coagulation abnormalities.[3] The presence of TIC in isolated TBI suggests that brain injury alone can activate systemic coagulopathy.[4]

Prothrombin complex concentrate (PCC) contains vitamin K-dependent clotting factors (II, VII, IX, and X) and is approved for the reversal of vitamin K antagonists.[5] Its off-label use has expanded in trauma settings for rapid international normalized ratio (INR) correction when fresh frozen plasma (FFP) is either unavailable or not feasible due to volume constraints.[6] The PROCOAG randomized controlled trial evaluated PCC in adult trauma patients with coagulopathy and active bleeding, and reported faster INR correction and reduced need for blood transfusion, although the impact on mortality or thromboembolic risk was not significant.[7]

While adult data support the haemostatic potential of PCC, paediatric evidence remains limited. Most reports are observational and describe heterogeneous populations, with no strong consensus on dose, timing, or monitoring.[8-10] Nonetheless, PCC has been used successfully to reverse TIC in children, particularly in the setting of congenital bleeding disorders, cardiac surgery, and isolated TBI.[7,9]

This report presents the use of PCC in a 1-year-old child with severe isolated TBI and profound coagulopathy. We discuss the timing, dosing, and clinical effects of PCC, contextualized by the limitations of monitoring and systemic complications that ultimately influenced the outcome.

CASE PRESENTATION

HISTORY AND EXAMINATION

A 1-year-old male with no prior illness fell from a third-floor on December 6, 2024. He was initially stabilized at a local hospital and transferred to a tertiary trauma centre by 9:29 PM.

ON ARRIVAL

The Glasgow Coma Scale was E1VTM1. He was hypotensive (blood pressure [BP] 50/20 mmHg), tachycardic (heart rate [HR] 120 bpm), with bilateral non-reactive pupils and absent motor response. Arterial blood gas (ABG) showed metabolic acidosis (pH 7.2, HCO_3^- 13.1), tissue hypoperfusion [elevated lactate (4.3 mmol/L)], hypernatremia (Na^+ 156 mmol/L), and poor oxygen saturation requiring mechanical ventilation.

CT of the head showed a right frontal contusion with subarachnoid haemorrhage (SAH), subdural haematoma (SDH), extradural haematoma (EDH), midline shift, and right parietal fracture. Abdominal imaging revealed a liver laceration (Grade III mild hemoperitoneum and right hemopneumothorax. No spinal or long bone injuries (Figure 10.5).

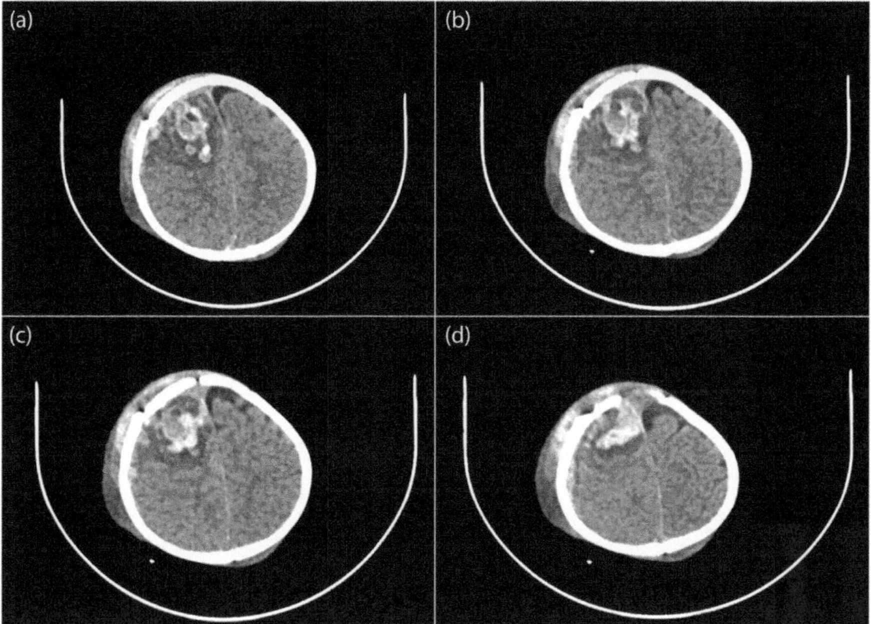

Figure 10.5 Axial non-contrast computed tomography (CT) brain images (Panels a–d) of a 1-year-old child following severe traumatic brain injury. (a) Hyperdense haemorrhagic contusions are noted in the right frontal lobe with surrounding edema and early midline shift. (b) Haemorrhage with coalescing haematomas, compression of the right lateral ventricle, and increasing midline shift. (c) Dense frontal haematoma, mass effect, and loss of grey-white matter differentiation. (d) Large extradural haematoma with associated skull fracture and marked effacement of cortical sulci, consistent with raised intracranial pressure.

Initial labs revealed severe coagulopathy (INR 5.1, activated partial thromboplastin time [aPTT] 126 sec), anaemia (Hb 4 g/dL), and acute hepatic injury (aspartate aminotransferase [AST] 3410 U/L, alanine aminotransferase [ALT] 1207 U/L). He was intubated and admitted to the ICU.

TREATMENT
Initial resuscitation included 1 unit each of FFP, packed red blood cells (PRBC), and random donor platelet (RDP) at ~9:42 PM on 6 December 2024. At 2:15 AM, on 7 December the patient received 100 mL PRBC and normal saline (NS). Approximately 10 hours post-injury (3:10 AM), the patient received intravenous vitamin K (1 mg), followed by PCC (human pro-thrombin complex, 350 IU ~35 IU/kg). By 5:00 AM, additional FFP (60 mL), RDP (70 mL), PRBCs (150 mL), and NS (100 mL) were infused. Intracranial pressure (ICP) monitoring showed sustained elevation (36–50 mmHg). Emergency decompression and SDH evacuation were performed at 8:30 AM (Table 10.3).

OUTCOME
Follow-up INR showed partial correction to 2.4 by 12:45 PM and 1.53 by 6:31 PM. aPTT also showed transient improvement (Table 10.4). Platelets increased to 1.7 lakh/mm^3, Hb to 12.2 g/dL. Renal parameters worsened (urea 158 mg/dL, creatinine 4.8 mg/dL). NPO (nothing by mouth) blood glucose level was 524 mg/dL. Despite 4 PRBC units, 3 FFP units, and 3 RDP units within 24 hours, the patient's ICP remained high, neurological status did not improve, and renal dysfunction worsened. The patient developed asystole by 11:00 PM.

Table 10.3 Timeline of haemostatic interventions: Blood product transfusions, vitamin K, and PCC administration

Date and time	Intervention	Details
6 December 2024, 9:42 PM	Initial transfusion	1 unit each of PRBC, FFP, and RDP
7 December 2024, 2:15 AM	PRBC and fluid support	100 mL PRBC + Normal saline
7 December 2024, 3:10 AM	Vitamin K	1 mg IV
7 December 2024, 3:50 AM	PCC (Prothrombin Complex Concentrate)	350 IU (~35 IU/kg)
7 December 2024, 5:00 AM	Additional transfusions	FFP (60 mL), PRBC (150 mL), RDP (70 mL)

Table 10.4 Laboratory parameters before and after PCC administration in a 1-year-old child following severe traumatic brain injury

Parameter (range[11])	Pre-PCC (6 December 2024, ~9:30 PM)	~6 Hours post-PCC (7 December 2024, 12:45 PM)	~15 Hours post-PCC (7 December 2024, 6:31 AM)
INR	5.06	2.4	1.53
PT (seconds)	—	31.3	20.6
aPTT (33.6–46.3 seconds)	126	61	69.4
Haemoglobin (10.9–15.0g/dL)	4	—	12.2
Platelets (150–450 × 10^9/L)	378	—	170
Urea (1–7 mg/dL)	26	140	158
Creatinine (0.04–0.33 mg/dL)	0.4	3.8	4.8
AST (16–60 U/L)	3410	368	—
ALT (5–55 U/L)	1207	115	—
Glucose (60–100 mg/dL)	292 (random)	—	524 (NOP)
Sodium (138–145 mmol/L)	143	157	—

Resuscitation failed. Death was declared at 11:30 PM; cause of death was hypovolemic shock with raised ICP secondary to severe TBI.

DISCUSSION

This case illustrates the early use of PCC in a 1-year-old child with isolated TBI complicated by TIC. Although PCC is increasingly included in adult trauma protocols, evidence for its use in paediatric neurotrauma remains limited, and its off-label application is guided primarily by clinical judgment and emerging case-based data.[5,6,11–13]

The patient received a PCC dose of 350 IU (~35 IU/kg) ~10 hours post-injury. This falls within the empiric range of 20–50 IU/kg of the previously reported paediatric case series.[8,14,15] INR serially reduced within 18 hours post-injury, indicating partial reversal of the coagulopathy. However, despite PCC administration and concurrent transfusion support, the patient succumbed within 24 hours due to refractory hypovolemic shock and raised ICP.

This outcome reflects a key limitation in isolated coagulation correction strategies in structural brain damage and advanced metabolic derangements and renal function deterioration.[3,14] The patient suffered extensive intracranial haemorrhages with midline shift, and the ICP values remained critically high prior to decompression. Neurological function never recovered, and renal dysfunction and hyperglycaemia suggested multiorgan dysfunction. These factors, collectively, contributed to a non-survivable condition, despite partial coagulation correction.

In settings where viscoelastic testing is not available, INR and aPTT remain the primary guides for PCC use, but they do not provide comprehensive insight into clot quality or fibrinolysis. The lack of TEG/ROTEM monitoring in this case underscores a common limitation in paediatric trauma care. Sribnick *et al.* reported successful PCC use guided by viscoelastic assays in a child with polytrauma and TBI, resulting in both safe surgery and neurological recovery.[9] Munlemvo *et al.* reviewed 53 reports of paediatric PCC use across trauma, congenital, and surgical indications, associating good haemostatic outcomes and low rates of adverse events with appropriately PCC dosage.[5] Karube *et al.* also supported its safety in paediatric trauma without reporting thrombotic complications.[14] Still, adult trauma studies note thromboembolic events in up to 35% of cases, especially with delayed or excessive dosing.[7]

Adding to these clinical challenges is the economic barrier. In India, a 500-IU vial of PCC may cost between ₹40,000 and ₹1,00,000 depending on brand and source, making routine use in paediatric trauma feasible only in well-resourced tertiary care centres. This restricts broader access and raises questions of sustainability unless public procurement, insurance support, or domestic manufacturing options are strengthened.

CONCLUSION

Early PCC administration can improve coagulation in paediatric TBI patients with TIC. However, its use alone is insufficient in the setting of extensive cerebral injury and systemic failure. Although PCC helped reduce the INR, the extent of cerebral damage had already caused irreversible neurological suppression. Rising ICP, multiorgan dysfunction, and persistent shock were not modifiable by coagulation correction alone. This case illustrates both the potential for rapid laboratory correction and the limitations of PCC in altering outcomes where irreversible damage has occurred. In those cases, PCC may buy time, but cannot salvage outcome in the setting of established critical intracranial pathology and failing physiology.

TAKE-HOME MESSAGE

PCC can correct coagulopathy rapidly in paediatric trauma when dosed appropriately, but it should be part of a broader management plan including timely surgical intervention and organ support. The normalization of INR is not equivalent to clinical recovery, especially in cases with established brain injury and secondary systemic dysfunction. Unavailability of viscoelastic testing limits the precision of PCC use in many paediatric trauma centres.

STATEMENT ON ETHICS AND CONSENT

This case report is based on retrospective data extracted from hospital medical records. No direct patient contact was involved. As the data were anonymized and analysed retrospectively, the requirement for informed patient consent was waived in accordance with institutional ethics guidelines.

REFERENCES

1. Di Battista AP, Rhind SG, Hutchison MG, Hassan S, Shiu MY, Inaba K. Inflammatory cytokine and chemokine profiles are associated with patient outcome and the hyperadrenergic state following acute traumatic brain injury. J Neuroinflammation. 2016;13(1): 40. doi: 10.1186/s12974-016-0500-3

2. Nakae R, Takayama Y, Kuwamoto K, Naoe Y, Sato H, Yokota H. Time course of coagulation and fibrinolytic parameters in patients with traumatic brain injury. J Neurotrauma. 2016;33(6):688–695. doi: 10.1089/neu.2015.4039

3. Kornblith LZ, Moore HB, Cohen MJ. Trauma-induced coagulopathy: The past, present, and future. J Thromb Haemost. 2019;17(6):852–862. doi:10.1111/jth.14418

4. Yuan Q, Sun YR, Wu X, Yu J, Li ZQ, Du ZY, *et al.* Coagulopathy in Traumatic Brain Injury and Its Correlation with Progressive Hemorrhagic Injury: A Systematic Review and Meta-Analysis. J Neurotrauma. 2016 Jul 15;33(14):1279–91. doi: 10.1089/neu.2015.4205.

5. Ghadimi K, Levy JH, Welsby IJ. Prothrombin complex concentrates for bleeding in the perioperative setting. Anesth Analg. 2016;122(5):1287–1300. doi: 10.1213/ANE.0000000000001188

6. Schöchl H, Voelckel W, Maegele M, Solomon C. Trauma-associated hyperfibrinolysis. Hamostaseologie. 2012;32(1):22–27. doi: 10.5482/ha-1178

7. Bouzat P, Charbit J, Abback PS, Huet-Garrigue D, Delhaye N; PROCOAG Study Group. Efficacy and Safety of Early Administration of 4-Factor Prothrombin Complex Concentrate in Patients With Trauma at Risk of Massive Transfusion: The PROCOAG Randomized Clinical Trial. JAMA. 2023 Apr 25;329(16):1367–1375. doi: 10.1001/jama.2023.4080.

8. Munlemvo DM, Hermans C, Lambermont B, Dive A, Maes N. Use of prothrombin complex concentrate in children: A narrative review. Transfus Clin Biol. 2022;29(3): 233–239. doi:10.1016/j.tracli.2022.03.003

9. Sribnick EA, Wenger N, Nicol K, Tobias JD. Use of viscoelastic monitoring and prothrombin complex concentrate in a pediatric patient with polytrauma and severe traumatic brain injury. BMJ Case Rep. 2020;13(12):e236608. doi:10.1136/bcr-2020-236608

10. Noga T, Bruce AA, Blain H, Nahirniak S. Four-factor prothrombin complex concentrates in pediatric patients: A retrospective case series. Vox Sang. 2016;110(3):253–257. doi:10.1111/vox.12353

11. Taketomo CK, Hodding JH, Kraus DM, eds. Pediatric and Neonatal Dosage *Handbook*. 21st ed. Hudson, OH: Lexicomp; 2014.

12. Hannadjas I, James A, Davenport R, Lindsay C, Brohi K, Cole E. Prothrombin complex concentrate (PCC) for treatment of trauma-induced coagulopathy: Systematic review and meta-analyses. Crit Care. 2023;27(1):422. doi:10.1186/s13054-023-04641-0

13. Moore EE, Moore HB, Kornblith LZ, *et al.* Trauma-induced coagulopathy. Nat Rev Dis Primers. 2021;7(1):30. doi:10.1038/s41572-021-00262-5

14. Karube T, Andersen C, Tobias JD. Single-Center Use of Prothrombin Complex Concentrate in Pediatric Patients. J Pediatr Intensive Care. 2020 Jun;9(2):106–112. doi: 10.1055/s-0039-1700953.

15. Ogiwara K, Nogami K, Mizumachi K, Nakagawa T, Noda N, Ohga S, *et al.* Hemostatic assessment of combined anticoagulant therapy using warfarin and PCC in severe protein C deficiency. Int J Hematol. 2019;109(6):650–656. doi:10.1007/s12185-019-02645-7

Case 5: Massive Transfusion in Trauma-Induced Coagulopathy: Case Report of a Polytrauma Patient

Radheshyam Meher, Arulselvi Subramanian, and Amit Gupta

INTRODUCTION

Massive transfusion is defined as replacement of one blood volume within 24 hours, transfusion of ≥10 packed red blood cell (PRBC) units in 24 hours, replacement of >50% blood volume in 3 hours, or transfusion of >4 PRBC units in 1 hour with ongoing haemorrhage.[1] Mortality after massive transfusion is reported to be ~30–40%.[2] Trauma is a leading cause of death in young adults, and trauma-induced coagulopathy (TIC) is a major contributor to poor outcomes in polytrauma patients. Activation of a Massive Transfusion Protocol (MTP) aims to prevent the lethal triad of acidosis, hypothermia, and coagulopathy.[3,4] We report a case of massive transfusion in a young polytrauma patient with TIC following a road traffic accident, with initial successful resuscitation in a resource-limited setting.

CASE

An 18-year-old previously healthy male was brought to the trauma centre following a high-velocity two-wheeler collision. He was a non-helmeted rider and presented in profound shock. On arrival, vitals were as follows: blood pressure (BP) 74/68 mmHg, heart rate (HR) 142 bpm, respiratory rate (RR) 24/min, temperature 35.8°C, and Glasgow Coma Scale (GCS) 15/15. He had multiple orthopaedic injuries (pelvic fracture, left humerus epicondyle fracture, right ankle swelling), and mesenteric tears involving the sigmoid colon and caecum. Clinically, the patient exhibited oozing from multiple venipuncture sites and hypothermia, indicating early signs of TIC. Laboratory values were prothrombin time (PT) 25.9 seconds, activated partial thromboplastin time (aPTT) 53 seconds, international normalized ratio (INR) 1.8, fibrinogen 1g/dL, platelet count 85,000/µL, base deficit of −19, lactate 9.6 mmol/L, and pH of 7.10. Focused Assessment with Sonography for Trauma (FAST) scan showed free fluid in the pelvis, and X-ray revealed bilateral superior and inferior pubic ramus fractures, while the pneumo-scan was negative. Computed tomography (CT) imaging was deferred due to hemodynamic instability. Initial resuscitation included warmed crystalloid boluses (1 L), administration of high-flow oxygen at 15 L/min, early use of tranexamic acid (1 g bolus followed by infusion), and activation of the MTP. He received 4 units each of PRBCs, random donor platelets (RDPs), and fresh frozen plasma (FFP) as an initial resuscitation, followed by an additional 8 PRBCs, 6 RDPs, 6 FFPs, and 4 cryoprecipitate units during the first 24 hours (Table 10.5). Calcium gluconate (10%) was administered with every 4 units of PRBCs. The patient underwent emergency damage control surgery, including bilateral internal iliac artery ligation, pre-peritoneal packing, and pelvic packing. Additional supportive measures included empiric antibiotics, vasopressors, and active warming. In total, he received 34 PRBCs, 53 RDPs, 31 FFPs, and 6 cryoprecipitate units during the hospital stay.

The patient stabilized hemodynamically within 4 hours of admission, with improvement in coagulopathy guided by laboratory and clinical parameters. He developed transient hypocalcaemia in the early hours, which was corrected with calcium gluconate infusion. However, during the hospital stay, he developed sepsis and progressive multiorgan dysfunction. Despite intensive supportive care, his condition deteriorated, and he expired on day 54.

Table 10.5 Transfusion of blood components during the hospital stay

	PRBC	RDP	FFP	Cryoprecipitate
1 hour	4	4	4	0
2-24 hours	8	6	6	4
After 24 hours	22	43	21	2
Total	**34**	**53**	**31**	**6**

DISCUSSION

Massive transfusion is a life-saving but high-risk intervention. It is associated with several complications, such as dilutional coagulopathy, hypothermia, metabolic disturbances, transfusion reactions, and logistic challenges.[3,4] In trauma, uncontrolled bleeding combined with TIC further worsen outcomes. TIC is now recognized as an early pathophysiological response involving endothelial injury, hypoperfusion, platelet dysfunction, and activation of anticoagulant pathways. Its presence is strongly correlated with higher transfusion requirements, multiple organ failure, and mortality.[5,6] In this case, early recognition of TIC based on clinical features and laboratory parameters prompted immediate activation of MTP with balanced transfusion of PRBCs, FFPs, and RDPs in a 1:1:1 ratio, in line with current recommendations.[7,8] Administration of tranexamic acid within 3 hours of injury is a proven mortality-reducing intervention, as supported by the CRASH-2 trial.[9] Calcium supplementation was also integrated, as hypocalcaemia is common during large volume transfusions and contributes to coagulopathy and myocardial depression. Furthermore, damage control surgery was a crucial adjunct to resuscitative efforts, enabling permissive hypotension, haemostatic resuscitation, and staged surgical interventions. Despite initial stabilization, delayed complications such as sepsis and multiorgan dysfunction contributed to mortality, consistent with the 'two-hit' model in trauma.[10,11] This underscores the importance of comprehensive trauma care extending beyond the emergency phase, encompassing prolonged intensive care, infection prevention, and organ support strategies. Another key lesson is the value of protocol-driven care and interdepartmental coordination. The availability of predefined MTP packages and timely communication between the clinical team and transfusion services minimized delays, optimized component use, and reduced wastage. In resource-limited settings, where viscoelastic assays like thromboelastography (TEG) or rotational thromboelastometry (ROTEM) may not be readily available, reliance on clinical judgement and conventional laboratory tests remains critical.[12]

CONCLUSION

Rapid activation of an MTP, early administration of tranexamic acid, balanced transfusion of blood components, correction of metabolic derangements, and timely damage control surgery were essential in achieving initial stabilization in a severely injured young patient. Despite these measures, late complications such as sepsis and multiorgan dysfunction contributed to mortality, underscoring the complex and evolving nature of post-trauma physiology. This case reinforces the need for coordinated, protocol-driven care and close communication between clinical and transfusion teams, especially in resource-limited settings where rapid decision-making and judicious use of laboratory parameters are vital.

TAKE-HOME MESSAGE

Early recognition of TIC and timely activation of an MTP with balanced component therapy are crucial for initial survival. However, long-term outcomes depend equally on coordinated critical care to address delayed complications such as sepsis and multiorgan dysfunction.

STATEMENT ON ETHICS AND CONSENT

This case report is based on retrospective data extracted from hospital medical records. No direct patient contact was involved. As the data were anonymized and analysed retrospectively, the requirement for informed patient consent was waived in accordance with institutional ethics guidelines.

REFERENCES

1. Pham HP, Shaz BH. Update on massive transfusion. Br J Anaesth. 2013;111(Suppl 1): i71–82.

2. Jain K, Jain S, Sood N, Puri A. Massive blood transfusion: A case report of transfusion of 70 units of blood and blood products in 24 hours. Glob J Transfus Med. 2018;3:68–71.

3. Kornblith LZ, Moore HB, Cohen MJ. Trauma-induced coagulopathy: The past, present, and future. J Thromb Haemost. 2019;17(6):852–62.

4. MacLeod JB, Lynn M, McKenney MG, Cohn SM, Murtha M. Early coagulopathy predicts mortality in trauma. J Trauma. 2003;55(1):39–44.

5. Hess JR, Brohi K, Dutton RP, Hauser CJ, Holcomb JB, Kluger Y, et al. The coagulopathy of trauma: A review of mechanisms. J Trauma. 2008;65(4):748–54.

6. Brohi K, Cohen MJ, Davenport RA. Acute coagulopathy of trauma: Mechanism, identification and effect. Curr Opin Crit Care. 2007;13(6):680–5.

7. Holcomb JB, Tilley BC, Baraniuk S, Fox EE, Wade CE, Podbielski JM, et al. Transfusion of plasma, platelets, and red blood cells in a 1:1:1 vs a 1:1:2 ratio and mortality in patients with severe trauma: The PROPPR randomized clinical trial. JAMA. 2015;313(5):471–82.

8. Cotton BA, Gunter OL, Isbell J, Au BK, Robertson AM, Morris JA Jr, et al. Damage control hematology: The impact of a trauma exsanguination protocol on survival and blood product utilization. J Trauma. 2008;64(5):1177–82.

9. Roberts I, Shakur H, Coats T, Hunt B, Balogun E, Barnetson L, et al. The CRASH-2 trial: A randomised controlled trial and economic evaluation of the effects of tranexamic acid on death, vascular occlusive events and transfusion requirement in bleeding trauma patients. Health Technol Assess. 2013;17(10):1–79.

10. Vincent JL, Marshall JC, Namendys-Silva SA, François B, Martin-Loeches I, Lipman J, et al. Assessment of the worldwide burden of critical illness: The intensive care over nations (ICON) audit. Lancet Respir Med. 2014;2(5):380–6.

11. Osuka A, Ogura H, Ueyama M, Shimazu T, Lederer JA. Immune response to traumatic injury: Harmony and discordance of immune system homeostasis. Acute Med Surg. 2014;1(2):63–9.

12. Hunt H, Stanworth S, Curry N, Woolley T, Cooper C, Ukoumunne O, et al. Thromboelastography (TEG) and rotational thromboelastometry (ROTEM) for trauma induced coagulopathy in adult trauma patients with bleeding. Cochrane Database Syst Rev. 2015;2015(2):CD010438.

INDEX

Note: Locators in *italics* represent figures and **bold** indicate tables in the text.

O

Obesity, in TIC, 39–40
Omics and transfusion strategies, 155–156

P

Packed red blood cell (PRBC) transfusion,
        122–123
Partial thromboplastin time (PTT), 3
PATCH trial, *see* Prehospital Tranexamic Acid
        for Severe Trauma trial
Pathophysiological mechanism of TIC, 11–12,
        12, 13
Pattern recognition receptors (PRRs), 27
PCC, *see* Prothrombin complex concentrate
PCS, *see* Platelet contribution to clot stiffness
PDW, *see* Platelet distribution width
PE, *see* Pulmonary embolism
Peripheral biomarkers in TIC, 83–84
Personalised coagulopathy management, 118
Plasma-based resuscitation, 117
Plasmin, 4–5
Plasminogen activator inhibitor, 5
        PAI-1, 24
Platelet activation and dysfunction, 56
        cellular and brain-derived microparticles
                (BDMPs), 57, *58*
        protein C pathway activation, 56
        thromboinflammation, 57–58
        tissue hypoperfusion, 57
Platelet contribution to clot stiffness (PCS), 88
Platelet distribution width (PDW), 74
Platelet dysfunction, 26
Platelet indices, clinical interpretation of, in
        trauma, **74**
Platelet-large cell ratio (P-LCR), 74
Platelet mapping assays, 80
Platelet transfusion, 123
P-LCR, *see* Platelet-large cell ratio
POCT, *see* Point-of-care testing
Point-of-care testing (POCT), 146, **147–150**
Post-trauma coagulopathy concept vs. the
        modern view of TIC, **21**
Pragmatic Randomized Optimal Platelet and
        Plasma Ratios (PROPPR) trial, 39
PRBC transfusion, *see* Packed red blood cell
        transfusion
Precision diagnostics using multiomics, 88
Pre-hospital and ED resuscitation, in TIC, 44
Pre-hospital care, of TIC, 113
Prehospital Tranexamic Acid for Severe Trauma
        (PATCH) trial, 115
Prognosis despite standard resuscitation,
        worsened, 137
Proinflammatory cytokines, 29
PROMMTT study, 113
PROPPR trial, *see* Pragmatic Randomized Optimal
        Platelet and Plasma Ratios trial
Protein C pathway, 7–8, *8*
        activation, 56

anticoagulation pathway, 7–8, *8*
        modulation, 117
Protein S, 7–8
Protein Z-dependent protease inhibitor (ZPI), 8
Proteometabolomic makers of TIC, 84
        RNA regulators (ceRNA network), 85–88
        "succinate-lipid-sheddase" axis, 84–85
Prothrombin complex concentrate (PCC), 113,
        124, 153
Prothrombin time (PT), 4, 58, 137
Prothrombin time ratio (PTr), 72
PRRs, *see* Pattern recognition receptors
PT, *see* Prothrombin time
PTr, *see* Prothrombin time ratio
PTT, *see* Partial thromboplastin time
Pulmonary embolism (PE), 21

Q

Quantra SEER sonorheometry, 88

R

RABT score, *see* Revised assessment of blood
                transfusion score
Randomised controlled trial (RCT), 113
Rapid TEG (r-TEG), 78
RCT, *see* Randomised controlled trial
RDCR, *see* Remote damage control resuscitation
Reactive oxygen species (ROS), 154
Recombinant activated coagulation factor VII
                (rFVIIa), 124
Rehabilitation and quality of life, impact of TIC
                on, 138–139
Remote damage control resuscitation (RDCR), 151
RETIC trial, *see* Reversal of Trauma Induced
                Coagulopathy trial
Reversal of Trauma Induced Coagulopathy
                (RETIC) trial, 116
Revised assessment of blood transfusion (RABT)
                score, 99–100
rFVIIa, *see* Recombinant activated coagulation
                factor VII
Risk factors and contributing elements to TIC,
                37, **42**
        clinical and physiological influences
                age, 38–39
                alcohol consumption, 40
                cirrhosis liver, 41
                comorbidities, 41
                gender, 39
                haemophilia, 41
                obesity, 39–40
                smoking, 40–41
        drugs, 41
                anticoagulants, 41–42
                antiplatelets, 42
                beta blockers, 42
                nonsteroidal anti-inflammatory drugs
                        (NSAIDs), 41
                statins, 42